Neurorehabilitation: Progress and Challenges

Neurorehabilitation: Progress and Challenges

Editors

Akiyoshi Matsugi
Naoki Yoshida
Hideki Nakano
Yohei Okada

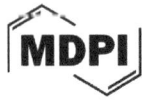

Basel • Beijing • Wuhan • Barcelona • Belgrade • Novi Sad • Cluj • Manchester

Editors

Akiyoshi Matsugi
Faculty of Rehabilitation
Osaka
Japan

Naoki Yoshida
Faculty of Health Sciences
Osaka
Japan

Hideki Nakano
Faculty of Health Sciences
Kyoto
Japan

Yohei Okada
Faculty of Health Sciences
Nara
Japan

Editorial Office
MDPI
St. Alban-Anlage 66
4052 Basel, Switzerland

This is a reprint of articles from the Special Issue published online in the open access journal *Journal of Clinical Medicine* (ISSN 2077-0383) (available at: https://www.mdpi.com/journal/jcm/special_issues/Neurorehabilitation_Progress_Challenges).

For citation purposes, cite each article independently as indicated on the article page online and as indicated below:

Lastname, A.A.; Lastname, B.B. Article Title. *Journal Name* **Year**, *Volume Number*, Page Range.

ISBN 978-3-7258-0295-1 (Hbk)
ISBN 978-3-7258-0296-8 (PDF)
doi.org/10.3390/books978-3-7258-0296-8

© 2024 by the authors. Articles in this book are Open Access and distributed under the Creative Commons Attribution (CC BY) license. The book as a whole is distributed by MDPI under the terms and conditions of the Creative Commons Attribution-NonCommercial-NoDerivs (CC BY-NC-ND) license.

Contents

Akiyoshi Matsugi, Naoki Yoshida, Hideki Nakano and Yohei Okada
The Neurorehabilitation of Neurological Movement Disorders Requires Rigorous and Sustained Research
Reprinted from: *J. Clin. Med.* 2024, *13*, 852, doi:10.3390/jcm13030852 1

Shuji Matsumoto, Megumi Shimodozono, Tomokazu Noma, Kodai Miyara, Tetsuya Onoda, Rina Ijichi, Takashi Shigematsu, and et al.
Effect of Functional Electrical Stimulation in Convalescent Stroke Patients: A Multicenter, Randomized Controlled Trial
Reprinted from: *J. Clin. Med.* 2023, *12*, 2638, doi:10.3390/jcm12072638 6

Seyoung Shin, Hwang-Jae Lee, Won Hyuk Chang, Sung Hwa Ko, Yong-Il Shin and Yun-Hee Kim
A Smart Glove Digital System Promotes Restoration of Upper Limb Motor Function and Enhances Cortical Hemodynamic Changes in Subacute Stroke Patients with Mild to Moderate Weakness: A Randomized Controlled Trial
Reprinted from: *J. Clin. Med.* 2022, *11*, 7343, doi:10.3390/jcm11247343 18

Corinna N. Gerber, Didier L. Gasser and Christopher John Newman
Hand Ownership Is Altered in Teenagers with Unilateral Cerebral Palsy
Reprinted from: *J. Clin. Med.* 2022, *11*, 4869, doi:10.3390/jcm11164869 32

Alberto Romano, Martina Favetta, Susanna Summa, Tommaso Schirinzi, Enrico Silvio Bertini, Enrico Castelli, Gessica Vasco and Maurizio Petrarca
Upper Body Physical Rehabilitation for Children with Ataxia through IMU-Based Exergame
Reprinted from: *J. Clin. Med.* 2022, *11*, 1065, doi:10.3390/jcm11041065 41

Mariusz Bedla, Paweł Pieta, Daniel Kaczmarski and Stanisław Deniziak
Estimation of Gross Motor Functions in Children with Cerebral Palsy Using Zebris FDM-T Treadmill
Reprinted from: *J. Clin. Med.* 2022, *11*, 954, doi:10.3390/jcm11040954 53

Emanuela Elena Mihai, Ilie Valentin Mihai and Mihai Berteanu
Effectiveness of Radial Extracorporeal Shock Wave Therapy and Visual Feedback Balance Training on Lower Limb Post-Stroke Spasticity, Trunk Performance, and Balance: A Randomized Controlled Trial
Reprinted from: *J. Clin. Med.* 2022, *11*, 147, doi:10.3390/jcm11010147 68

Yu-Sheng Yang, Chi-Hsiang Tseng, Wei-Chien Fang, Ia-Wen Han and Shyh-Chour Huang
Effectiveness of a New 3D-Printed Dynamic Hand–Wrist Splint on Hand Motor Function and Spasticity in Chronic Stroke Patients
Reprinted from: *J. Clin. Med.* 2021, *10*, 4549, doi:10.3390/ jcm10194549 84

Yoshiki Tamaru, Akiyoshi Yanagawa and Akiyoshi Matsugi
Sensory Nerve Conduction Velocity Predicts Improvement of Hand Function with Nerve Gliding Exercise Following Carpal Tunnel Release Surgery
Reprinted from: *J. Clin. Med.* 2021, *10*, 4121, doi:10.3390/jcm10184121 98

Tae-sung In, Jin hwa Jung, May Kim, Kyoung-sim Jung and Hwi-young Cho
Effect of Posterior Pelvic Tilt Taping on Pelvic Inclination, Muscle Strength, and Gait Ability in Stroke Patients: A Randomized Controlled Study
Reprinted from: *J. Clin. Med.* 2021, *10*, 2381, doi:10.3390/jcm10112381 109

Carmen Adella Sîrbu, Dana-Claudia Thompson, Florentina Cristina Plesa, Titus Mihai Vasile, Dragoș Cătălin Jianu, Marian Mitrica, Daniela Anghel, and et al.
Neurorehabilitation in Multiple Sclerosis—A Review of Present Approaches and Future Considerations
Reprinted from: *J. Clin. Med.* **2022**, *11*, 7003, doi:10.3390/jcm11237003 117

Selena Marcos-Antón, María Dolores Gor-García-Fogeda and Roberto Cano-de-la-Cuerda
An sEMG-Controlled Forearm Bracelet for Assessing and Training Manual Dexterity in Rehabilitation: A Systematic Review
Reprinted from: *J. Clin. Med.* **2022**, *11*, 3119, doi:10.3390/jcm11113119 143

Gustavo Rodríguez-Fuentes, Lucía Silveira-Pereira, Pedro Ferradáns-Rodríguez and Pablo Campo-Prieto
Therapeutic Effects of the Pilates Method in Patients with Multiple Sclerosis: A Systematic Review
Reprinted from: *J. Clin. Med.* **2022**, *11*, 683, doi:10.3390/jcm11030683 159

Editorial

The Neurorehabilitation of Neurological Movement Disorders Requires Rigorous and Sustained Research

Akiyoshi Matsugi [1,*], Naoki Yoshida [2], Hideki Nakano [3] and Yohei Okada [4]

1. Faculty of Rehabilitation, Shijonawate Gakuen University, Osaka 574-0011, Japan
2. Faculty of Health Sciences, Kansai University of Health Sciences, Osaka 590-0433, Japan; ysd@rehalab.jpn.org
3. Department of Physical Therapy, Faculty of Health Sciences, Kyoto Tachibana University, Kyoto 607-8175, Japan; nakano-h@tachibana-u.ac.jp
4. Faculty of Health Science, Kio University, Nara 635-0832, Japan; y.okada@kio.ac.jp
* Correspondence: a-matsugi@reha.shijonawate-gakuen.ac.jp

1. Introduction

Movement disorders that stem from neurological conditions such as stroke, cerebral palsy, multiple sclerosis (MS), Parkinson's disease (PD), and spinocerebellar degeneration (SCD) can significantly impair a person's activities of daily living (ADL). Neurorehabilitation aims to mitigate the impact of these movement disorders, alleviate constraints on the ADL, and promote increased social participation [1]. The advancements in neurorehabilitation necessitate a thorough exploration of the underlying mechanisms of movement disorders, the formulation of pathological hypotheses, and the development of new clinical interventions and assessments, including outcome measure studies. This Special Issue collects contributions from a wide range of domains, including fundamental research that elucidates the intricacies of movement disorders and advancements in evaluation measurement technologies, innovative interventional studies, and prediction of clinical outcome studies.

These studies are expected to augment the recent developments in the field of neurorehabilitation. In this editorial, we review these findings and discuss the future of, as well as the remaining issues in, this field.

2. An Overview of the Published Articles

The RALLY Trial, led by Shuji Matsumoto et al., investigated the Walkaide® device's effectiveness at enhancing the walking ability of post-stroke patients with foot drop (Contribution 1). Despite the lack of significant improvement in the primary outcome measure—the distance covered during a 6-min walk test—this study provides valuable insights into the role of functional electrical stimulation (FES) in Japanese stroke patients during their convalescent phase.

Shin et al. conducted a randomized controlled trial (RCT) to assess the impact of the RAPAEL® Smart Glove digital training system on the upper extremity function and cortical hemodynamic changes in patients with subacute stroke (Contribution 2). This study highlights the potential of game-based virtual reality training to improve motor function and cortical activation, which is consistent with previous studies [2].

Gerber et al. explored hand ownership in teenagers with unilateral cerebral palsy, revealing the difference in their experiences compared to those of typically developing teenagers (Contribution 3). This study emphasizes the importance of understanding the subjective experience of hand ownership and provides insights into early intervention strategies.

Romano et al. (Contribution 4) presented a novel approach that used exergame-based exercise training for children with ataxia. This study demonstrated improvements in their hand dexterity, emphasizing the potential of exergaming to engage children during effective upper-body rehabilitation.

Bedla et al. proposed a novel method for estimating the Gross Motor Function Measure (GMFM) of children with cerebral palsy using the Zebris FDM-T treadmill (Contribution 5). This approach offers a promising alternative for objective diagnostics through its reduction in assessment time and enhanced accessibility.

Mihai et al. investigated the combined effects of radial extracorporeal shock wave therapy and visual feedback balance training on lower limb post-stroke spasticity, trunk performance, and balance (Contribution 6). This study demonstrates the ability of a comprehensive approach to address multiple aspects of post-stroke rehabilitation.

Yang et al. introduced a 3D-printed dynamic hand–wrist splint for chronic stroke patients, and demonstrated how it improved hand dexterity (Contribution 7). This innovative intervention offers a personalized and effective solution for at-home rehabilitation.

Tamaru et al. explored the effects of nerve gliding exercises following carpal tunnel release surgery, emphasizing the importance of the conduction velocity of sensory nerves in predicting hand function improvement (Contribution 8). This study provides valuable insights into postoperative rehabilitation strategies.

In et al. investigated the effects of posterior pelvic tilt taping on the pelvic inclination, muscle strength, and gait ability of stroke patients (Contribution 9). This study highlights the potential benefits of taping as an adjunctive intervention to enhance the postural control and gait of stroke survivors.

A comprehensive review, written by Sîrbu et al., assesses current neurorehabilitation approaches to multiple sclerosis, emphasizing the need for personalized strategies to address the varied symptoms of this prevalent neurological disorder (Contribution 10).

Marcos-Antón et al. conducted a systematic review of the use of the MYO Armband® for assessing and training manual dexterity in individuals with upper limb impairment (Contribution 11). Their work provides a comprehensive overview of the accuracy and clinical effects of this technology and offers valuable guidance for practitioners.

Rodríguez-Fuentes et al. systematically reviewed the therapeutic effects of the Pilates method for patients with multiple sclerosis (Contribution 12). While highlighting positive outcomes in terms of balance, gait, and physical functional conditions, this review emphasizes the need for larger-scale studies with well-defined protocols.

3. Knowledge Gaps and Further Study

In summation, the impairments addressed by these neurological disease studies are gait disturbance, balance impairment, and upper extremity utility. These are in line with the unmet rehabilitation needs most sought after by neurological disorder patients. The studies published in this Special Issue have made valuable contributions to the field of neurorehabilitation; however, they also reveal persistent knowledge gaps that require further exploration. Key areas for future investigation include more robust large-scale clinical trials that encompass diverse participant populations. Additionally, long-term follow-up studies are necessary to evaluate the sustained effects of these interventions. Comparative effectiveness research is needed to identify the most efficacious rehabilitation strategies, while the exploration and integration of innovative technologies into neurorehabilitation practices are promising for generating advancements in the field. Furthermore, a comprehensive understanding of individualized rehabilitation plans based on patient-specific factors is essential for tailoring interventions to meet diverse patient needs and optimize their outcomes. For example, in this SI, there was no positive effect found in the functional electrical stimulation of ankle muscle on gait speed, despite a well-controlled study (Contribution 1). However, this intervention study should be conducted other view such as other outcome, other population, and other stimulation conditions.

Selecting optimal outcomes is crucial to advancing clinical reasoning, just as clinical research is to selecting optimal interventions. In this SI, upper limb functions were measured in a number of important studies, in patients with cerebral palsy, peripheral nerve injury, and post stroke (Contributions 2, 3, 4, 7, 8, and 11). However, there is no internationally agreed-upon outcome to be obtained for these diseases, which hinders the future consolidation of these findings. Core outcome sets (COSs) are necessary to advance clinical research [3]; however, their development is lacking for certain conditions, even for common incurable neurological diseases, such as SCD and PD, which are targets of neurorehabilitation. We must also initiate the development of COSs for the treatment of neurological diseases.

While the narrative and literature reviews reported in this SI (Contribution 7) are important in establishing the efficacy of neurorehabilitation treatments, more systematic reviews should also to be conducted to proactively examine the effectiveness of rehabilitation interventions in conditions such as stroke [4], PD [5], and SCD [6]. Furthermore, guidelines [7] must be developed so that physicians, physical therapists, occupational therapists, and patients worldwide can choose the evidence-based treatment that will lead to the best outcome. Additionally, clinicians must be educated on how to utilize the findings of systematic reviews.

Neuromodulation technology plays an important role in promoting neurorehabilitation [8]. Transcranial electrical stimulation and repetitive transcranial magnetic stimulation are now being validated for stroke [9], SCD [10], and PD [11]. However, there are few RCTs of this technology, and parameter selection methods for the population conditions and individual cases that are expected to find this technology effective remain unclear. In addition to conventional physical and occupational therapies, we must continue to examine the efficacy of neuromodulation.

Neuroregenerative medicine [12] for spinal cord injuries [13], stroke, and neurodegenerative diseases, such as PD and SCD, is expected in the near future. Neurorehabilitation after structural regeneration may be effective in restoring function to patients, and this issue should be addressed in the future.

4. Conclusions

The field of neurorehabilitation continues to evolve, with innovative interventions being accompanied by outcome studies aimed at addressing the complex challenges posed by various neurological conditions. While advancements in wearable technology, such as virtual reality and noninvasive brain stimulation, offer promising avenues for rehabilitation, the multifaceted nature of neurological disorders requires continuous research and collaboration to optimize treatment strategies. This editorial underscores the progress that has been made and highlights the avenues for future exploration within the dynamic landscape of neurorehabilitation.

Author Contributions: Writing—original draft preparation, A.M.; writing—review and editing, A.M., N.Y., H.N. and Y.O. All authors have read and agreed to the published version of the manuscript.

Acknowledgments: We thank English language editing service and the fee for editing was covered by JSPS KAKENHI (grant number: 23K10418).

Conflicts of Interest: The authors declare no conflicts of interest.

List of Contributions

1. Matsumoto, S.; Shimodozono, M.; Noma, T.; Miyara, K.; Onoda, T.; Ijichi, R.; Shigematsu, T.; Satone, A.; Okuma, H.; Seto, M.; et al. Effect of Functional Electrical Stimulation in Convalescent Stroke Patients: A Multicenter, Randomized Controlled Trial. *J. Clin. Med.* **2023**, *12*, 2638. https://doi.org/10.3390/jcm12072638.
2. Shin, S.; Lee, H.J.; Chang, W.H.; Ko, S.H.; Shin, Y.I.; Kim, Y.H. A Smart Glove Digital System Promotes Restoration of Upper Limb Motor Function and Enhances Cortical Hemodynamic Changes in Subacute Stroke Patients with Mild to Moderate Weakness: A Randomized Controlled Trial. *J. Clin. Med.* **2022**, *11*, 7343. https://doi.org/10.3390/jcm11247343.
3. Gerber, C.N.; Gasser, D.L.; Newman, C.J. Hand Ownership Is Altered in Teenagers with Unilateral Cerebral Palsy. *J. Clin. Med.* **2022**, *11*, 4869. https://doi.org/10.3390/jcm11164869.

4. Romano, A.; Favetta, M.; Summa, S.; Schirinzi, T.; Bertini, E.S.; Castelli, E.; Vasco, G.; Petrarca, M. Upper Body Physical Rehabilitation for Children with Ataxia through IMU-Based Exergame. *J. Clin. Med.* **2022**, *11*, 1065. https://doi.org/10.3390/jcm11041065.
5. Bedla, M.; Pieta, P.; Kaczmarski, D.; Deniziak, S. Estimation of Gross Motor Functions in Children with Cerebral Palsy Using Zebris FDM-T Treadmill. *J. Clin. Med.* **2022**, *11*, 954. https://doi.org/10.3390/jcm11040954.
6. Mihai, E.E.; Mihai, I.V.; Berteanu, M. Effectiveness of Radial Extracorporeal Shock Wave Therapy and Visual Feedback Balance Training on Lower Limb Post-Stroke Spasticity, Trunk Performance, and Balance: A Randomized Controlled Trial. *J. Clin. Med.* **2021**, *11*, 147. https://doi.org/10.3390/jcm11010147.
7. Yang, Y.S.; Tseng, C.H.; Fang, W.C.; Han, I.W.; Huang, S.C. Effectiveness of a New 3D-Printed Dynamic Hand-Wrist Splint on Hand Motor Function and Spasticity in Chronic Stroke Patients. *J. Clin. Med.* **2021**, *10*, 4549. https://doi.org/10.3390/jcm10194549.
8. Tamaru, Y.; Yanagawa, A.; Matsugi, A. Sensory Nerve Conduction Velocity Predicts Improvement of Hand Function with Nerve Gliding Exercise Following Carpal Tunnel Release Surgery. *J. Clin. Med.* **2021**, *10*, 4121. https://doi.org/10.3390/jcm10184121.
9. In, T.S.; Jung, J.H.; Kim, M.; Jung, K.S.; Cho, H.Y. Effect of Posterior Pelvic Tilt Taping on Pelvic Inclination, Muscle Strength, and Gait Ability in Stroke Patients: A Randomized Controlled Study. *J. Clin. Med.* **2021**, *10*, 2381. https://doi.org/10.3390/jcm10112381.
10. Sirbu, C.A.; Thompson, D.C.; Plesa, F.C.; Vasile, T.M.; Jianu, D.C.; Mitrica, M.; Anghel, D.; Stefani, C. Neurorehabilitation in Multiple Sclerosis—A Review of Present Approaches and Future Considerations. *J. Clin. Med.* **2022**, *11*, 7003. https://doi.org/10.3390/jcm11237003.
11. Marcos-Anton, S.; Gor-Garcia-Fogeda, M.D.; Cano-de-la-Cuerda, R. An sEMG-Controlled Forearm Bracelet for Assessing and Training Manual Dexterity in Rehabilitation: A Systematic Review. *J. Clin. Med.* **2022**, *11*, 3119. https://doi.org/10.3390/jcm11113119.
12. Rodriguez-Fuentes, G.; Silveira-Pereira, L.; Ferradans-Rodriguez, P.; Campo-Prieto, P. Therapeutic Effects of the Pilates Method in Patients with Multiple Sclerosis: A Systematic Review. *J. Clin. Med.* **2022**, *11*, 683. https://doi.org/10.3390/jcm11030683.

References

1. Khan, F.; Amatya, B.; Galea, M.P.; Gonzenbach, R.; Kesselring, J. Neurorehabilitation: Applied neuroplasticity. *J. Neurol.* **2017**, *264*, 603–615. [CrossRef] [PubMed]
2. Hao, J.; Xie, H.; Harp, K.; Chen, Z.; Siu, K.C. Effects of Virtual Reality Intervention on Neural Plasticity in Stroke Rehabilitation: A Systematic Review. *Arch. Phys. Med. Rehabil.* **2022**, *103*, 523–541. [CrossRef] [PubMed]
3. Kirkham, J.J.; Williamson, P. Core outcome sets in medical research. *BMJ Med.* **2022**, *1*, e000284. [CrossRef] [PubMed]
4. Calabro, R.S.; Sorrentino, G.; Cassio, A.; Mazzoli, D.; Andrenelli, E.; Bizzarini, E.; Campanini, I.; Carmignano, S.M.; Cerulli, S.; Chisari, C.; et al. Robotic-assisted gait rehabilitation following stroke: A systematic review of current guidelines and practical clinical recommendations. *Eur. J. Phys. Rehabil. Med.* **2021**, *57*, 460–471. [CrossRef] [PubMed]
5. Okada, Y.; Ohtsuka, H.; Kamata, N.; Yamamoto, S.; Sawada, M.; Nakamura, J.; Okamoto, M.; Narita, M.; Nikaido, Y.; Urakami, H.; et al. Effectiveness of Long-Term Physiotherapy in Parkinson's Disease: A Systematic Review and Meta-Analysis. *J. Parkinsons Dis.* **2021**, *11*, 1619–1630. [CrossRef]
6. Matsugi, A.; Ohtsuka, H.; Bando, K.; Kondo, Y.; Kikuchi, Y. Effects of non-invasive brain stimulation for degenerative cerebellar ataxia: A protocol for a systematic review and meta-analysis. *BMJ Open* **2023**, *13*, e073526. [CrossRef] [PubMed]
7. Gittler, M.; Davis, A.M. Guidelines for Adult Stroke Rehabilitation and Recovery. *JAMA* **2018**, *319*, 820–821. [CrossRef]
8. Antal, A.; Luber, B.; Brem, A.K.; Bikson, M.; Brunoni, A.R.; Cohen Kadosh, R.; Dubljevic, V.; Fecteau, S.; Ferreri, F.; Floel, A.; et al. Non-invasive brain stimulation and neuroenhancement. *Clin. Neurophysiol. Pract.* **2022**, *7*, 146–165. [CrossRef] [PubMed]
9. Kim, W.J.; Rosselin, C.; Amatya, B.; Hafezi, P.; Khan, F. Repetitive transcranial magnetic stimulation for management of post-stroke impairments: An overview of systematic reviews. *J. Rehabil. Med.* **2020**, *52*, 1–10. [CrossRef] [PubMed]
10. Qiu, Y.T.; Chen, Y.; Tan, H.X.; Su, W.; Guo, Q.F.; Gao, Q. Efficacy and Safety of Repetitive Transcranial Magnetic Stimulation in Cerebellar Ataxia: A Systematic Review and Meta-analysis. *Cerebellum* **2023**. [CrossRef] [PubMed]
11. Zhang, W.; Deng, B.; Xie, F.; Zhou, H.; Guo, J.F.; Jiang, H.; Sim, A.; Tang, B.; Wang, Q. Efficacy of repetitive transcranial magnetic stimulation in Parkinson's disease: A systematic review and meta-analysis of randomised controlled trials. *EClinicalMedicine* **2022**, *52*, 101589. [CrossRef] [PubMed]

12. Rando, T.A.; Ambrosio, F. Regenerative Rehabilitation: Applied Biophysics Meets Stem Cell Therapeutics. *Cell Stem Cell* **2018**, *22*, 306–309. [CrossRef] [PubMed]
13. Tashiro, S.; Nakamura, M.; Okano, H. Regenerative Rehabilitation and Stem Cell Therapy Targeting Chronic Spinal Cord Injury: A Review of Preclinical Studies. *Cells* **2022**, *11*, 685. [CrossRef] [PubMed]

Disclaimer/Publisher's Note: The statements, opinions and data contained in all publications are solely those of the individual author(s) and contributor(s) and not of MDPI and/or the editor(s). MDPI and/or the editor(s) disclaim responsibility for any injury to people or property resulting from any ideas, methods, instructions or products referred to in the content.

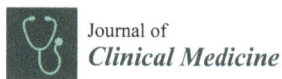

Article

Effect of Functional Electrical Stimulation in Convalescent Stroke Patients: A Multicenter, Randomized Controlled Trial

Shuji Matsumoto [1,2,*], Megumi Shimodozono [3], Tomokazu Noma [4], Kodai Miyara [5], Tetsuya Onoda [6], Rina Ijichi [7], Takashi Shigematsu [8], Akira Satone [9], Hidenobu Okuma [10], Makiko Seto [11], Masanori Taketsuna [12], Hideaki Kaneda [12], Miyuki Matsuo [12], Shinsuke Kojima [12] and the RALLY Trial Investigators [†]

1. Center of Medical Education, Faculty of Health Sciences, Ryotokuji University, Chiba 279-8567, Japan
2. Department of Rehabilitation and Physical Medicine, Mito Clinical Education and Training Center, University of Tsukuba Hospital, Mito 310-0015, Japan
3. Department of Rehabilitation and Physical Medicine, Graduate School of Medical and Dental Sciences, Kagoshima University, Kagoshima 890-8544, Japan
4. Department of Rehabilitation, Faculty of Health Science, Nihon Fukushi University, Aichi 470-3295, Japan
5. Department of Rehabilitation, Kagoshima University Hospital, Kagoshima 890-0075, Japan
6. Department of Rehabilitation, Kirishima Medical Center, Kagoshima 899-5112, Japan
7. Department of Rehabilitation, Kirishima Sugiyasu Hospital, Kagoshima 899-4201, Japan
8. Department of Rehabilitation, Hamamatsu City Rehabilitation Hospital, Shizuoka 433-8511, Japan
9. Department of Rehabilitation, Tokachi Rehabilitation Center, Hokkaido 080-0835, Japan
10. Department of Rehabilitation, Kumamoto Takumadai Rehabilitation Hospital, Kumamoto 862-0924, Japan
11. Department of Rehabilitation, Nagasaki Kita Hospital, Nagasaki 851-2103, Japan
12. Translational Research Center for Medical Innovation, Kobe 650-0047, Japan
* Correspondence: shushusa71@yahoo.co.jp; Tel.:+81-29-231-2371
† The list of the RALLY trial Investigators and Committees is provided in the Appendix B.

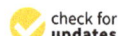

Citation: Matsumoto, S.; Shimodozono, M.; Noma, T.; Miyara, K.; Onoda, T.; Ijichi, R.; Shigematsu, T.; Satone, A.; Okuma, H.; Seto, M.; et al. Effect of Functional Electrical Stimulation in Convalescent Stroke Patients: A Multicenter, Randomized Controlled Trial. J. Clin. Med. 2023, 12, 2638. https://doi.org/10.3390/jcm12072638

Academic Editors: Akiyoshi Matsugi, Naoki Yoshida, Hideki Nakano and Yohei Okada

Received: 22 February 2023
Revised: 29 March 2023
Accepted: 30 March 2023
Published: 1 April 2023

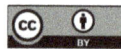

Copyright: © 2023 by the authors. Licensee MDPI, Basel, Switzerland. This article is an open access article distributed under the terms and conditions of the Creative Commons Attribution (CC BY) license (https://creativecommons.org/licenses/by/4.0/).

Abstract: Background: We evaluated whether the Walkaide® device could effectively improve walking ability and lower extremity function in post-stroke patients with foot drop. Patients aged 20–85 years with an initial stroke within ≤6 months and a functional ambulation classification score of 3 or 4 were eligible. Materials and Methods: Patients were randomly allocated to the functional electrical stimulation (FES) or control group at a 1:1 ratio. A 40 min training program using Walkaide was additionally performed by the FES group five times per week for 8 weeks. The control group received the 40 min training program without FES. Results: A total of 203 patients were allocated to the FES (n = 102) or control (n = 101) groups. Patients who did not receive the intervention or whose data were unavailable were excluded. Finally, the primary outcome data of 184 patients (n = 92 in each group) were analyzed. The mean change in the maximum distance during the 6-MWT (primary outcome) was 68.37 ± 62.42 m and 57.50 ± 68.17 m in the FES and control groups (difference: 10.86 m; 95% confidence interval: −8.26 to 29.98, p = 0.26), respectively. Conclusions: In Japanese post-stroke patients with foot drop, FES did not significantly improve the 6 min walk distance during the convalescent phase. The trial was registered at UMIN000020604.

Keywords: electrical stimulation; gait; stroke; lower extremity; walking

1. Introduction

While age-standardized rates of stroke mortality have decreased worldwide in the past two decades, both the absolute number of people experiencing a stroke every year and the number of stroke survivors have been increasing [1]. Stroke survivors, often with disabilities, cannot actively dorsiflex the foot during the swing phase of gait (known as foot drop). Foot drop is a common disorder following stroke and is associated with severe motor impairment, weakness or lack of voluntary control of the dorsiflexor muscles of the ankle joint, and increased spasticity of the plantar flexor muscles [2]. Foot drop is classified as the inability to dorsiflex the foot and is most commonly caused by weakness of the dorsiflexors (and abductor muscles) and/or overactivity of the plantar flexor muscle group (and adductor muscles) [3]. Foot drop decreases gait velocity and limits functional mobility. Traditionally, an ankle-foot orthosis (AFO) is used for foot drop [4]; however, the effects of the AFO attachment include an increase in walking speed and stride [5].

Functional electrical stimulation (FES)—an alternative to foot drop treatment—is designed to restore motor function in paralyzed limbs by electrically stimulating the neuromuscular system during ambulation [6]. Several randomized trials have demonstrated that FES devices have similar benefits as AFOs for key walking measures in patients with foot drop caused by stroke [7–10]. However, only a few studies have exclusively focused on convalescent stroke patients (≤6 months post-stroke). Furthermore, most studies of FES were conducted in Europe and the U.S., where lifestyles are very different from those in Japan and shoes are worn even indoors [11–13]. In Japan, people do not usually wear shoes indoors. Hence, whether FES devices would be effective for Japanese convalescent stroke patients with foot drop remains unclear.

Walkaide® (Innovative Neurotronics, Reno, NV, USA) is an FES device suitable for walking with bare feet as it has a tilt sensor [8]. The Walkaide® FES system is a self-contained FES device with built-in tilt sensor that attaches with a cuff to the leg below the knee. When the leg is tilted back at the end of stance, stimulation of the common peroneal nerve is initiated, producing dorsiflexion of the ankle to facilitate leg clearance during swing. When the leg is tilted forward at the end of the swing phase, stimulation is terminated. In this trial, we examined whether the Walkaide® FES system effectively improves walking ability and lower extremity function in Japanese patients with unstable gait from foot drop post-stroke.

2. Materials and Methods

2.1. Study Design

We performed a randomized, controlled, open-label trial enrolling patients with post-stroke hemiplegic gait disorder (foot drop) from 30 rehabilitation centers across Japan (study sites and trial investigators are provided in Appendix B). The study protocol was approved by the ethics committees of all participating institutions. This study was conducted in accordance with the tenets of the Declaration of Helsinki. A detailed description of the study design and the methods has been published previously, with a brief summary provided here [14]. The trial was registered with ClinicalTrials.gov, registration number was NCT02898168 (https://clinicaltrials.gov/ct2/show/NCT02898168) (accessed on 22 March 2023).

2.2. Participants

Patients aged 20–85 years were eligible for inclusion if they had an initial stroke within ≤6 months with a functional ambulation classification (FAC) score of 3 or 4 (FAC is a scale of 0–5, where 3 indicates supervision or standby guarding and 4 indicates independent on level surfaces) prior to providing consent for this study [15]. Patients who could not complete the rehabilitation program due to comorbidities (including severe osteoarthritis, liver, kidney, or cardiovascular dysfunction) were excluded. In addition, the exclusion criteria included the following: contraindication to the device (e.g., metallic implant, implanted medical electrical device, past or current epilepsy, and uncontrolled seizure disorder); neuromuscular disorders (excluding stroke); mental disorder; severe edema of a lower extremity; evidence of deep venous thrombosis or thromboembolism; severe atherosclerosis of the lower extremities; or musculoskeletal systems that would potentially affect gait; and a high risk of falling. Patients with other conditions that may affect the outcome were also excluded (e.g., use of FES or a robot suit within 1 month, botulinum toxin injections or phenol nerve block injection within 6 months, or severe sensory dysfunction or higher brain dysfunction before consenting to this study).

After the enrolled patients provided written informed consent, the treating physician and physical therapists evaluated FES compatibility for a screening period of up to 7 days.

Patients were excluded if any of the following was observed: (1) unresponsiveness to the FES device, (2) intolerance to continuous stimulation, and (3) gait function improved significantly during the screening period. The full eligibility criteria are provided in the previous paper [14].

2.3. Randomization and Masking

After the screening period, the enrolled patients were randomly allocated to either the FES or control group (1:1 ratio) with a minimization method using an electronic data capturing system—eClinical Base (Translational Research Center for Medical Innovation) (https://www.tri-kobe.org/support/tools/, accessed on 22 March 2023). The allocation was centralized using web-based randomization software (eClinical Base). Randomization was stratified according to the following factors: FAC score 3 or 4, age < 65 years, type of stroke (ischemic or hemorrhagic), and institution.

This was an open-label trial with both patients and physicians unblinded to the treatment allocation. However, all outcomes except the examinations with FES and questionnaires were evaluated by investigators blinded to the treatment allocation. The 10 m walk tests (10-MWT) were videotaped, and gait disturbance was evaluated by an independent central adjudication committee [14].

2.4. Procedures

A 60 min usual physiotherapy treatment was provided to both the FES and control groups 5 days a week over 8 weeks (40 days), consisting of basic activity training as follows: (1) mat exercise, (2) standing up and sitting down, (3) ambulation with assistive devices or manual support, and/or range of motion (ROM) training, and/or gait training using an AFO (if the patient had already used it at the time of recruitment). In addition to the usual rehabilitation training, the patients included in this study received their allocated program (FES or control). Any rehabilitation programs initiated before this trial were continued under the condition that the intervals, duration, or contents remained the same throughout the trial [14]. The study participants received the allocated program (FES or control) in addition to the usual training. To ensure homogeneity of treatment at the 30 facilities, an educational program was implemented in advance

2.4.1. FES Group

The participants in the FES group underwent a 40 min training program 5 days a week for 8 weeks with Walkaide® (Teijin Pharma Ltd., Tokyo, Japan) (the stimulation parameters have been detailed previously [14]). WalkAide electrical stimulation was performed by applying electrodes to the peroneal nerve bifurcation and the tibialis anterior muscle using an asymmetrical biphasic pulse. Stimulation was performed at voltages ranging from 121 V at 1 KΩ to 150 V at 1 MΩ, and the electrodes were fixed at the voltage at which appropriate ankle dorsiflexion for walking was obtained. After appropriate dorsiflexion was obtained, the pulse width (25–300 µs) and stimulation period (maximum 3 s) were adjusted to set the appropriate stimulation pattern for each subject [14]. The therapeutic electrical stimulation (TES) mode was used in patients with an FAC score of 3. In contrast, the HAND mode (manual electrical stimulation) and TILT mode (electrical stimulation delivered in the swing phase based on a tilt sensor) were used in patients with an FAC score of 4. Treatment modes were selected to be adjusted by qualified program providers. The use of AFO was prohibited during FES training. All training was overviewed by physicians or physical therapists.

2.4.2. Control Group

A 40 min training program without FES was provided 5 days a week for 8 weeks. For patients with an FAC score of 3, self-stretching and foot dorsiflexion ROM training (triple foot triceps stretch training to extend the foot dorsiflexion ROM) was added; for patients with an FAC score of 4, gait training using AFO was added.

2.5. Outcomes

The primary outcome was the mean change in the distance covered during the 6 min walk test (6-MWT), defined as the difference in the distances (meters) during a 6-MWT performed barefoot at week 0 (pretreatment period) and until week 8 [16]. The secondary outcomes included the changes in the 10-MWT [17,18], performed at a comfortable walking speed, of which the average value of two measurements was calculated [16,19,20]. Other secondary outcome measures included were as follows: (1) the 6-MWT with an AFO or FES; (2) the Fugl–Meyer assessment score; (3) the modified Ashworth scale score; (4) the active and passive ROM for ankle dorsiflexion; (5) the Timed Up and Go test; (6) Stroke Impact Scale score; (7) patient-reported outcome measures (questionnaire); and (8) gait evaluation by the care providers (videotaped). All outcomes were collected during week 0 and week 8. For the safety assessment, any adverse events (AEs) were collected regardless of their severity.

2.6. Statistical Analysis

The planned study population comprised 200 patients (100 in each group). With 200 patients, a difference of 43.8 m in the 6-MWT was detectable with a statistical power of 80%, based on the assumption that the standard deviation (SD) was 110 m. Two-sample t-tests were performed to compare the change in the 6-MWT distance between the groups. All analyses were predefined in the statistical analysis plan before locking the database and were conducted using SAS version 9.4 (SAS Institute Inc., Cary, NC, USA). Data are expressed as means with SDs for continuous variables and frequencies and percentages for discrete variables unless specifically mentioned. The significance level was set at $p < 0.05$ (two-tailed). As the primary analysis was conducted in accordance with the modified intention-to-treat principle, the analysis excluded patients whose intervention was not initiated, but included patients whose intervention was prematurely discontinued, as prespecified in the protocol.

3. Results

The study was conducted with enrolment from May 2016 to December 2018. A total of 203 patients were randomly assigned to the FES ($n = 102$) or control group ($n = 101$) (Figure 1). Eighty-four patients in the FES group and 85 patients in the control group completed the intervention. After excluding 19 patients who did not receive the intervention or whose data were not available, the data of the primary outcomes of 184 patients (92 in each group) were analyzed. The baseline characteristics of the two groups were similar (Table 1). The mean age at recruitment was 64 (SD: 11) years. A total of 138 (75%) patients were men. A total of 102 patients (55%) had cerebral infarction, while 101 patients (55%) had an FAC score of 3.

The primary outcome (mean change in the maximum distance during the 6-MWT (barefoot) from the baseline to the end of the trial) was 68.37 (SD: 62.42) m in the FES group and 57.50 (SD: 68.17) m in the control group (Tables 2 and A1). There was no statistically significant difference between the groups (10.86 m; 95% CI: −8.26 to 29.98, $p = 0.26$).

In the secondary outcomes (Table 2), no statistically significant difference was observed between the groups other than the active dorsiflexion ROM, patient-reported outcome measures, and gait analysis (barefoot). Other outcomes of examinations with FES are presented in Appendix A. $p = 0.26$).

There were seven (7%) cases and two (2%) cases of AEs in the FES and control groups, respectively (Table 3). The most frequent AE was falling (five events in three patients in the FES group), with mild severity in all cases, and no events were related to the trial device. One case of a serious AE occurred in the FES group (femur fracture, one event), whereas no such AEs were reported in the control group. In one patient in the FES group, the device malfunctioned due to Bluetooth and application failure, which was resolved through inspection and replacement of the device.

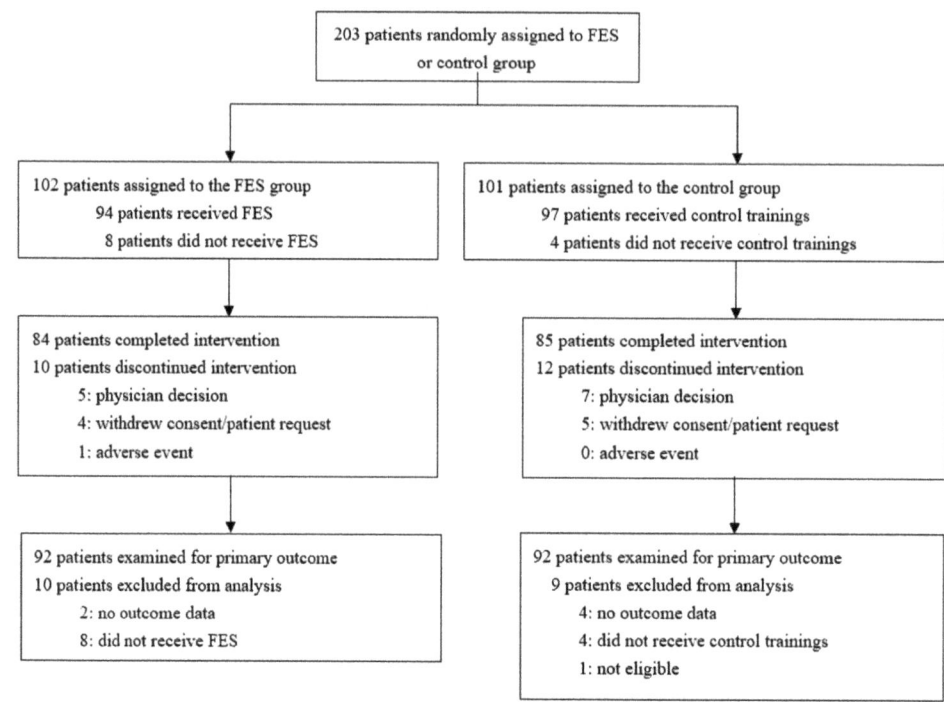

Figure 1. Trial profile. Abbreviation: FES, functional electrical stimulation.

Table 1. Baseline characteristics by treatment allocation. Data are presented as means (SDs) or n (%). Abbreviations: FAC, functional ambulation classification; MAS, modified Ashworth scale; SD, standard deviation.

		FES (n = 92)	Control (n = 92)
Age, years		63.5 (10.5)	64.3 (11.8)
Sex (male)		70 (76)	68 (74)
Body weight, kg		62.6 (10.9)	61.4 (12.0)
Time since stroke onset, days		59.5 (32.6)	63.7 (30.4)
Cause of hemiplegia	Cerebral hemorrhage	42 (46)	40 (43)
	Cerebral infarction	50 (54)	52 (57)
FAC category	3	49 (53)	52 (57)
	4	43 (47)	40 (43)
MAS score of plantar flexor muscles, knee extended	0	10 (11)	14 (15)
	1	28 (30)	27 (29)
	1+	32 (35)	31 (34)
	2	17 (18)	18 (20)
	3	5 (5)	1 (1)
	4	0 (0)	0 (0)
MAS score of plantar flexor muscles, knee flexed	0	21 (23)	21 (23)
	1	34 (37)	34 (37)
	1+	24 (26)	25 (27)
	2	11 (12)	10 (11)
	3	2 (2)	1 (1)
	4	0 (0)	0 (0)
Dorsiflexion range of motion	Active	5.5 (5.5)	7.6 (7.6)
	Passive, knee extended	7.0 (6.1)	6.0 (7.6)
	Passive, knee flexed	13.6 (6.6)	14.7 (7.5)

Table 2. Primary and secondary outcomes. Data are presented as means (SDs). No conclusions can be made regarding differences in secondary outcomes because of the lack of planned adjustment for multiple comparisons. Abbreviations: 6-MWT, 6 min walk test; AFO, ankle-foot orthosis; FMA, Fugl–Meyer Assessment.

		FES (n = 92)			Control (n = 92)			
		Baseline	Follow-Up	Change	Baseline	Follow-Up	Change	p-Value
6-MWT (barefoot) distance, m		164.21 (105.99)	232.57 (122.88)	68.37 (62.42)	153.87 (113.96)	211.37 (126.89)	57.50 (68.17)	0.26
6-MWT (with AFO) distance, m		179.46 (92.66)	238.24 (97.87)	58.78 (55.66)	178.61 (109.96)	245.00 (123.76)	66.40 (55.25)	0.39
10-m walk test (barefoot) speed, m/s		0.55 (0.29)	0.76 (0.31)	0.21 (0.18)	0.51 (0.3)	0.68 (0.37)	0.17 (0.17)	0.16
10-m walk test (with AFO) speed, m/s		0.54 (0.25)	0.71 (0.28)	0.17 (0.16)	0.55 (0.28)	0.71 (0.33)	0.16 (0.14)	0.86
Lower extremity FMA score		25.65 (4.87)	27.31 (4.33)	1.66 (2.49)	25.16 (5.14)	26.43 (5.29)	1.28 (2.9)	0.34
MAS score of plantar flexor muscles	Knee extended	1.36 (0.69)	1.21 (0.68)	−0.15 (0.67)	1.24 (0.66)	1.06 (0.67)	−0.18 (0.61)	0.76
	Knee flexed	1.06 (0.71)	1.07 (0.72)	0.01 (0.68)	1.04 (0.68)	0.90 (0.65)	−0.14 (0.65)	0.15
Dorsiflexion range of motion	Active	5.46 (5.57)	8.54 (6.54)	3.08 (4.21)	7.73 (7.6)	8.33 (8.7)	0.61 (4.25)	0.001
	Passive, knee flexed	13.62 (6.59)	14.66 (6.37)	1.03 (5.51)	14.72 (7.48)	15.06 (7.74)	0.34 (5.58)	0.41
Timed up and go test (barefoot), s	At comfortable speed	28.52 (15.88)	19.18 (10.09)	−9.34 (10.23)	31.29 (18.84)	22.84 (16.66)	−8.45 (10.71)	0.58
	At maximum speed	23.32 (13.07)	16.30 (9.82)	−7.03 (8.61)	27.02 (17.83)	18.99 (13.66)	−8.03 (10.24)	0.49
Timed up and go test (with AFO), s	At comfortable speed	27.81 (16.77)	20.12 (11.69)	−7.68 (12.45)	29.68 (19.66)	21.48 (15.65)	−8.20 (10.8)	0.78
	At maximum speed	23.32 (13.07)	16.30 (9.82)	−7.03 (8.61)	27.02 (17.83)	18.99 (13.66)	−8.03 (10.24)	0.49
Stroke Impact Scale	Mobility	53.49 (21.26)	76.17 (17.61)	22.69 (21.61)	52.17 (21.11)	71.71 (23.03)	19.54 (21.52)	0.33
	Total score	54.32 (12.17)	64.50 (13.84)	10.18 (11.92)	54.15 (13.32)	62.92 (14.3)	8.77 (10.9)	0.41
Patient-reported	Burden in raising the foot during barefoot walking	40.76 (22.23)	59.42 (20.57)	18.66 (23.44)	37.35 (23.73)	51.45 (22.76)	14.10 (24.32)	0.20
	Spasticity while walking bare-footed	50.53 (28.79)	67.58 (26.64)	17.05 (33.84)	57.49 (32.74)	60.08 (28.12)	2.59 (33.37)	0.005
	Stability in bare-footed walking	41.85 (24.93)	64.25 (23.22)	22.41 (22.69)	40.19 (25.36)	54.55 (26.79)	14.35 (24.91)	0.02
Gait disturbance evaluated by the care providers (barefoot)	At stance phase	3.15 (12.54)	9.38 (12.34)	6.23 (6.96)	1.99 (11.85)	6.05 (12.97)	4.06 (6.32)	0.04
	At swing phase	2.42 (10.23)	7.12 (10.26)	4.70 (5.45)	1.77 (9.79)	4.68 (10.53)	2.90 (4.71)	0.02
	At all phases	5.57 (22.69)	16.50 (22.52)	10.93 (12.17)	3.76 (21.55)	10.73 (23.44)	6.96 (10.79)	0.03
Gait disturbance (AFO)	At stance phase	2.76 (9.49)	8.28 (10.13)	5.53 (5.71)	2.79 (10.23)	6.87 (10.98)	4.08 (6.62)	0.15
	At swing phase	1.81 (7.99)	6.26 (8.26)	4.45 (4.38)	1.90 (8.48)	5.19 (9.02)	3.29 (5.09)	0.13
	At all phases	4.57 (17.37)	14.54 (18.31)	9.97 (9.81)	4.69 (18.63)	12.06 (19.94)	7.37 (11.53)	0.13

Table 3. Adverse events. Data are presented as n (%).

	FES (n = 94)	Control (n = 96)	p-Value
Any adverse event	7 (7)	2 (2)	0.10
Adverse events related to treatment	0	0	-
Any serious adverse event	1 (1)	0	0.49

4. Discussion

To the best of our knowledge, this was the first large-scale randomized, controlled trial conducted to evaluate the effectiveness of FES in Japanese convalescent post-stroke patients with hemiplegic gait disorder. Previous studies with smaller sizes have shown that FES improves the quality of gait in non-Japanese patients with foot drop [7–10]. However, the effect of the FES device is expected to be different from that in Western patients because of the Japanese lifestyle, which is often spent barefoot, requiring complex muscle movements due to the instability of the ankle joint. In this trial, FES did not significantly improve the distance covered by post-stroke patients with foot drop in the barefoot 6-MWT, which was the primary outcome.

Only a few studies with small sample sizes ($n < 30$) have focused on convalescent stroke patients [21,22]. In our trial ($n = 184$), the mean duration of the convalescent period was 61.6 days. In general, considering the plasticity of the brain, the paralysis of lower limb function is best improved within 3 months after onset. As this trial focused on such a convalescent phase important for recovery from paralysis, it could offer valuable information. Previous studies have shown the effectiveness of FES in improving receptivity to gait [21] and improving ankle paralysis [22,23], but all of these studies were conducted with small numbers of patients. On the other hand, there are also reports that FES did not improve ankle paralysis [24], which may depend on the number of cases, the time since stroke onset, and the paralysis assessment scale. In the FES group in this study, there were no group differences in walking speed, cadence, or FAC grade, though there was a tendency toward improved receptivity to gait (Appendix A). The ROM for ankle dorsiflexion and Fugl–Meyer assessment were used to assess paralysis in our study. Although no improvement was observed with the Fugl–Meyer assessment, there was an improvement in the ankle dorsiflexion ROM. These findings suggest that the device selection, frequency of use, and study endpoint should be carefully considered in future studies.

As it is usual to walk indoors with bare feet in Japan, we chose the 6-MWT (barefoot) as the primary outcome measure for our trial. Wearing Walkaide® enables patients to comfortably walk indoors with bare feet while feeling the ground with the soles of the foot. Everaert et al. [8] conducted a randomized, controlled, crossover trial with three parallel arms ($n = 121$) to compare the effectiveness of Walkaide® and AFO in post-stroke patients within 1 year from onset (convalescent phase plus chronic phase, mean: 6.4 months; SD: 3.6 months). A large but non-significant difference in improvement was observed in walking speed (barefoot) when comparing Walkaide® and AFO. Similarly, no significant difference was observed in either the 10-MWT (barefoot) or 6-MWT (barefoot) in our trial. In the trial of Everaert et al. [8], AFO was not used in the control group, which may have affected the difference. In many trials, FES was shown to be non-superior to AFO [10,25,26]. In particular, we speculated that allowing the control group to use AFO might have masked the effectiveness of FES in this study. In contrast, a significant difference was observed in the gait evaluation, when walking barefoot, by care providers and was better in the FES group. This suggests that FES can make patients walk correctly and cleanly, as reported by Sheffler et al. [22], although walking speed and distance were unchanged.

We analyzed the walking speed, stride length, gait, and walking distance within a specified time, as in the 6-MWT, 3-MWT, and 10-MWT, and observed significant improvements after the FES intervention in the 6-MWT (barefoot, FES, AFO), 10-MWT (barefoot, FES, AFO), and timed up and go test (degree of comfort in a maximum of barefoot, FES, AFO). However, as mentioned before, there is a possibility that the effectiveness of FES was unexpectedly masked because AFO use was allowed in the control group in our trial. Moreover, it was noteworthy that the barefoot gait evaluation in the stance phase, swing phase, and all phases showed a significant difference between the groups. In the previous reports, the evaluation methods were diverse, and the results varied depending on the equipment used for the intervention and the intervention methodology (frequency, duration, control, etc.). Generally, FES is not superior to AFO, and improvements with FES are similar to those with AFO in various walking evaluation methods. According to the report by Everaert et al. [8], significantly more patients preferred Walkaide® as a supportive device after the study. The study by Salisbury et al. [21] also reported that the FES device tended to improve the patient's receptivity to walking. Thus, patients experienced comfort while walking with the FES support, which did not change the walking speed or distance; this was reflected by the differences between the groups in the three patient-reported outcomes assessed. Post-stroke patients preferred Walkaide® as a supportive device.

Study Limitations

This study had some limitations. First, the inclusion criteria should have been broader, including patients with an earlier onset or lower walking ability. Second, more consideration should be given to the use of AFO in the control group to avoid affecting the results. Third, we should have promoted the selection of the TILT mode more actively because Walkaide® is originally intended for use in the TILT mode. In future studies, these limitations should be considered when planning the study design. Lastly, gait disorders are complex in nature, involving not only weakness of the legs, but also spatio-temporal patterns, joint position sense [27], and other coordination disorders [28] that affect the nature of movement. Although we have tried to eliminate, as much as possible, the influence on gait, other than that of stroke, in the eligibility criteria, it is important to try to analyze in detail and stratify the data of the gait condition recordings conducted in this study.

5. Conclusions

FES did not significantly improve the distance covered during the barefoot 6-MWT performed by Japanese convalescent stroke patients with hemiplegic gait disorder (foot drop). A similar study design, the PLEASURE study [29] of chronic stroke patients, found that the magnitude of improvement in gait ability and ankle-specific body function in the FES group was similar to that in the control group, as did the results of this study. Electrical stimulation to promote ankle dorsiflexion with the WalkAide did not show efficacy in the treatment of Japanese convalescent stroke patients with drooping legs, but future work is needed to investigate the therapeutic effects of the device or stimulation conditions.

Author Contributions: All authors have read and approved the final version of this report and have final responsibility for the decision to submit it for publication. S.M. and M.S. (Megumi Shimodozono) contributed to the conceptualization, investigation, and supervision. T.N. and K.M. contributed to the investigation and supervision. T.O., R.I., T.S., A.S., H.O. and M.S. (Makiko Seto) contributed to the investigation. M.T. contributed to the formal analysis and software. H.K., M.M. and S.K. contributed to the Writing–review & editing and visualization. RALLY Trial Investigators contributed to interventions and evaluations throughout the study. All authors have read and agreed to the published version of the manuscript.

Funding: The RALLY study was supported by Teijin Pharma Ltd. (Tokyo, Japan).

Institutional Review Board Statement: The study was conducted in accordance with the Declaration of Helsinki and approved by the Ethics Committees of all participating institutions (https://www.umin.ac.jp/ctr, UMIN000020604).

Informed Consent Statement: Informed consent was obtained from all subjects involved in the study.

Data Availability Statement: The data that support the findings of this study are available from the corresponding author, [S.M.], upon reasonable request.

Acknowledgments: We would like to thank all of the individuals that participated in this study, without whom this study would not be possible. The RALLY trial investigators and committees are presented in the Appendix B. All individuals associated with this study have agreed to the acknowledgements.

Conflicts of Interest: The authors declare that there is no conflict of interest. The funder, Teijin Pharma Ltd., had no involvement in the study design, data collection, management, analysis, interpretation, manuscript preparation, or the decision to submit the manuscript for publication. However, the company was informed of the progress of the study. No confidentiality agreement regarding the data was signed.

Appendix A

Table A1. Outcomes of examinations with FES. Data are presented as means (SDs). 6-MWT, 6 min walk test; FES, functional electrical stimulation.

		FES (n = 92)		
		Baseline	Follow-Up	Change
6-MWT distance, m		193.07 (108.05)	257.08 (110.47)	64.01 (61.99)
10 m walk test speed, m/s		0.58 (0.27)	0.78 (0.29)	0.20 (0.15)
Timed up and go test, s	At comfortable speed	25.78 (18.92)	18.18 (9.58)	−7.61 (16.8)
	At maximum speed	21.71 (18.12)	15.35 (8.12)	−6.37 (16.23)
Gait disturbance at 10 m walk test	At stance phase	6.27 (11.31)	11.83 (11.1)	5.56 (5.99)
	At swing phase	4.67 (9.24)	9.08 (8.91)	4.41 (4.69)
	At all phases	10.94 (20.48)	20.91 (19.96)	9.97 (10.51)

Appendix B

The RALLY trial investigators and committees

Principal Investigator:
Shuji Matsumoto, Center of Medical Education, Faculty of Health Sciences, Ryotokuji University, Japan.

Vice Principal Investigator:
Megumi Shimodozono, Department of Rehabilitation and Physical Medicine, Graduate School of Medical and Dental Sciences, Kagoshima University, Japan.
Ryuji Miyata, Department of Rehabilitation and Physical Medicine, Graduate School of Medical and Dental Sciences, Kagoshima University, Japan.
Data And Safety Monitoring Committee.
Toyoko Asami, Department of Rehabilitation Medicine, Saga University Hospital, Japan.
Akihiko Oowatashi, School of Health Sciences, Faculty of Medicine, Kagoshima University, Japan.
Saburo Omine, Faculty of Rehabilitation, Kyusyu Nutrition Welfare University.

Blinded Independent Central Review Board (Fugl–Meyer assessment, gait evaluation):
Rina Ijichi, Department of Rehabilitation, Kirishima Sugiyasu Hospital, Japan.
Tetsuya Onoda, Department of Rehabilitation, Kirishima Medical Center, Japan.

Trial Statistician:
Masanori Taketsuna, Translational Research Center for Medical Innovation, Japan.

Study sites and trial investigators:
Jun Ohkawara, Department of Rehabilitation, Ohkawara Neurosurgical Hospital.
Takashi Shigematsu, Shintaro Iio, Tetsuya Suzuki, Department of Rehabilitation, Hamamatsu City Rehabilitation Hospital.
Akira Satone, Keisuke Ono, Senshuu Abe, Eri Tanita, Department of Rehabilitation, Tokachi Rehabilitation Center.
Hidenobu Okuma, Hironori Fujisaki, Department of Rehabilitation, Kumamoto Takumadai Rehabilitation Hospital.
Makiko Seto, Junya Sasahara, Hiroyuki Yamamoto, Department of Rehabilitation, Nagasaki Kita Hospital.
Shigeatsu Natsume, Masamori Fujiwara, Department of Rehabilitation, Eishokai Medical Corporation, Yoshida Hospital Cerebrovascular Research Institute.
Norihito Kimura, Department of Rehabilitation, Caress Sapporo Tokeidai Memorial Hospital.
Hirokazu Kawano, Department of Rehabilitation, Junwakai Memorial Hospital.
Osamu Kira, Yousuke Miyanaga, Department of Rehabilitation Therapy, Junwakai Memorial Hospital.
Kenji Matsumoto, Makiko Hayakawa, Department of Rehabilitation, Kansai Rehabilitation Hospital.
Yuji Hashimoto, Department of Rehabilitation, Sapporo Shiroishi Memorial Hospital.

Yasuhide Kido, Osamu Yamazaki, Yuuichi Suzuki, Department of Rehabilitation, Matsuyama Rehabilitation Hospital.
Megumi Shimodozono, Rintaro Ohama, Ryuji Miyata, Department of Rehabilitation and Physical Medicine, Graduate School of Medical and Dental Sciences, Kagoshima University.
Tomohiro Uema, Department of Rehabilitation, Kagoshima University Hospital.
Makoto Ide, Koichiro Tobinaga, Tsutomu Asou, Shun Kumamoto, Department of Rehabilitation, St Mary's Healthcare Center.
Keizo Shigenobu, Yumeko Amano, Department of Rehabilitation, Kohshinkai Ogura Hospital.
Toshihiro Nakamura, Kota Homan, Department of Rehabilitation, Acras Central Hospital.
Yuki Onishi, Atsushi Manji, Kazuki Ogashira, Department of Rehabilitation, Saitama Misato General Rehabilitation Hospital.
Tojiro Yanagi, Tetuya Noda, Horoki Fukuda, Department of Rehabilitation, Yame Rehabili Hospital.
Katsuhiro Harada, Yuki Nakama, Keisuke Shibuya, Department of Rehabilitation, Fujimoto Kamimachi Hospital.
Kanjiro Suzuki, Nobuaki Oshikawa, Tatsuya Yamashita, Department of Rehabilitation, Nichinan Municipal Chubu Hospital.
You Ikegami, Kouhei Totiki, Department of Rehabilitation, Yohkoh Rehabilitation Hospital.
Taisuke Arai, Kenji Ogushi, Shinya Nakagawa, Department of Rehabilitation, Shin Yachiyo Hospital.
Rintaro Ohama, Yuji Sakashita, Kazutoshi Tomioka, Sota Araki, Department of Rehabilitation, Tarumizu Municipal Medical Center, Tarumizu Central Hospital.
Yuko Takiyoshi, Hirohisa Oyadomari, Wakako Omine, Sayoko Hirayama, Department of Rehabilitation, Nambu Tokushukai Hospital.
Shoichi Tanaka, Keisuke Sato, Takafumi Miyagi, Department of Rehabilitation, Chuzan Hospital.
Masahiko Toshima, Kazuhiro Yanai, Naoki Shoji, Yuto Yamamoto. Department of Rehabilitation, Hokusei Memorial Hospital. Makoto Kawasaki, Sakurajyuji Hospital.
Satoru Matayoshi, Department of Rehabilitation, Okinawa Rehabilitation Center Hospital.
Keisuke Horinouchi, Department of Rehabilitation, Kajikionsen Hospital.
Yuichi Komaba, Daiki Ooshima, Department of Rehabilitation, Hakujikai Memorial Hospital.
Taro Ogawa, Department of Rehabilitation, Sapporo Keijinkai Rehabilitation Hospital.
Jun Takeshita, Department of Rehabilitation, IMS Itabashi Rehabilitation Hospital.
Data Center:
Translational Research Center for Medical Innovation.
Satoshi Nakagawa, Project Manager.
Kuniko Hosokawa, Data Manager.
Yoko Nakagawa, Statistical Programmer.

References

1. Feigin, V.L.; Forouzanfar, M.H.; Krishnamurthi, R.; Mensah, G.A.; Connor, M.; Bennett, D.A.; Moran, A.E.; Sacco, R.L.; Anderson, L.; Truelsen, T.; et al. Global and Regional Burden of Stroke During 1990–2010: Findings From the Global Burden of Disease Study 2010. *Lancet* **2014**, *383*, 245–254. [CrossRef]
2. Da Cunha, M.J.; Rech, K.D.; Salazar, A.P.; Pagnussat, A.S. Functional electrical stimulation of the peroneal nerve improves post-stroke gait speed when combined with physiotherapy. A systematic review and meta-analysis. *Ann. Phys. Rehabil. Med.* **2021**, *64*, 101388. [CrossRef] [PubMed]
3. Prenton, S.; Hollands, K.L.; Kenney, P.J.L. Functional electrical stimulation versus ankle foot orthoses for foot-drop: A meta-analysis of orthotic effects. *J. Rehabil. Med.* **2016**, *48*, 646–656. [CrossRef] [PubMed]
4. Ohata, K.; Yasui, T.; Tsuboyama, T.; Ichihashi, N. Effects of an Ankle-Foot Orthosis with Oil Damper on Muscle Activity in Adults After Stroke. *Gait. Posture* **2011**, *33*, 102–107. [CrossRef]
5. Shahabi, S.; Shabaninejad, H.; Kamali, M.; Jalali, M.; Ahmadi Teymourlouy, A. The Effects of Ankle-Foot Orthoses on Walking Speed in Patients with Stroke: A Systematic Review and Meta-analysis of Randomized Controlled Trials. *Clin. Rehabil.* **2020**, *34*, 145–159. [CrossRef]

6. Gil-Castillo, J.; Alnajjar, F.; Koutsou, A.; Torricelli, D.; Moreno, J.C. Advances in Neuroprosthetic Management of Foot Drop: A Review. *J. Neuroeng. Rehabil.* **2020**, *17*, 46. [CrossRef] [PubMed]
7. Kluding, P.M.; Dunning, K.; O'Dell, M.W.; Wu, S.S.; Ginosian, J.; Feld, J.; McBride, K. Foot Drop Stimulation Versus Ankle Foot Orthosis After Stroke: 30-Week Outcomes. *Stroke* **2013**, *44*, 1660–1669. [CrossRef]
8. Everaert, D.G.; Stein, R.B.; Abrams, G.M.; Dromerick, A.W.; Francisco, G.E.; Hafner, B.J.; Huskey, T.N.; Munin, M.C.; Nolan, K.J.; Kufta, C.V. Effect of a Foot-Drop Stimulator and Ankle-Foot Orthosis on Walking Performance After Stroke: A Multicenter Randomized Controlled Trial. *Neurorehabil. Neural Repair.* **2013**, *27*, 579–591. [CrossRef]
9. Sheffler, L.R.; Taylor, P.N.; Gunzler, D.D.; Buurke, J.H.; IJzerman, M.J.; Chae, J. Randomized Controlled Trial of Surface Peroneal Nerve Stimulation for Motor Relearning in Lower Limb Hemiparesis. *Arch. Phys. Med. Rehabil.* **2013**, *94*, 1007–1014. [CrossRef] [PubMed]
10. Bethoux, F.; Rogers, H.L.; Nolan, K.J.; Abrams, G.M.; Annaswamy, T.M.; Brandstater, M.; Browne, B.; Burnfield, J.M.; Feng, W.; Freed, M.J.; et al. The Effects of Peroneal Nerve Functional Electrical Stimulation Versus Ankle-Foot Orthosis in Patients with Chronic Stroke: A Randomized Controlled Trial. *Neurorehabil. Neural Repair* **2014**, *28*, 688–697. [CrossRef]
11. Miyai, I.; Sonoda, S.; Nagai, S.; Takayama, Y.; Inoue, Y.; Kakehi, A.; Kurihara, M.; Ishikawa, M. Results of New Policies for Inpatient Rehabilitation Coverage in Japan. *Neurorehabil. Neural Repair* **2011**, *25*, 540–547. [CrossRef]
12. Reed, S.D.; Blough, D.K.; Meyer, K.; Jarvik, J.G. Inpatient Costs, Length of Stay, and Mortality for Cerebrovascular Events in Community Hospitals. *Neurology* **2001**, *57*, 305–314. [CrossRef] [PubMed]
13. Gillum, R.F.; Kwagyan, J.; Obisesan, T.O. Ethnic and Geographic Variation in Stroke Mortality Trends. *Stroke* **2011**, *42*, 3294–3296. [CrossRef] [PubMed]
14. Matsumoto, S.; Shimodozono, M.; Noma, T. Rationale and Design of the theRapeutic Effects of Peroneal Nerve functionAl Electrical stimuLation for Lower Extremity in Patients with Convalescent Poststroke Hemiplegia (RALLY) Study: Study Protocol for a Randomised Controlled Study. *BMJ Open* **2019**, *9*, e026214. [CrossRef] [PubMed]
15. Holden, M.K.; Gill, K.M.; Magliozzi, M.R.; Nathan, J.; Piehl-Baker, L. Clinical Gait Assessment in the Neurologically Impaired: Reliability and Meaningfulness. *Phys. Ther.* **1984**, *64*, 35–40. [CrossRef]
16. Solway, S.; Brooks, D.; Lacasse, Y.; Thomas, S. A Qualitative Systematic Overview of the Measurement Properties of Functional Walk Tests Used in the Cardiorespiratory Domain. *Chest* **2001**, *119*, 256–270. [CrossRef]
17. Wade, D.T.; Wood, V.A.; Heller, A.; Maggs, J.; Langton Hewer, R. Walking after Stroke. Measurement and Recovery Over the First 3 Months. *Scand. J. Rehabil. Med.* **1987**, *19*, 25–30.
18. Street, T.; Taylor, P.; Swain, I. Effectiveness of Functional Electrical Stimulation on Walking Speed, Functional Walking Category, and Clinically Meaningful Changes for People with Multiple Sclerosis. *Arch. Phys. Med. Rehabil.* **2015**, *96*, 667–672. [CrossRef] [PubMed]
19. Graham, J.E.; Ostir, G.V.; Fisher, S.R.; Ottenbacher, K.J. Assessing Walking Speed in Clinical Research: A Systematic Review. *J. Eval. Clin. Pract.* **2008**, *14*, 552–562. [CrossRef]
20. Stein, R.B.; Everaert, D.G.; Thompson, A.K.; Chong, S.L.; Whittaker, M.; Robertson, J.; Kuether, G. Long-Term Therapeutic and Orthotic Effects of a Foot Drop Stimulator on Walking Performance in Progressive and Nonprogressive Neurological Disorders. *Neurorehabil. Neural Repair* **2010**, *24*, 152–167. [CrossRef]
21. Salisbury, L.; Shiels, J.; Todd, I.; Dennis, M. A Feasibility Study to Investigate the Clinical Application of Functional Electrical Stimulation (FES), for Dropped Foot, During the Sub-acute Phase of Stroke-A Randomized Controlled Trial. *Physiother. Theory Pract.* **2013**, *29*, 31–40. [CrossRef]
22. Sheffler, L.R.; Taylor, P.N.; Bailey, S.N.; Gunzler, D.D.; Buurke, J.H.; IJzerman, M.J.; Chae, J. Surface Peroneal Nerve Stimulation in Lower Limb Hemiparesis: Effect on Quantitative Gait Parameters. *Am. J. Phys. Med. Rehabil.* **2015**, *94*, 341–357. [CrossRef] [PubMed]
23. Mesci, N.; Ozdemir, F.; Kabayel, D.D.; Tokuc, B. The Effects of Neuromuscular Electrical Stimulation on Clinical Improvement in Hemiplegic Lower Extremity Rehabilitation in Chronic Stroke: A Single-Blind, Randomised, Controlled Trial. *Disabil. Rehabil.* **2009**, *31*, 2047–2054. [CrossRef] [PubMed]
24. Wilkinson, I.A.; Burridge, J.; Strike, P.; Taylor, P. A Randomised Controlled Trial of Integrated Electrical Stimulation and Physiotherapy to Improve Mobility for People Less Than 6 Months Post Stroke. *Disabil. Rehabil. Assist. Technol.* **2015**, *10*, 468–474. [CrossRef]
25. Bethoux, F.; Rogers, H.L.; Nolan, K.J.; Abrams, G.M.; Annaswamy, T.; Brandstater, M.; Browne, B.; Burnfield, J.M.; Feng, W.; Freed, M.J.; et al. Long-Term Follow-Up to a Randomized Controlled Trial Comparing Peroneal Nerve Functional Electrical Stimulation to an Ankle Foot Orthosis for Patients with Chronic Stroke. *Neurorehabil. Neural Repair* **2015**, *29*, 911–922. [CrossRef]
26. Bosch, P.R.; Harris, J.E.; Wing, K.; American Congress of Rehabilitation Medicine (ACRM) Stroke Movement Interventions Subcommittee. Review of Therapeutic Electrical Stimulation for Dorsiflexion Assist and Orthotic Substitution from the American Congress of Rehabilitation Medicine Stroke Movement Interventions Subcommittee. *Arch. Phys. Med. Rehabil.* **2014**, *95*, 390–396. [CrossRef] [PubMed]
27. Li, S.; Francisco, G.E.; Zhou, P. Post-stroke Hemiplegic Gait: New Perspective and Insights. *Front. Physiol.* **2018**, *9*, 1021. [CrossRef]

28. Dean, J.C.; Kautz, S.A. Foot placement control and gait instability among people with stroke. *J. Rehabil. Res. Dev.* **2015**, *52*, 577–590. [CrossRef]
29. Hachisuka, K.; Ochi, M.; Kikuchi, T.; Saeki, S. Clinical effectiveness of peroneal nerve functional electrical stimulation in chronic stroke patients with hemiplegia (PLEASURE): A multicentre, prospective, randomised controlled trial. *Clin Rehabil.* **2021**, *35*, 367–377. [CrossRef]

Disclaimer/Publisher's Note: The statements, opinions and data contained in all publications are solely those of the individual author(s) and contributor(s) and not of MDPI and/or the editor(s). MDPI and/or the editor(s) disclaim responsibility for any injury to people or property resulting from any ideas, methods, instructions or products referred to in the content.

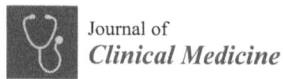 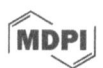

Article

A Smart Glove Digital System Promotes Restoration of Upper Limb Motor Function and Enhances Cortical Hemodynamic Changes in Subacute Stroke Patients with Mild to Moderate Weakness: A Randomized Controlled Trial

Seyoung Shin [1,†], Hwang-Jae Lee [2,†], Won Hyuk Chang [1], Sung Hwa Ko [3], Yong-Il Shin [3,4,*] and Yun-Hee Kim [1,5,*]

1. Department of Physical and Rehabilitation Medicine, Center for Prevention and Rehabilitation, Heart Vascular Stroke Institute, Samsung Medical Center, Sungkyunkwan University School of Medicine, Seoul 06351, Republic of Korea
2. Robot Business Team, Samsung Electronics, Suwon 16677, Republic of Korea
3. Department of Rehabilitation Medicine, Pusan National University School of Medicine, Pusan National University Yangsan Hospital, Yangsan 50612, Republic of Korea
4. Research Institute of Convergence for Biomedical Science and Technology, Pusan National University Yangsan Hospital, Yangsan 50612, Republic of Korea
5. Department of Health Science and Technology, Department of Medical Devices Management and Research, Department of Digital Healthcare, SAIHST, Sungkyunkwan University, Seoul 06355, Republic of Korea
* Correspondence: rmshin01@gmail.com (Y.-I.S.); yun1225.kim@samsung.com (Y.-H.K.); Tel.: +82-51-360-2872 (Y.-I.S.); +82-2-3410-2824 (ext. 2818) (Y.-H.K.); Fax: +82-2-3410-0388 (Y.-H.K.)
† These authors contributed equally to this work.

Abstract: This study was a randomized controlled trial to examine the effects of the RAPAEL® Smart Glove digital training system on upper extremity function and cortical hemodynamic changes in subacute stroke patients. Of 48 patients, 20 experimental and 16 controls completed the study. In addition to conventional occupational therapy (OT), the experimental group received game-based digital hand motor training with the RAPAEL® Smart Glove digital system, while the control group received extra OT for 30 min. The Fugl-Meyer assessment (UFMA) and Jebsen-Tayler hand function test (JTT) were assessed before (T0), immediately after (T1), and four weeks after intervention (T2). Cortical hemodynamics (oxyhemoglobin [OxyHb] concentration) were measured by functional near-infrared spectroscopy. The experimental group had significantly better improvements in UFMA (T1-T0 mean [SD]; Experimental 13.50 [7.49]; Control 8.00 [4.44]; $p = 0.014$) and JTT (Experimental 21.10 [20.84]; Control 5.63 [5.06]; $p = 0.012$). The OxyHb concentration change over the ipsilesional primary sensorimotor cortex during the affected wrist movement was greater in the experimental group (T1, Experimental 0.7943×10^{-4} µmol/L; Control -0.3269×10^{-4} µmol/L; $p = 0.025$). This study demonstrated a beneficial effect of game-based virtual reality training with the RAPAEL® Smart Glove digital system with conventional OT on upper extremity motor function in subacute stroke patients.

Keywords: stroke; upper extremity; motor function; cortical neuroplasticity; virtual reality

1. Introduction

Stroke is a leading cause of morbidity and the main cause of sensory-motor impairment worldwide. Several studies have reported that more than 65% of chronic stroke patients have had motor and sensory problems in the hemiparetic upper extremity [1,2]. Hand function is required for many activities of daily living (ADL), such as manipulating objects, eating, and computer and telephone use. Loss of hand function is a serious, common result of a cortical lesion from a cerebrovascular attack [3]. Therefore, recovery of hand function is of primary importance in the neurorehabilitation of stroke survivors. Furthermore, timing must be considered when planning neurorehabilitation focused on neuroplasticity following a stroke [4]. Previous studies have demonstrated that earlier rehabilitation leads to greater neuroplasticity in cortical areas controlling hand function in the lesioned hemispheres [5,6].

Previous evidence suggests that intensive repeated training is likely to be necessary to modify neural organization and promote recovery of hand motor skills in stroke patients [7,8]. Conventional rehabilitation for hand function and neuroplasticity, such as constraint-induced movement therapy [9], high-intensity training, and repetitive task-oriented training [10] often has unsatisfactory results due to insufficient patient motivation. In this regard, game-based virtual reality (VR) training is becoming a promising technology to promote motor recovery by providing high-intensity and repeated task-oriented rehabilitation with three-dimensional game programs involving patient body movement [11–14]. A 2017 Cochrane Review suggested that addition of VR to conventional care produced a significant difference between intervention and control groups in upper limb function [15]. A recent meta-analysis of 17 studies confirmed the feasibility of VR in early stroke rehabilitation and also suggested that VR intervention showed similar outcomes in upper extremity and ADL function to dose-matched conventional therapy [16].

Additionally, robotic rehabilitation was posited to have a positive effect on attention; reduce the effort needed to enhance motor control, specifically in the hand; boost motivation; boost adherence to treatment; and boost sensorimotor integration [17]. Consequently, robotic rehabilitation may complement standard rehabilitation for restoring hand function [18]. However, despite these advantages, common problems with robotic devices are their high cost, large size, and rigid components. Most devices are designed for hospital use and are too complex for patients to use on their own at home. A sensor-based, soft, smart glove device can allow multiple degrees of freedom and complex motions with soft components [19–21]. There are several smart gloves with varying features from exoskeletal gloves to fabric or strip type gloves [22]. Commercial smart gloves have been used in many fields including motion capture, video games, industrial training, and medicine. In this study, we used the RAPAEL® Smart Glove digital system with game-based VR developed by Neofect (Yong-in, Republic of Korea) for task-oriented hand training with interactive motion recognition of user movement. A task-specific, interactive, game-based VR system combined with a soft smart glove can be used for motor recovery in stroke patients [21]. The RAPAEL® Smart Glove digital system with game-based VR system for post stroke patients showed that the smart glove group had greater improvement in upper extremity motor functions than did a conventional occupational therapy group [21,23]. Similar results were demonstrated in a study with cerebral palsy patients [24]. These studies reported consistent results for effectiveness of smart glove systems for upper extremity rehabilitation. However, no study examined cortical biosignals induced by the intervention. The most reliable and repeatable cortical hemodynamic response following motor stimulation consists of increase in oxygenated hemoglobin (OxyHb) coupled with a decrease in deoxygenated hemoglobin (deOxy Hb) [25]. Functional near-infrared spectroscopy (fNIRS) is a useful and non-invasive tool for measuring blood hemodynamic changes by recording the density of cerebral blood oxygenation in real-time [26]. fNIRS is more convenient, less expensive, and more tolerant of patient movement compared to functional magnetic resonance imaging (fMRI) and is more resistant to artifacts than electroencephalography (EEG) [26,27]. Although more evidence is required on the reliability and repeatability of fNIRS data, previous studies suggested fNIRS for localizing cortical activity by measuring hemodynamic changes [25,28].

The aim of this study was to examine the superiority of RAPAEL® Smart Glove digital training compared with conventional occupational therapy (OT) alone on upper extremity function in subacute stroke patients and cortical hemodynamic changes in a small sub-sample of patients.

2. Materials and Methods

2.1. Participants

A sample size of 40 patients (20 in each of groups) was deemed sufficient to detect a clinically significant difference of 10 points for the Fugl-Meyer assessment (UFMA), assuming a standard deviation of 10.73 points, using a two-sample two-sided t-test of mean difference, a power of 80%, and a significance level of 5%. The calculation is based on the assumption that the measurements on UFMA are normally distributed, and the calculations were performed with G*Power software (version 3.1). This study enrolled 48 in-patients with upper limb functional deficits caused by stroke, who presented at Samsung Medical Center of Seoul or Pusan National University Yangsan Hospital of Yangsan-si, Republic of Korea. Participants were eligible for inclusion if they met the following requirements: (1) age between 20 and 85 years, (2) >3 weeks and <3 months after stroke onset, (3) active range of motion (ROM) in the wrist >10 degrees, and (4) unilateral upper limb deficit with a 66 > Fugl-Myer Assessment score >22. Exclusion criteria were (1) history of preexisting neurological or psychiatric disorder, (2) multiple or bilateral stroke lesions, (3) Korean Mini-Mental State Exam (K-MMSE) score <17, (4) aphasia, and (5) pregnancy. Ethics approval was granted by the Ethics Committees of Samsung Medical Center of Seoul and Pusan National University Yangsan Hospital, and written informed consent was obtained from all participants before the study. This study was retrospectively registered at ClinicalTrials.gov (accessed on 1 May 2015, NCT02431390).

2.2. Study Design

A randomized, controlled, parallel group trial with a single, blinded evaluator design was performed to test the effectiveness of hand motor training with the RAPAEL® Smart Glove digital system and game-based VR in subacute stroke patients. Eligible participants were randomly placed in either the experimental group with hand motor training with the RAPAEL® Smart Glove digital system or in the control group with conventional OT for the same amount of time. All participants were assigned a code number, and a lottery method was used for simple randomization. The clinical research coordinator assigned each patient to one of the two groups after the lottery. The patients were assigned to occupational therapists who conducted the intervention. To ensure blinding of the evaluator, patients were instructed not to share their allocation. The independent examiner who measured the outcomes and the occupational therapists who managed the intervention sessions were experts in their respective fields.

2.3. RAPAEL® Smart Glove Digital System

The RAPAEL® Smart Glove digital system was designed to provide repetitive task-oriented training to induce neuroplasticity of the motor system controlling hand function in stroke patients. The system has two types of embedded sensors to collect information on individual motions in real time. From those sensors, the system provides real-time active and passive ROM of the wrist and fingers during movement. Additionally, the system provides information about game-based VR training progress and patient achievements. By applying a 'Learning Schedule Algorithm' to game-like exercises, the RAPAEL® Smart Glove can create ADL-related tasks compatible with an individual's functional level.

2.4. Intervention Protocols

All participants were treated with 20 intervention sessions over 4 weeks, 5 times per week, 1 h per day. The experimental group received game-based VR hand motor training with the RAPAEL® Smart Glove digital system. If participants missed any training during the intervention period, additional sessions were offered at another time during the week or during an optional additional week at the end of the intervention period. For VR treatment, the occupational therapist observed each patient and selected the appropriate content and game level. The participants were required to successfully perform tasks related to a specific intended movement to obtain a high score.

In the training protocol, the average time per session was 1 h, divided into 30 min with the VR training program and 30 min of conventional OT. The intervention structure was customized to participant hand function level. As the sessions progressed, the training intensity gradually increased by changing the VR game level. The control group had 1-h sessions of conventional OT alone without VR hand motor training.

2.5. Outcome Measures

We performed the following assessments before intervention (T0), immediately after the intervention (T1), and 4 weeks after the intervention (T2). During outcome measurements, the examiners were blinded to participant group.

2.5.1. Primary Outcome: Motor Function

An occupational therapist performed upper extremity UFMA for motor impairment of the affected side and the Jebsen-Taylor hand function test (JTT) at T0, T1, and T2. The UFMA consists of 33 items (3-point ordinal scale; range, 0–66), with higher scores indicating less impairment [29]. The JTT assesses hand function according to ADL with a series of 7 timed subtests of writing, simulated page turning, picking up small objects, simulated feeding, stacking checkers, picking up large light objects, and picking up large heavy objects [30]. In the original JTT, a subtest is considered missing if it is not completed within a certain amount of time. To overcome this limitation of the original JTT scoring system, we adopted a modified system presented in a previous study. According to this modification, each subtest is scored from 0 to 15, and the total score is the sum of all subtest scores and ranges from 0 to 105 [31].

2.5.2. Secondary Outcome: Cortical Activation Changes in the Motor Cortical Regions

To investigate cortical hemodynamic changes, we measured OxyHb concentration using the NIRSscout® system (NIRx Medical Technology, Berlin, Germany), which is a multimodal, compatible, fNIRS platform. This system has optodes of 16 sources and 16 detectors, which cover the primary sensorimotor cortex (SMC), the premotor cortex (PMC), and the supplementary motor area (SMA), using 45 channels of interest (Supplementary Figure S1). The NIRSscout® uses two wavelengths (760 nm and 850 nm) with a sampling rate of 3.91 Hz. The optodes were positioned according to the international 10/20 system, and the channel distance (i.e., distance between the source and detector) was 3.0 cm. Cortical hemodynamic responses were recorded for 700 s at T0 and T1. Baseline OxyHb concentration data were collected during the first 300 s, followed by 400 s of affected wrist and hand movement. This movement consisted of five blocks of 80 s (80 s × 5 times = 400 s), each with 30 s of rest, 10 s of wrist flexion-extension, 30 s of rest, and 10 s of hand grasp task.

Amount of change in OxyHb concentration over the ipsilesional SMC was the secondary outcome. Change in OxyHb concentration was calculated as OxyHb concentration during wrist/hand movement minus OxyHb concentration during rest (ΔOxyHb = OxyHb rest − OxyHb during wrist or hand task). The OxyHb concentration was analyzed by the NIRS-SPM (Near Infrared Spectroscopy-Statistical Parametric Mapping) software package in MATLAB (The Mathworks, MA, USA) [32]. To investigate cortical hemodynamics in the affected side of the brain, the left-brain lesions were flipped from left to right during data preprocessing, so all included lesions were set on the right. We used a modified Beer-Lambert law to calculate OxyHb level following change in cortical concentration [33]. The international 10/20 system was used to position optodes with the cranial vertex (Cz) located beneath the first source. The nasion, left ear, right ear, and inion were identified in each subject. A stand-alone application was used for spatial registration of the 49 functional channels on a Montreal Neurological Institute brain.

Gaussian smoothing with a 2s full width at half maximum (FWHM) was applied to correct noise from the fNIRS system. A wavelet discrete cosine transform (DCT)-based detrending algorithm was used to correct signal distortion due to breathing or movement, and a general linear model (GLM) analysis with a canonical hemodynamic response curve was performed to model the hypothesized OxyHb response under the experimental conditions [32]. To investigate changes in cortical hemodynamics during the affected wrist and hand movements, we selected five regions of interest (ROIs), defined by Brodmann's area (BA) or anatomical markers: the SMC (BA 1, 2, 3, and 4), the PMC (BA 6), and the SMA (anterior boundary: vertical line to the anterior commissure, posterior boundary: anterior margin of the SMC, medial boundary: midline between the right and left hemispheres, lateral boundary: 15 mm lateral to the midline between the right and the left hemispheres).

2.6. Statistical Analysis

We performed per-protocol (PP) analysis of the data of participants who completed the experiments. All statistical analyses were performed with SPSS version 27.0 (version 27; SPSS, Inc., Chicago, IL, USA), and the significance level was set at 0.05. The Shapiro-Wilk test was used to confirm that all outcome variables were normally distributed. The Chi-square test was used for binary parameters to compare baseline characteristics between groups. For between-group analysis, the independent t-test and the Mann-Whitney U test were appropriately used. The paired t-test or Wilcoxon signed rank test with Bonferroni's correction was used for comparing the three time points (T0, T1, and T2). For measuring time x group interaction in UFMA and JTT, repeated measures analysis of variance (RMANOVA) was performed.

For comparing ΔOxyHb, statistical parametric mapping (SPM) t-statistic maps were computed for group analyses and were considered significant at an uncorrected threshold of $p < 0.05$. Median, interquartile range (IQR), and p value from the Mann-Whitney U test were provided to depict the change within each group.

3. Results

3.1. Participants Characteristics

A total of 48 subacute stroke patients were screened for this study from December 2015 to May 2017. Among 48 patients, six did not meet the inclusion criteria. We allocated 42 patients into experimental and control groups, each with 21 patients. During the study, one participant from the experimental group and five from the control group dropped out for reasons of: (1) patient choice (one patient), (2) failure to complete the interventions (three patients), and (3) follow-up loss (two patients). Finally, a total of 36 participants completed the 20-session intervention program and followed up until four weeks after intervention completion. These patients were included for the PP analysis. Figure 1 provides a consort flow diagram of participant recruitment and retention through this study. General characteristics of the 36 participants are shown in Table 1. No significant differences in general characteristics or dependent variables were observed between groups.

Table 1. Baseline characteristics of the study population.

Characteristic	Experimental Group (n = 20)	Control Group (n = 16)	p-Value
Sex (male: female)	10:10	7:9	0.709 [b]
Age (years)	57.00 (12.78)	63.69 (8.58)	0.070 [a]
Stroke onset duration (days)	24.70 (16.26)	34.00 (25.49)	0.336 [c]
Stroke type			
Ischemic: Hemorrhagic	11:09	13:03	0.097 [b]
Side of stroke			
Right: left	13:07	9:07	0.593 [b]
Upper extremity function			
UFMA, total	41.30 (8.90)	37.13 (12.84)	0.258 [a]
JTT, total	12.00 (15.29)	8.25 (11.93)	0.290 [c]
Spasticity of upper extremity			
MAS 0: MAS 1	18:02	15:01	0.585 [b]
K-MMSE	24.95 (3.97)	25.31 (3.57)	0.778 [a]

Continuous values are expressed as mean (standard deviation). UFMA, Fugl-Meyer assessment of upper extremity; JTT, Jebsen-Taylor hand function test; MAS, Modified Ashworth Scale; K-MMSE, Korean version of the Mini-Mental State Exam. [a] Independent t-test; [b] Chi-square test; [c] Mann-Whitney test.

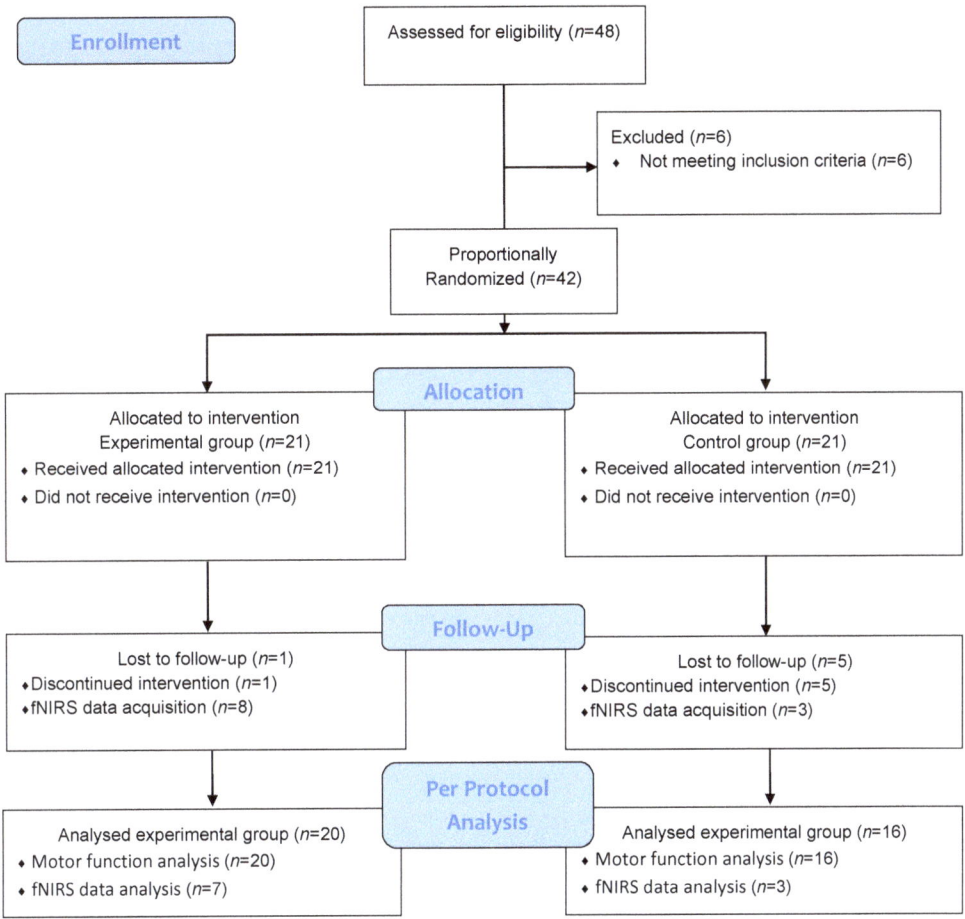

Figure 1. Consort flow diagram. fNIRS: functional near-infrared spectroscopy.

3.2. Primary Outcome Results

The UFMA raw scores before and after intervention are presented in Table 2 (Supplementary Table S1 for median and IQR and Supplementary Table S2 for within-group *p*-value) and Figure 2. The changes in the UFMA scores in the two groups are compared in Table 3. After the intervention, the experimental group showed larger improvement in the UFMA total (mean [SD]; Experimental 13.50 [7.49]; Control 8.00 [4.44]; *p* = 0.014) and subscores in wrist (Experimental 3.35 [2.25]; Control 1.38 [1.36]; *p* = 0.024), hand (Experimental 4.60 [3.68]; Control 2.13 [1.86]; *p* = 0.043), and coordination/speed (Experimental 1.40 [1.14]; Control 0.69 [0.79]; *p* = 0.048) than the control group. In the subsequent four weeks, there were significant differences between the two groups only in UFMA wrist (Experimental 0.20 [1.15]; Control 1.75 [1.44]; *p* = 0.001) subscore. In addition, the UFMA total score had a significant group × time interaction such that the experimental group had greater improvement ($p < 0.05$). Among the UFMA subscores, the wrist and hand items had a significant group × time interaction such that the experimental group showed greater improvement ($p < 0.05$).

Table 2. Assessment scores for the affected upper extremity in the experimental and control groups.

Variables	Experimental Group (n = 20)			Control Group (n = 16)			Time × Group Interaction
	T0	T1	T2	T0	T1	T2	p-Value
UFMA, total	41.30 (8.90)	54.80 (8.27) [a]	58.70 (7.53) [b,c]	37.13 (12.84)	45.13 (10.44) [a]	49.32 (10.98) [b,c]	0.027 *
UFMA, subscore							
Shoulder/Elbow/Forearm	27.00 (4.95)	32.20 (3.73) [a]	33.85 (3.54) [b,c]	26.25 (6.10)	30.38 (3.85) [a]	31.19 (4.31) [b]	0.148
Wrist	4.70 (2.41)	8.05 (2.48) [a]	8.25 (2.45) [b]	3.31 (2.98)	4.69 (2.63) [a]	6.44 (2.87) [b,c]	0.010 *
Hand	6.15 (3.34)	10.75 (3.09) [a]	11.85 (2.48) [b,c]	5.56 (3.85)	7.69 (3.75) [a]	8.81 (3.54) [b,c]	0.019 *
Coordination/Speed	2.40 (1.14)	3.80 (1.51) [a]	4.35 (1.42) [b,c]	1.69 (1.85)	2.38 (1.78) [a]	2.88 (1.45) [b]	0.052
JTT, total	12.00 (15.29)	33.10 (21.12) [a]	40.90 (23.52) [b,c]	8.25 (11.93) [a]	13.88 (14.62)	18.00 (15.41) [b,c]	0.004 **
JTT, subscore							
Writing	3.05 (4.32)	7.50 (5.24) [a]	8.85 (5.13) [b]	1.81 (3.43)	4..38 (4.02) [a]	5.38 (4.47) [b,c]	0.180
Simulated page turning	0.45 (0.76)	1.90 (1.78) [a]	2.95 (2.06) [b,c]	0.63 (1.54)	1.01 (1.77) [a]	1.38 (1.89) [b]	0.003 **
Picking up small objects	0.75 (1.77)	3.55 (3.19) [a]	4.75 (3.70) [b,c]	0.69 (1.30)	1.19 (1.80)	1.69 (2.12) [b]	0.004 **
Simulated feeding	1.90 (2.97)	5.90 (4.25) [a]	7.40 (4.80) [b,c]	1.50 (2.81)	2.13 (3.61)	2.69 (3.57) [b]	0.001 **
Stacking checkers	1.90 (2.59)	5.75 (3.88) [a]	6.75 (3.93) [b]	1.63 (2.96)	2.25 (3.59)	2.88 (3.67) [b]	0.002 **
Picking up large light objects	1.90 (3.11)	4.45 (3.49) [a]	5.35 (4.17) [b,c]	0.94 (1.48)	1.38 (1.71) [a]	1.88 (2.00) [b]	0.008 **
Picking up large heavy objects	2.05 (3.10)	4.05 (3.44) [a]	4.85 (3.83) [b]	1.06 (1.53)	1.50 (1.79) [a]	2.13 (1.89) [b]	0.038 *

All values are presented as mean (SD). T0: before the intervention; T1: immediately after the intervention; T2: four weeks after the intervention; UFMA: Fugl-Meyer assessment of upper extremity; JTT: Jebsen-Taylor hand function test. * $p < 0.05$, ** $p < 0.01$ for time x group interaction by repeated measurement analysis of variance (RMANOVA). [a] $p < 0.05$ for T1-T0, [b] $p < 0.05$ for T2-T0, [c] $p < 0.05$ for T2-T1 within-group comparisons by paired t-test or Wilcoxon signed rank test as appropriate after Bonferroni's correction. The uncorrected and corrected p-values are described in Supplementary Table S2.

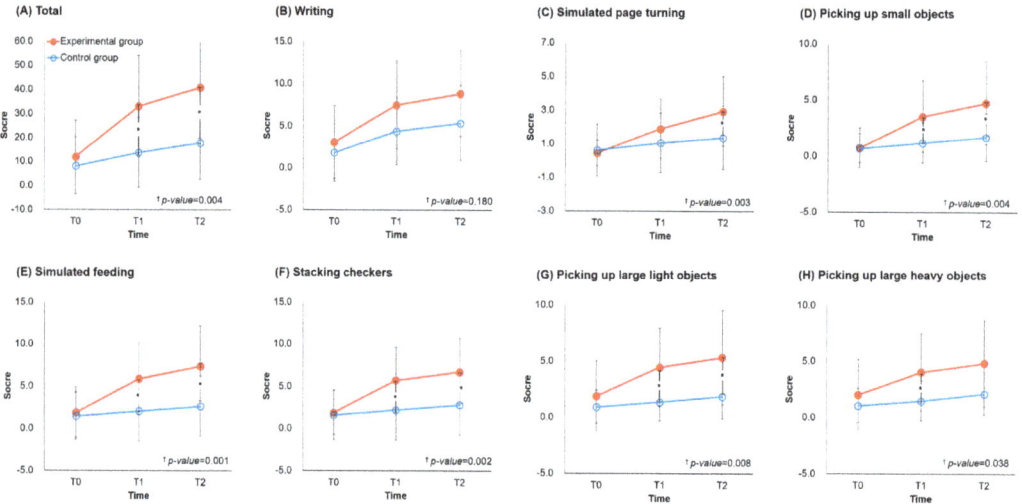

Figure 2. Fugl-Meyer assessment of upper extremity in experimental and control groups. T0, before the intervention; T1, immediately after the intervention; T2, four weeks after the intervention. * $p < 0.05$ between-group comparisons according to independent t-test or Mann-Whitney U test for continuous variables as appropriate after Bonferroni's correction. † p-value according to repeated measure analysis of variance.

The JTT raw scores before and after intervention are presented in Table 2 and Figure 3. The changes in JTT scores in the two groups are compared in Table 3. The changes of JTT total (Experimental 21.10 [20.84]; Control 5.63 [5.06]; $p = 0.012$) and subscores in picking up small objects (Experimental 2.80 [3.16]; Control 0.50 [1.10]; $p = 0.004$), simulated feeding (Experimental 4.00 [4.12]; Control 0.63 [1.26]; $p = 0.003$), stacking checkers (Experimental 3.85 [4.04]; Control 0.63 [1.50]; $p = 0.001$), and picking up large light (Experimental 2.55 [2.72]; Control 0..44 [0.51]; $p = 0.004$) and heavy objects (Experimental 2.00 [2.68]; Control

0.44 [0.51]; $p = 0.041$) showed significant differences between groups immediately after the intervention. In the subsequent four weeks, there were significant differences between the two groups only in JTT picking up small objects subscore (Experimental 1.20 [1.15]; Control 0.50 [0.73]; $p = 0.044$). In addition, the JTT total score had a significant group × time interaction such that the experimental group demonstrated greater improvement ($p < 0.05$). More interestingly, for each individual JTT component (simulated page turning, picking up small objects, simulated feeding, stacking checkers, picking up large light objects, and picking up large heavy objects) except for writing, the experimental group showed significantly greater improvement than the control group ($p < 0.05$), according to RMANOVA.

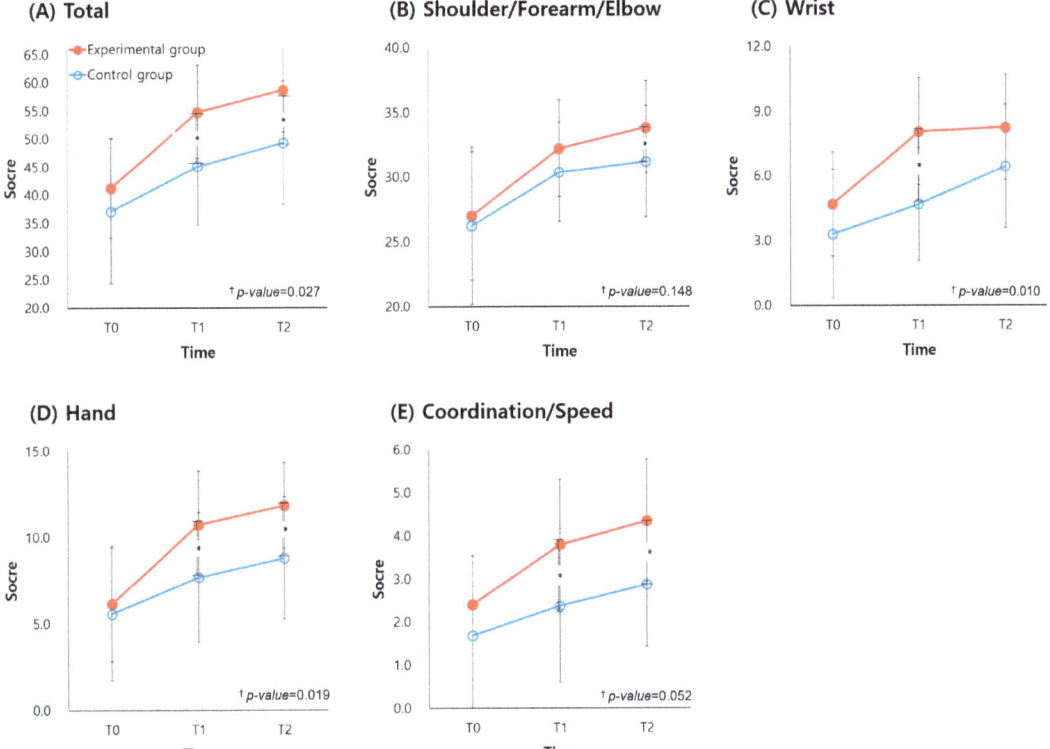

Figure 3. Group analysis of Jebsen-Taylor hand function test in experimental and control groups. T0, before the intervention; T1, immediately after the intervention; T2, four weeks after the intervention. * $p < 0.05$ between-group comparisons according to independent *t*-test or Mann-Whitney U test for continuous variables as appropriate after Bonferroni's correction. † *p*-value according to repeated measure analysis of variance.

Table 3. Changes in assessment scores for the affected upper extremity in the experimental and control groups.

Variables	T1-T0			T2-T1		
	Experimental	Control	p-Value	Experimental	Control	p-Value
UFMA, total	13.50 (7.49)	8.00 (4.44)	0.014 *	3.90 (2.55)	4.19 (3.71)	0.488
UFMA, subscore						
Shoulder/Elbow/Forearm	5.20 (3.22)	4.13 (2.75)	0.297	1.65 (1.79)	0.81 (1.91)	0.362
Wrist	3.35 (2.25)	1.38 (1.36)	0.024 *	0.20 (1.15)	1.75 (1.44)	0.001 **
Hand	4.60 (3.68)	2.13 (1.86)	0.043 *	1.10 (1.33)	1.13 (1.09)	0.716
Coordination/Speed	1.40 (1.14)	0.69 (0.79)	0.048 *	0.55 (0.69)	0.50 (0.89)	0.587
JTT, total	21.10 (20.84)	5.63 (5.06)	0.012 *	7.80 (6.21)	4.13 (3.84)	0.073
JTT, subscore						
Writing	4.45 (5.06)	2.56 (3.24)	0.374	1.35 (1.53)	1.00 (1.10)	0.519
Simulated page turning	1.45 (1.85)	0.44 (0.51)	0.083	1.05 (1.36)	0.31 (0.60)	0.075
Picking up small objects	2.80 (3.16)	0.50 (1.10)	0.004 **	1.20 (1.15)	0.50 (0.73)	0.044 *
Simulated feeding	4.00 (4.12)	0.63 (1.26)	0.003 **	1.50 (1.82)	0.56 (1.21)	0.067
Stacking checkers	3.85 (4.04)	0.63 (1.50)	0.001 **	1.00 (1.81)	0.63 (0.96)	0.647
Picking up large light objects	2.55 (2.72)	0.44 (0.51)	0.004 **	0.90 (1.33)	0.50 (0.73)	0.451
Picking up large heavy objects	2.00 (2.68)	0.44 (0.51)	0.041 *	0.80 (1.32)	0.63 (1.15)	0.713

All values are presented as mean (SD). T0: before the intervention; T1: immediately after the intervention; T2: four weeks after the intervention; UFMA: Fugl-Meyer assessment of upper extremity; JTT: Jebsen-Taylor hand function test. * $p < 0.05$, ** $p < 0.01$ for between-group comparisons by independent t-test or Mann-Whitney U test as appropriate.

3.3. Secondary Outcome Results

fNIRS data were gathered from 11 consenting participants (eight experimental and three control). One patient from the experimental group was excluded from the final analysis because of background noise. In total, seven participants from the experimental group and three from the control group were included for analysis. Statistical parametric mapping revealed t-statistic maps for ΔOxyHb concentration during wrist and hand movement.

Immediately after the intervention (T1), ΔOxyHb concentration in the affected SMC was greater in the experimental group than the control group during affected wrist movement (median values; Experimental group, 0.7943×10^{-4} μmol/L; Control group, -0.3269×10^{-4} μmol/L; $p = 0.025$) (Figure 4). On the other hand, ΔOxyHb values showed no significant differences in any cortical area during finger movement or in the unaffected SMC, bilateral PMC, or SMA during wrist movement (Supplementary Table S3).

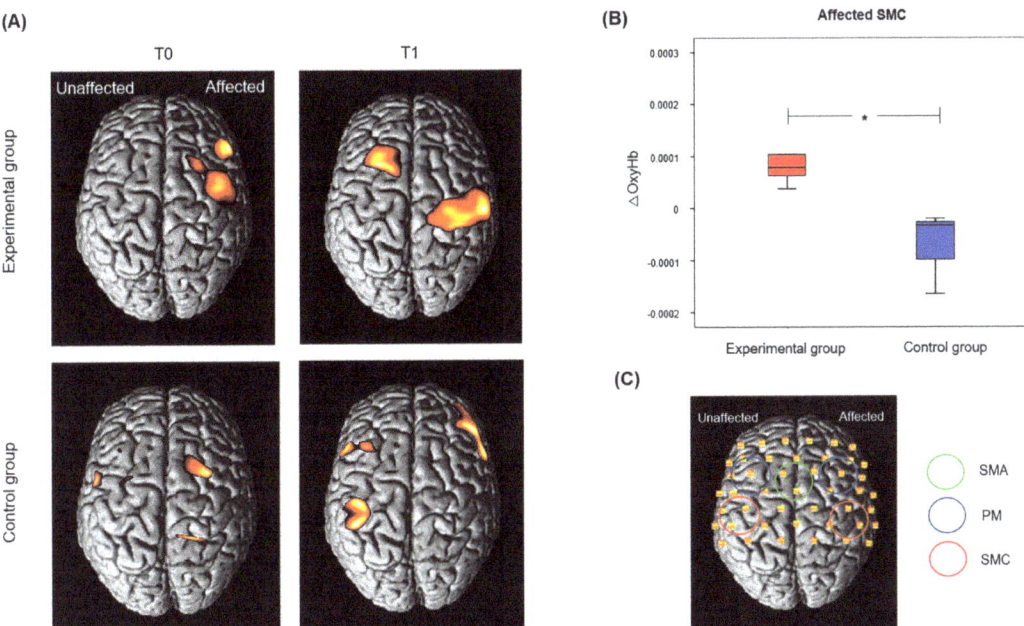

Figure 4. The results of group analysis of oxygenated hemoglobin in experimental and control groups during affected wrist movement. (**A**) Group-average activation map of OxyHb. (**B**) Changes in oxygenated hemoglobin concentration (ΔOxyHb) in the affected primary sensorimotor cortex at T1. (**C**) fNIRS channel montage and affected cortical areas. T0: before the intervention; T1: immediately after the intervention; OxyHb: oxygenated hemoglobin; SMC: primary sensorimotor cortex; PMC: premotor cortex; SMA: supplementary motor area. * $p < 0.01$ for between-group comparison (Mann-Whitney U test).

4. Discussion

The current study was conducted to examine the effects of neurorehabilitation with the RAPAEL® Smart Glove digital system on upper extremity motor function in subacute stroke patients. The findings from this study suggest that convergent VR training with the RAPAEL® Smart Glove digital system combined with conventional OT has some key benefits in terms of upper extremity neurorehabilitation compared with conventional OT only. The game contents used in this study were closely related to ADLs and might provide a positive effect not only on motor function, but also on ADL performance. More importantly, recovery in upper extremity motor function and ADLs was maintained for four weeks after the intervention.

It is well known that activation of the contralesional hemisphere could be an obstacle for motor recovery of the affected hand in the early or subacute stage of stroke [34,35]. On the other hand, activation of the ipsilesional hemisphere is a main therapeutic strategy for motor recovery. Successful rehabilitation and neurostimulation have been shown to increase ipsilesional cortical activation [36]. In other words, suppressing cortical activity of the unaffected areas and facilitating cortical activity of the affected areas are key for motor recovery after stroke. In this study, fNIRS data of sub-samples of the study population showed that game-based VR training with the RAPAEL® Smart Glove digital system can possibly increase hemodynamic changes of the affected SMC. Although this is weak evidence because of the limited participants, the results suggest that game-based VR training can induce positive cortical hemodynamic changes in subacute stroke patients. This finding must be verified in a larger study population.

In general, cortical changes result from changes in behavioral patterns, an important finding in neurorehabilitation [37]. Intensive rehabilitation training in subacute stroke patients induced changes in cortical sensorimotor maps and maximized improvement in motor function [38]. A previous functional magnetic resonance imaging (fMRI) study reported that activation of the affected SMC was significantly increased in a virtual environment [39]. VR stimulation also induced differences in connectivity of brain cortices in healthy participants [40]. A recent review article introduced several studies using VR for upper limb rehabilitation in stroke patients, since it is a promising tool for encouraging active engagement of participants to lead to good outcomes [41]. However, one study showed only low to moderate results of VR techniques in subacute stroke patients [42]. Our results indicate not only positive effects of the RAPAEL® Smart Glove digital system on upper limb function, but also possible evidence for underlying cortical hemodynamic changes detected by fNIRS.

In a previous study, robot-assisted therapy showed a comparable effect to conventional therapy, while VR showed no superiority to conventional therapy when provided alone [42]. However, both new techniques showed significantly better functional improvement when they were added to conventional therapy [18,42,43]. The RAPAEL® Smart Glove digital system collects haptic data from a human body and provides real-time ROM information. The intervention protocol of this study was a combined therapy of a smart glove with VR and conventional occupational therapy which provides evidence of the usefulness of such combination therapy protocol.

In rehabilitation, patient motivation and convenience are important in achieving a positive clinical outcome [44]. User-friendly equipment will foster patient use. A smart glove has the advantages of convenience, light weight, availability for haptic stimulation, and remote control. A smart glove can be used in an unsupervised environment such as the home to allow telerehabilitation [45]. The RAPAEL® Smart Glove digital system is wearable, lightweight, and flexible for hand movement [19]. None of the participants in this study who completed 20 training sessions with the RAPAEL® Smart Glove digital system experienced adverse events. This result indicates that this system does not pose a risk or cause discomfort to patients, while increasing their motivation. Therefore, the RAPAEL® Smart Glove digital system has a potential to be applied safely both in and out of the clinic.

This study had some limitations. First, the number of participants used in analysis was relatively small. Although we allocated enough participants after sample size calculation, PP analysis was performed for a smaller number of patients due to drop-out (Figure 1). Second, fNIRS analyses were performed in a small number of participants, contributing to a low statistical power of cortical hemodynamic results. The numbers in the experimental and control groups showed discrepancies and did not follow a normal distribution. Therefore, caution is needed when generalizing these results to all subacute stroke patients. Nevertheless, our study has the advantage of real-time biosignal measurements of cortical hemodynamic changes, which provides a clue for further investigation of brain activity related through VR devices. Future research should confirm the neuroplastic effect of the RAPAEL® Smart Glove digital system in a sufficient number of participants. The usability of the VR-based smart glove for home-based rehabilitation also needs to be examined to expand its usefulness for upper extremity dysfunction in stroke patients.

5. Conclusions

This study demonstrated a beneficial effect of combined game-based VR training with the RAPAEL® Smart Glove digital system with conventional OT on upper extremity motor function in subacute stroke patients. In addition, the VR-based smart glove combined with conventional rehabilitation showed a possibility of increasing cortical hemodynamic changes in the affected SMC of these patients.

Supplementary Materials: The following supporting information can be downloaded at: https://www.mdpi.com/article/10.3390/jcm11247343/s1. Table S1. Median scores of the Fugl-Meyer assessments for affected upper extremity in the experimental and control groups. Table S2. Uncorrected and corrected *p*-values of within-group analysis. Table S3. Changes in oxygenated hemoglobin concentration in brain cortices. Figure S1. Arrangement of channels in functional near-infrared analysis.

Author Contributions: Conceptualization, Y.-H.K. and Y.-I.S.; methodology, Y.-H.K., Y.-I.S., W.H.C., S.S., H.-J.L. and S.H.K.; formal analysis, S.S. and H.-J.L.; resources, Y.-H.K., Y.-I.S., W.H.C., S.S., H.-J.L. and S.H.K.; data curation, Y.-H.K., Y.-I.S., W.H.C., S.S., H.-J.L. and S.H.K.; writing, original draft preparation, S.S. and H.-J.L.; writing review and editing, Y.-H.K. and Y.-I.S.; supervision, Y.-H.K., Y.-I.S., W.H.C., and S.H.K.; funding acquisition, Y.-H.K. and Y.-I.S. All authors have read and agreed to the published version of the manuscript.

Funding: This study was supported by a grant of the Korea Health Technology R&D Project through the Korea Health Industry Development Institute (KHIDI) funded by the Ministry of Health & Welfare, Republic of Korea (Grant No.: HI15C0570) and by the Ministry of Science and ICT, Republic of Korea, under the ICT Creative Consilience program (IITP-2021-2020-0-01821) supervised by the Institute for Information & Communications Technology Planning & Evaluation. Also supported by The Korea Medical Device Development Fund grant funded by the Korea government (the Ministry of Science and ICT, the Ministry of Trade, Industry and Energy, the Ministry of Health & Welfare, the Ministry of Food and Drug Safety) (Project Number: KMDF-RS-2022-00140478).

Institutional Review Board Statement: Ethics approval was granted by the Ethics Committees of Samsung Medical Center of Seoul (2015-01-095) and of Pusan National University Yangsan Hospital (PNUYH-03-2015-002). This study was retrospectively registered at ClinicalTrials.gov (accessed on 1 May 2015, NCT02431390).

Informed Consent Statement: Informed consent was obtained from all participants before the study.

Data Availability Statement: The data that support the findings of this study are available from the corresponding author on reasonable request.

Acknowledgments: We thank all participants for their participation in this study.

Conflicts of Interest: The authors declare no conflict of interest.

References

1. Kernan, W.N.; Ovbiagele, B.; Black, H.R.; Bravata, D.M.; Chimowitz, M.I.; Ezekowitz, M.D.; Fang, M.C.; Fisher, M.; Furie, K.L.; Heck, D.V.; et al. Guidelines for the prevention of stroke in patients with stroke and transient ischemic attack: A guideline for healthcare professionals from the American Heart Association/American Stroke Association. *Stroke* **2014**, *45*, 2160–2236. [CrossRef] [PubMed]
2. Colomer, C.; Baldovi, A.; Torrome, S.; Navarro, M.D.; Moliner, B.; Ferri, J.; Noe, E. Efficacy of Armeo(R) Spring during the chronic phase of stroke. Study in mild to moderate cases of hemiparesis. *Neurologia* **2013**, *28*, 261–267. [CrossRef] [PubMed]
3. Sale, P.; Lombardi, V.; Franceschini, M. Hand robotics rehabilitation: Feasibility and preliminary results of a robotic treatment in patients with hemiparesis. *Stroke Res.Treat.* **2012**, *2012*, 820931. [CrossRef] [PubMed]
4. Zeiler, S.R.; Krakauer, J.W. The interaction between training and plasticity in the poststroke brain. *Curr. Opin. Neurol.* **2013**, *26*, 609–616. [CrossRef]
5. Bernhardt, J.; Godecke, E.; Johnson, L.; Langhorne, P. Early rehabilitation after stroke. *Curr. Opin. Neurol.* **2017**, *30*, 48–54. [CrossRef]
6. Coleman, E.R.; Moudgal, R.; Lang, K.; Hyacinth, H.I.; Awosika, O.O.; Kissela, B.M.; Feng, W. Early Rehabilitation After Stroke: A Narrative Review. *Curr. Atheroscler. Rep.* **2017**, *19*, 59. [CrossRef]
7. Nudo, R.J. Neural bases of recovery after brain injury. *J. Commun. Disord.* **2011**, *44*, 515–520. [CrossRef]
8. Song, G.B. The effects of task-oriented versus repetitive bilateral arm training on upper limb function and activities of daily living in stroke patients. *J. Phys. Ther. Sci.* **2015**, *27*, 1353–1355. [CrossRef]
9. Giuliani, C. Constraint-induced movement therapy early after stroke improves rate of upper limb motor recovery but not long-term motor function. *J. Physiother.* **2015**, *61*, 95. [CrossRef]
10. Kim, J.; Yim, J. Effects of High-Frequency Repetitive Transcranial Magnetic Stimulation Combined with Task-Oriented Mirror Therapy Training on Hand Rehabilitation of Acute Stroke Patients. *Med. Sci. Monit.* **2018**, *24*, 743–750. [CrossRef]
11. Choi, Y.H.; Paik, N.J. Mobile Game-based Virtual Reality Program for Upper Extremity Stroke Rehabilitation. *J. Vis. Exp.* **2018**, *133*, e56241. [CrossRef] [PubMed]

12. Lee, M.M.; Lee, K.J.; Song, C.H. Game-Based Virtual Reality Canoe Paddling Training to Improve Postural Balance and Upper Extremity Function: A Preliminary Randomized Controlled Study of 30 Patients with Subacute Stroke. *Med. Sci. Monit.* **2018**, *24*, 2590–2598. [CrossRef]
13. Lee, S.; Kim, Y.; Lee, B.H. Effect of Virtual Reality-based Bilateral Upper Extremity Training on Upper Extremity Function after Stroke: A Randomized Controlled Clinical Trial. *Occup. Ther. Int.* **2016**, *23*, 357–368. [CrossRef] [PubMed]
14. Wang, Z.R.; Wang, P.; Xing, L.; Mei, L.P.; Zhao, J.; Zhang, T. Leap Motion-based virtual reality training for improving motor functional recovery of upper limbs and neural reorganization in subacute stroke patients. *Neural Regen. Res.* **2017**, *12*, 1823–1831. [CrossRef] [PubMed]
15. Laver, K.E.; Lange, B.; George, S.; Deutsch, J.E.; Saposnik, G.; Crotty, M. Virtual reality for stroke rehabilitation. *Cochrane Database Syst. Rev.* **2017**, *11*, CD008349. [CrossRef] [PubMed]
16. Hao, J.; Yao, Z.; Harp, K.; Gwon, D.Y.; Chen, Z.; Siu, K.C. Effects of virtual reality in the early-stage stroke rehabilitation: A systematic review and meta-analysis of randomized controlled trials. *Physiother. Theory Pract.* **2022**, 1–20. [CrossRef] [PubMed]
17. Nef, T.; Mihelj, M.; Riener, R. ARMin: A robot for patient-cooperative arm therapy. *Med. Biol. Eng. Comput.* **2007**, *45*, 887–900. [CrossRef] [PubMed]
18. Masiero, S.; Celia, A.; Rosati, G.; Armani, M. Robotic-assisted rehabilitation of the upper limb after acute stroke. *Arch. Phys. Med. Rehabil.* **2007**, *88*, 142–149. [CrossRef]
19. Yap, H.K.; Lim, J.H.; Nasrallah, F.; Yeow, C.H. Design and Preliminary Feasibility Study of a Soft Robotic Glove for Hand Function Assistance in Stroke Survivors. *Front. Neurosci.* **2017**, *11*, 547. [CrossRef]
20. Biggar, S.; Yao, W. Design and Evaluation of a Soft and Wearable Robotic Glove for Hand Rehabilitation. *IEEE Trans. Neural Syst. Rehabil. Eng. A Publ. IEEE Eng. Med. Biol. Soc.* **2016**, *24*, 1071–1080. [CrossRef]
21. Shin, J.H.; Kim, M.Y.; Lee, J.Y.; Jeon, Y.J.; Kim, S.; Lee, S.; Seo, B.; Choi, Y. Effects of virtual reality-based rehabilitation on distal upper extremity function and health-related quality of life: A single-blinded, randomized controlled trial. *J. Neuroeng. Rehabil.* **2016**, *13*, 17. [CrossRef] [PubMed]
22. Caeiro-Rodríguez, M.; Otero-González, I.; Mikic-Fonte, F.A.; Llamas-Nistal, M. A Systematic Review of Commercial Smart Gloves: Current Status and Applications. *Sensors* **2021**, *21*, 2667. [CrossRef] [PubMed]
23. Lee, H.S.; Lim, J.H.; Jeon, B.H.; Song, C.S. Non-immersive Virtual Reality Rehabilitation Applied to a Task-oriented Approach for Stroke Patients: A Randomized Controlled Trial. *Restor. Neurol. Neurosci.* **2020**, *38*, 165–172. [CrossRef] [PubMed]
24. Chang, H.J.; Ku, K.H.; Park, Y.S.; Park, J.G.; Cho, E.S.; Seo, J.S.; Kim, C.W.; O, S.H. Effects of Virtual Reality-Based Rehabilitation on Upper Extremity Function among Children with Cerebral Palsy. *Healthcare* **2020**, *8*, 391. [CrossRef] [PubMed]
25. Leff, D.R.; Orihuela-Espina, F.; Elwell, C.E.; Athanasiou, T.; Delpy, D.T.; Darzi, A.W.; Yang, G.Z. Assessment of the cerebral cortex during motor task behaviours in adults: A systematic review of functional near infrared spectroscopy (fNIRS) studies. *NeuroImage* **2011**, *54*, 2922–2936. [CrossRef]
26. Jalalvandi, M.; Riyahi Alam, N.; Sharini, H.; Hashemi, H.; Nadimi, M. Brain Cortical Activation during Imagining of the Wrist Movement Using Functional Near-Infrared Spectroscopy (fNIRS). *J. Biomed. Phys. Eng.* **2021**, *11*, 583–594. [CrossRef]
27. Cui, X.; Bray, S.; Bryant, D.M.; Glover, G.H.; Reiss, A.L. A quantitative comparison of NIRS and fMRI across multiple cognitive tasks. *NeuroImage* **2011**, *54*, 2808–2821. [CrossRef]
28. Lloyd-Fox, S.; Blasi, A.; Elwell, C.E. Illuminating the developing brain: The past, present and future of functional near infrared spectroscopy. *Neurosci. Biobehav. Rev.* **2010**, *34*, 269–284. [CrossRef]
29. Lundquist, C.B.; Maribo, T. The Fugl-Meyer assessment of the upper extremity: Reliability, responsiveness and validity of the Danish version. *Disabil. Rehabil.* **2017**, *39*, 934–939. [CrossRef]
30. Allgower, K.; Hermsdorfer, J. Fine motor skills predict performance in the Jebsen Taylor Hand Function Test after stroke. *Clin. Neurophysiol.* **2017**, *128*, 1858–1871. [CrossRef]
31. Kim, J.H.; Kim, I.S.; Han, T.R. New Scoring System for Jebsen Hand Function Test. *J. Korean Acad. Rehabil. Med.* **2007**, *31*, 623–629.
32. Ye, J.C.; Tak, S.; Jang, K.E.; Jung, J.; Jang, J. NIRS-SPM: Statistical parametric mapping for near-infrared spectroscopy. *NeuroImage* **2009**, *44*, 428–447. [CrossRef] [PubMed]
33. Cope, M.; Delpy, D.T. System for long-term measurement of cerebral blood and tissue oxygenation on newborn infants by near infra-red transillumination. *Med. Biol. Eng. Comput.* **1988**, *26*, 289–294. [CrossRef] [PubMed]
34. Hensel, L.; Tscherpel, C.; Freytag, J.; Ritter, S.; Rehme, A.K.; Volz, L.J.; Eickhoff, S.B.; Fink, G.R.; Grefkes, C. Connectivity-Related Roles of Contralesional Brain Regions for Motor Performance Early after Stroke. *Cereb. Cortex* **2021**, *31*, 993–1007. [CrossRef] [PubMed]
35. Lotze, M.; Markert, J.; Sauseng, P.; Hoppe, J.; Plewnia, C.; Gerloff, C. The role of multiple contralesional motor areas for complex hand movements after internal capsular lesion. *J. Neurosci.* **2006**, *26*, 6096–6102. [CrossRef]
36. Oujamaa, L.; Relave, I.; Froger, J.; Mottet, D.; Pelissier, J.Y. Rehabilitation of arm function after stroke. Literature review. *Ann. Phys. Rehabil. Med.* **2009**, *52*, 269–293. [CrossRef]
37. Bergfeldt, U.; Jonsson, T.; Bergfeldt, L.; Julin, P. Cortical activation changes and improved motor function in stroke patients after focal spasticity therapy–an interventional study applying repeated fMRI. *BMC Neurol.* **2015**, *15*, 52. [CrossRef]
38. Kaelin-Lang, A.; Luft, A.R.; Sawaki, L.; Burstein, A.H.; Sohn, Y.H.; Cohen, L.G. Modulation of human corticomotor excitability by somatosensory input. *J. Physiol.* **2002**, *540*, 623–633. [CrossRef]

39. Merians, A.S.; Tunik, E.; Adamovich, S.V. Virtual reality to maximize function for hand and arm rehabilitation: Exploration of neural mechanisms. *Stud. Health Technol. Inform.* **2009**, *145*, 109–125.
40. Forlim, C.G.; Bittner, L.; Mostajeran, F.; Steinicke, F.; Gallinat, J.; Kuhn, S. Stereoscopic Rendering via Goggles Elicits Higher Functional Connectivity During Virtual Reality Gaming. *Front. Hum. Neurosci.* **2019**, *13*, 365. [CrossRef]
41. Kim, W.S.; Cho, S.; Ku, J.; Kim, Y.; Lee, K.; Hwang, H.J.; Paik, N.J. Clinical Application of Virtual Reality for Upper Limb Motor Rehabilitation in Stroke: Review of Technologies and Clinical Evidence. *J. Clin. Med.* **2020**, *9*, 3369. [CrossRef] [PubMed]
42. Everard, G.; Declerck, L.; Detrembleur, C.; Leonard, S.; Bower, G.; Dehem, S.; Lejeune, T. New technologies promoting active upper limb rehabilitation after stroke. An overview and network meta-analysis. *Eur. J. Phys. Rehabil. Med.* **2022**, *58*, 530–548. [CrossRef] [PubMed]
43. Morone, G.; Cocchi, I.; Paolucci, S.; Iosa, M. Robot-assisted therapy for arm recovery for stroke patients: State of the art and clinical implication. *Expert Rev. Med. Devices* **2020**, *17*, 223–233. [CrossRef] [PubMed]
44. Maclean, N.; Pound, P.; Wolfe, C.; Rudd, A. Qualitative analysis of stroke patients' motivation for rehabilitation. *BMJ* **2000**, *321*, 1051–1054. [CrossRef] [PubMed]
45. Lansberg, M.G.; Legault, C.; MacLellan, A.; Parikh, A.; Muccini, J.; Mlynash, M.; Kemp, S.; Buckwalter, M.S.; Flavin, K. Home-based virtual reality therapy for hand recovery after stroke. *PM&R* **2022**, *14*, 320–328. [CrossRef]

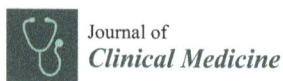

Article

Hand Ownership Is Altered in Teenagers with Unilateral Cerebral Palsy

Corinna N. Gerber, Didier L. Gasser and Christopher John Newman *

Paediatric Neurology and Neurorehabilitation Unit, Department of Paediatrics, Lausanne University Hospital and Lausanne University, 1011 Lausanne, Switzerland
* Correspondence: christopher.newman@chuv.ch; Tel.: +41-21-314-96-07

Abstract: We explored hand ownership in teenagers with unilateral cerebral palsy (UCP) compared with typically developing teenagers. Eighteen participants with UCP and 16 control teenagers participated. We used the rubber hand illusion to test hand ownership (HO). Both affected/non-affected hands (UCP) and dominant/non-dominant hands (controls) were tested during synchronous and asynchronous strokes. HO was assessed by measuring the proprioceptive drift toward the fake hand (as a percentage of arm length) and conducting a questionnaire on subjective HO. Both groups had significantly higher proprioceptive drift in the synchronous stroking condition for both hands. Teenagers with UCP showed a significantly higher proprioceptive drift when comparing their paretic hand (median 3.4% arm length) with the non-dominant hand of the controls (median 1.7% arm length). The questionnaires showed that synchronous versus asynchronous stroking generated a robust change in subjective HO in the control teenagers, but not in the teenagers with UCP. Teenagers with UCP have an altered sense of HO and a distorted subjective experience of HO that may arise from the early dysfunction of complex sensory–motor integration related to their brain lesions. HO may influence motor impairment and prove to be a target for early intervention.

Keywords: cerebral palsy; hemiplegia; teenager; body ownership; rubber hand illusion; proprioceptive drift

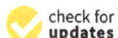

Citation: Gerber, C.N.; Gasser, D.L.; Newman, C.J. Hand Ownership Is Altered in Teenagers with Unilateral Cerebral Palsy. *J. Clin. Med.* **2022**, *11*, 4869. https://doi.org/10.3390/jcm11164869

Academic Editors: Naoki Yoshida, Hideki Nakano, Yohei Okada and Akiyoshi Matsugi

Received: 21 July 2022
Accepted: 18 August 2022
Published: 19 August 2022

Publisher's Note: MDPI stays neutral with regard to jurisdictional claims in published maps and institutional affiliations.

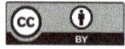

Copyright: © 2022 by the authors. Licensee MDPI, Basel, Switzerland. This article is an open access article distributed under the terms and conditions of the Creative Commons Attribution (CC BY) license (https://creativecommons.org/licenses/by/4.0/).

1. Introduction

In children with unilateral cerebral palsy (UCP), the use of the affected hand in daily life, referred to as performance, is often below its use in a clinical environment, referred to as capacity [1,2]. This underuse is associated with developmental disregard [3] and is hypothesised to be due to the disproportional amount of attention required to use the affected limb in daily life [4]. Anecdotally, children with UCP report experiences that hint at potential issues with hand ownership (HO), described with phrases such as "I forget my hand" or "It's as if my hand wasn't there". Appropriate HO is a prerequisite for the production of adapted voluntary movements [5]. Alterations in HO may impair affected hand use in UCP.

Body ownership relies on the spatial and temporal binding between perceptual events and is grounded in the brain's ability to integrate multiple sources of sensory information [6]. The importance of visual–tactile integration in establishing HO is evidenced in the rubber hand illusion (RHI) [7], in which multisensory conflicts induce the self-attribution of a rubber hand. Viewing someone stroking a rubber hand (seen, not felt) while the viewer's own hand, which is occluded from view, is being stroked synchronously (felt, not seen) induces a sense of ownership for the rubber hand, with the illusion of feeling the strokes being applied to it [8]. The viewer's own hand is perceived in a position displaced towards the fake hand, a phenomenon named proprioceptive drift (PD). Illusory ownership and PD decrease or disappear when strokes are applied asynchronously to the rubber and real hands [9].

Illusory ownership can be induced in healthy adults [7] and typically developing (TD) children. Applying the RHI in children demonstrated that the multisensory processes underlying body representations are different in children aged 4 to 9 years compared with adults [10]. For HO, these younger children rely more strongly on the sight of their hands and less on their proprioception than adults. A further study in 10- to 13-year-olds [11] showed that pointing responses reached adult levels at 10 to 11 years, showing that, from this age, children integrate their hands by using an adult-like balance of sensory cues.

Adults with unilateral stroke seem to have a looser sense of HO and experience stronger illusory effects on the affected hand [12]. The effects of early brain anomalies on the development of HO are unknown. It is likely that the early damage to the motor and sensory cortex and pathways typically encountered in UCP disrupts the development of HO, which is important for both hand integration and motor function; however, to this date, body ownership has not been explored in cerebral palsy. In this study, we aimed to explore HO in teenagers with UCP compared with TD controls, questioning whether hand ownership is altered in UCP. We hypothesised that RHI could be induced in both groups, and that the RHI would have stronger effects on the affected hand in youngsters with UCP.

2. Materials and Methods

2.1. Study Design and Setting

This pilot case–control study was approved by the regional ethics committee (CER-VD decision 2017-0208) and was conducted between July 2018 and July 2019 at Lausanne University Hospital (CHUV), Switzerland.

2.2. Participants

We aimed to include a minimal convenience sample of 15 participants in each group (UCP and TD), in line with previous studies on the RHI [13]. Youngsters aged 10–20 years old were included in the study, based on the previous study on TD children who were shown to reach an adult perception of the bodily self by 10 years [11].

Participants with UCP were recruited from the paediatric neurorehabilitation clinic of Lausanne University Hospital. The inclusion criteria were: (i) UCP diagnosed by a paediatric neurologist, (ii) age 10 to 20 years, (iii) hand use classified as Manual Ability Classification System (MACS) level I-III, and (iv) ability to hold each hand, palm down, on a table.

We recruited controls among the acquaintances of the study participants and children of Lausanne University Hospital's paediatric department's collaborators. The inclusion criteria for TD controls were: (i) age 10 to 20 years, (ii) no known history of brain lesions or disorders, and (iii) no known sensory and/or motor impairment of the upper extremities.

The exclusion criteria for all participants were: (i) surgery at the trunk or upper limb level within the last six months before inclusion in the study; (ii) botulinum toxin injections in the upper limbs within the three months before inclusion in the study; (iii) any clinically significant disease (e.g., renal failure, hepatic dysfunction, and cardiovascular disease); (iv) known or suspected non-compliance; (v) inability to follow the procedures of the study, for example, due to language problems or behavioural issues; (vi) cognitive age estimated below 10 years; and (vii) severe visual impairments, including hemianopsia.

The TD controls had one test session during which the RHI experiment was conducted, and participants with UCP had an additional session to assess secondary outcomes. Written informed consent was obtained from participants older than 14 years and from their legal guardians if they were younger than 18 years.

2.3. Procedure

The RHI experiment followed the protocol established by Cowie et al. [11]. We used distances relative to the participant's arm length for the setup (Figure 1) and the measurement of PD. To account for different hand appearances, we selected, from three pairs of fake hands (silicon prosthetics), the one most resembling the participant's hand: adult female, adult male, and child (Ortho Kern SA, Lausanne, Switzerland).

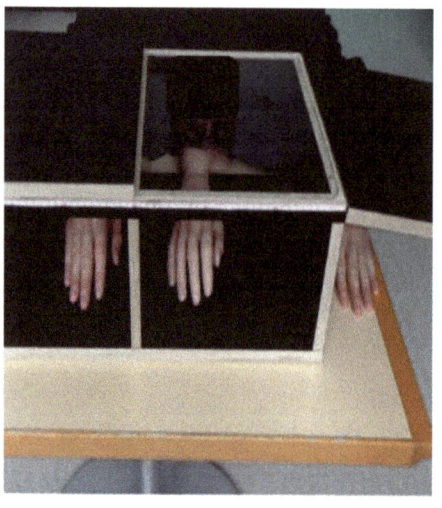
(a)

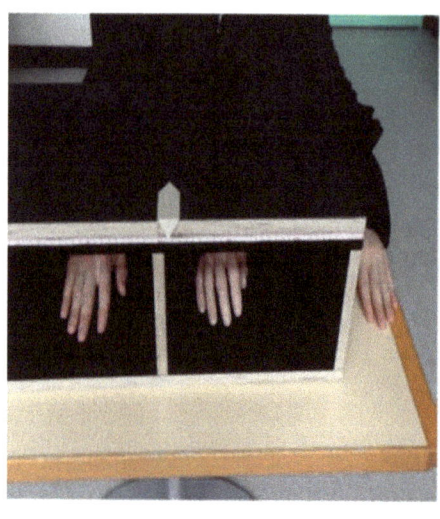
(b)

Figure 1. Rubber hand illusion experimental setup. (**a**) Stimulation phase: during the stroking with a paintbrush, the participant sees a rubber hand while their real hand (here, the right hand) is hidden. (**b**) Measurement condition. Both the real and the rubber hands are hidden. The participant indicates where he feels the index finger of his (in this case, right) hand by instructing the experimenter to move the cursor to the right or to the left.

To induce the RHI illusion, the experimenter stroked the visible fake hand and the hidden real hand of the participant with two identical paint brushes in two different stroking conditions (synchronously and asynchronously).

The affected hand (UCP) or the non-dominant hand (TD) was tested first, and the two stroking conditions were applied randomly. For each side and condition, the experiment consisted of four baseline measures with the fake and real hands hidden in the box, followed by a stimulation phase (2 min) and four post-stimulation phases (each 20 s), where the fake hand was visible while the real hand was hidden in the box. After each baseline, stimulation, and post-stimulation phase, both hands were hidden for the PD measurement.

2.4. Outcome Measures

We measured PD as a primary outcome to quantify the RHI. To avoid visual cues (e.g., the midline of the box), a black sheet of paper was placed over it before each measurement. The experimenter then moved a cursor (Figure 1) along the box following the participant's instruction of "left" or "right" until the participant felt confident that the ruler indicated the position of their index finger. The distance of the indicated position from the midline was measured in millimetres.

The PD was normalised to arm length and calculated as follows:

$$PD = \frac{\left(\frac{\sum BL_i}{4}\right) - \frac{Stim + \sum Post_i}{5}}{L} * 100$$

in which BL is the baseline measure, $Stim$ is the stimulation phase, $Post$ is the post-stimulation phase, L is the arm length of the participant, and i is the number of measurements.

The subjective sense of ownership of the rubber hand was assessed as a secondary outcome with a 6-statement questionnaire adapted from Botvinick and Cohen [9] and Burin et al. [12]. Three statements explored the predicted phenomena: (i) I felt the touch of the paintbrush where I saw the rubber hand was touched; (ii) It seemed as if the touch I felt was caused by the paintbrush touching the rubber hand; and (iii) It felt as if the rubber hand was my hand. The three control statements with no expected effect were: (i) I felt my hand drifting towards the rubber hand; (ii) It seemed as if the touch I was feeling came from somewhere between my own hand and the rubber hand; (iii) It felt as if my real hand was turning rubbery. Participants responded on a 7-point Likert scale with the following coding: no, definitely not (-3); no (-2); no, not really (-1); neither yes nor no (0); yes, a little (1); yes, a lot (2); and yes, really a lot (3).

We measured the motor function and capacity, as well as sensory functioning, of participants with UCP as potential co-factors of HO. For this purpose, we used the second version of the Melbourne Assessment of Unilateral Upper Limb Function (MA2), the Assisting Hand Assessment (AHA), 2-point discrimination, and a joint-position sense test.

The MA2 and AHA were both video recorded with video-based scorings. The MA2 is a valid and reliable measure of upper limb function in children with central motor disorders [14]. Sub-scores on a scale from 0–100 are provided for the range of motion, dexterity, fluency, and accuracy. The AHA measures the spontaneous use of the more-affected hand during bimanual activities. The 22 items describe actions under the following sub-headings: general use, arm use, grasp and release, fine motor adjustments, coordination, and pace. We used two versions of the AHA: the kids-AHA [15] for participants under 12 years old, and the Ad-AHA [16] for adolescents aged 13 years or older.

We measured sensory function according to the protocol described by Cooper et al. [17]. Static 2-point discrimination was measured with an aesthesiometer (Baseline, Fabrication Enterprise Inc., White Plains, NY, USA) on the palmar side of the distal phalanx of both index fingers with pressure to the point of skin blanching. The minimal distance of the two pressure points that the patient actually perceived (with eyes closed) as two distinct points was recorded. To measure joint position sense, a component of proprioception, the tester fixed the proximal and middle phalanges, held the patient's distal phalanges of the index finger, and moved the latter up and down passively. The patient had to detect the direction of movement (up/down) with their eyes closed, and the correct answers out of five trials were recorded.

2.5. Statistical Analyses

Due to the small sample size, non-parametric tests were used. We compared the synchronous and asynchronous stroking conditions using the Wilcoxon Signed Ranks Test for both hands of both groups separately. Subsequently, we performed a Mann–Whitney test to compare the PD of the participants with UCP's affected hand with the controls' non-dominant hand and of the participants with UCP's non-affected hand with the controls' dominant hand for the synchronous stroking condition.

Spearman correlations were calculated to investigate associations between the difference in perceived hand position (i.e., PD) after the synchronous stroking of the affected hand with clinical co-factors.

Statistical analyses were performed with SPSS 26 (IBM, Armonk, NY, USA). Alpha was set at 0.05, and Bonferroni corrections were applied where necessary.

3. Results

Eighteen participants with UCP (mean age: 13 y 10 m; SD 2 y 10 m, six females) and sixteen TD controls (age 14 y 1 m; SD: 3 y 0 m, 6 females) were included. Half (nine) of the participants with UCP had right-sided hemiparesis, half had left-sided hemiparesis, and nine participants were at MACS level I, five at MACS level II, and four at MACS level III. None had previously participated in an RHI study.

The difference in PD between the synchronous and asynchronous conditions was significant in both groups and for both hands (Figure 2).

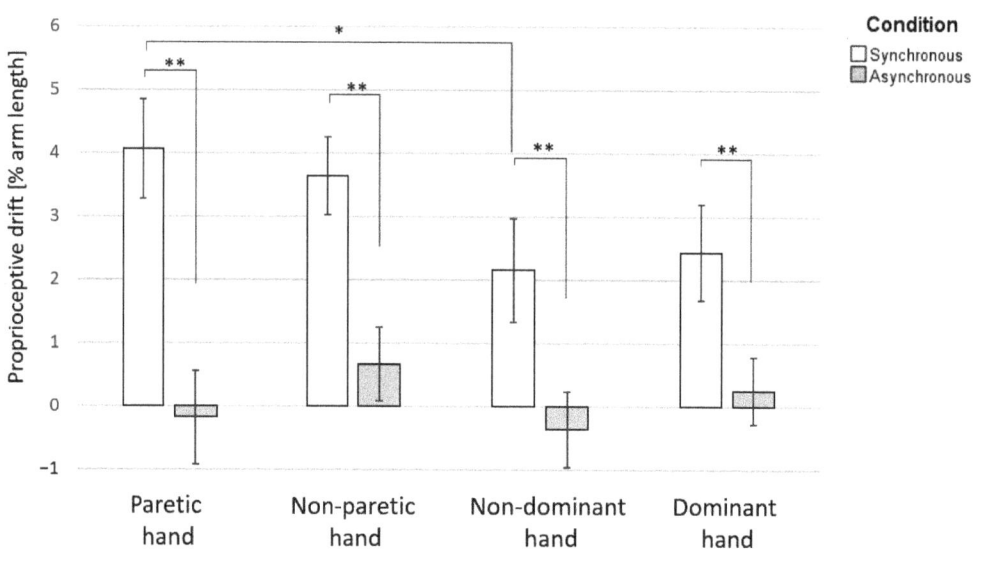

Figure 2. Proprioceptive drift in teenagers with unilateral cerebral palsy and typically developing teenagers. A positive value of proprioceptive drift indicates a drift of the felt index finger location towards the rubber hand, while a negative value shows a drift away from the rubber hand. Significant differences are indicated as follows: * $p < 0.05$, and ** $p < 0.01$.

For group analyses of the PD after the synchronous stroking condition, we found a significant difference between the affected hand of participants with UCP and the non-dominant hand of TD participants (median PD of affected hands: 3.4% arm length; median PD of non-dominant hands: 1.7% arm length; the distributions in the two groups differed significantly, Mann–Whitney U = 201, n1 = 18, n2 = 16, $p = 0.049$ two-tailed). However, no difference was observed between the unaffected and dominant hands (median PD of unaffected hands: 3.5% arm length; median PD of dominant hands: 2.0% arm length; the distributions in the two groups differed significantly, Mann–Whitney U = 189, n1 = 18, n2 = 16, $p = 0.121$, two-tailed).

The HO questions showed that the controls had a significantly higher subjective experience of HO over the fake hand after the synchronous stroking condition of their non-dominant hand (3/3 statements), whereas no effect was found for the control questions (0/3 statements). In children with CP, the results for the subjective experience of HO were inconsistent for the questions regarding their affected hand (Figure 3).

The results of the clinical co-factors are displayed in Table 1. There were no significant correlations between the clinical co-factors and PD.

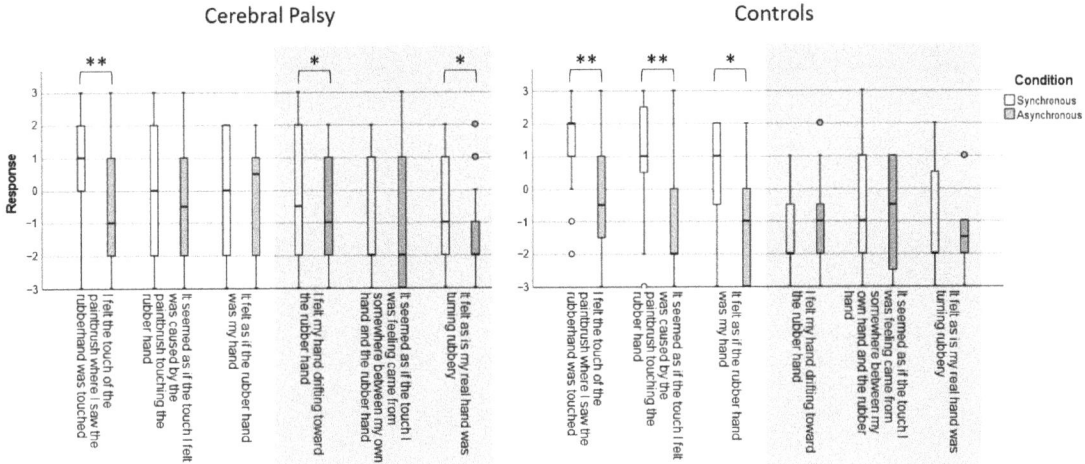

Figure 3. Subjective ratings of hand ownership in teenagers with unilateral cerebral palsy and typically developing teenagers. Responses to statements on subjective body ownership were given on a 7-point Likert scale ranging from "do completely agree" +3 to "do not agree at all" −3, where 0 corresponded to neither agreeing nor disagreeing. Greyed areas indicate control statements. Significant differences are indicated as follows: * $p < 0.05$, and ** $p < 0.01$.

Table 1. Clinical measures of motor and sensory function and correlations with proprioceptive drift of the affected hand in teenagers with unilateral cerebral palsy.

		AHA_Score (%)	Melbourne Assessment 2				TPD (mm)	JPS (N)
			RoM (%)	Precision (%)	Dexterity (%)	Fluidity (%)		
Proprioceptive Drift (synchronous stroking)	Mean (SD)	69.7 (22.0)	77.6 (23.5)	90.4 (16.2)	71.6 (24.2)	71.9 (25.5)	1.5 (2.6)	4.3 (0.8)
	Correlation Coefficient	−0.011	−0.227	−0.339	−0.094	−0.142	−0.007	−0.236
	p	0.964	0.364	0.169	0.712	0.573	0.978	0.345
	N	18	18	18	18	18	16	18

Abbreviations: AHA, Assisting hand assessment; RoM, Range of motion; TPD, Two-point discrimination; JPS, joint position sense; p, p-value; N, number.

4. Discussion

Teenagers with UCP were responsive to the RHI, whereas, for TD teenagers, the RHI effects were dependent on the synchronicity of the stroking. The effects of the RHI on teenagers with UCP demonstrated that they had an altered sense of ownership of their paretic hands. The RHI experiment generated a significantly higher PD of their paretic hand towards the rubber hand than for the non-dominant hand in TD controls. Synchronous versus asynchronous stroking generated a robust change in subjective hand ownership in TD teenagers, but not in teenagers with UCP.

In TD children, the perceived hand position, which requires implicit hand ownership, seems to mature during late childhood. In a study that applied the RHI to children, Cowie et al. [10] showed that, during the first decade, children had consistently higher levels of PD than during the second decade, when PD approached adult levels. This was in contrast to the explicit hand ownership (the phenomenological experience in which the ownership of the hand is experienced consciously) that was measured through questions on the subjective experience of ownership, which is present from early childhood and demonstrates no significant development between 4 years of age and adulthood. This developmental trajectory of hand ownership was attributed to an early reliance on visual–tactile integration to develop a perception of bodily layout and propriety, followed by later developing visual–proprioceptive processes to consolidate the perception and ownership of body parts [10].

In teenagers with UCP, both processes seem to be disrupted. The persistence of a significantly higher PD for the paretic hand throughout the teenage years into adulthood most likely demonstrates a prolonged reliance on visual input to contribute to hand ownership, with a potential failure in the expected maturation of visual–proprioceptive processes. In contrast, subjective ownership was distorted in teenagers with UCP compared with TD teenagers, with an atypical pattern of responses to the questionnaire. Among the statements that were devised to detect illusory ownership, there was a clear dissociation between the positive response to the sensory illusion ("I felt the touch of the paintbrush where I saw the rubber hand was touched") and the negative response to the ownership illusion ("It felt as if the rubber hand was my hand"). This contrasts with findings in adults after stroke, who experience a change in the belief of ownership over the rubber hand [12], pointing towards a specific influence of early injury in the maldevelopment of subjective body ownership. For the statements with no expected effect, teenagers with UCP were more likely to report that they felt their hand drifting towards the rubber hand, and that they felt their real hand turning rubbery.

The complex construct of subjective hand and bodily ownership relies on the interplay of brain areas, including the fronto-parietal network and temporo-parietal junction, as demonstrated by functional MRI [18–21] and transcranial magnetic stimulation [22] experiments conducted during the RHI. Early anomalies in frontal, fronto-parietal, or larger brain areas, which are implicated in sensory–motor processing and are classically affected in cerebral palsy, may limit these children's ability to develop a typical sense of body ownership for their affected body parts, as demonstrated in our findings regarding the paretic hand of teenagers with UCP.

The effects of atypical HO on the development of hand motor skills in children with UCP and, conversely, the effects of manual motor impairment on the development of HO remain to be determined. We were unable to demonstrate any association between impairment in HO, as measured by PD, and measures of motor or sensory function. Voluntary movements have been suggested as important in supporting proper multisensory integration and, therefore, for subjective body ownership [12,23]. In adults with paresis, the decrease in the number of movement-related signals, which disrupts the normal integration of afferent and efferent signals for the arm, weakens body ownership. However, there is also evidence that atypical body ownership can lead to motor difficulties. A small case series of adults with right brain damage and hemiplegia, affected by an atypical form of hemisomatoagnosia, revealed that the pathological self-attribution of an alien hand directly affected the patients' motor programme by modifying motor awareness, sense of agency, and action execution [24]. Hence, distorted HO due to early brain damage might hinder optimal motor development and performance in people with CP.

Could HO become a target for therapy? Mirror therapy is an approach based on the manipulation of hand ownership [25]. In mirror therapy, patients look at the reflection of their non-impaired upper limbs on a mirror placed at their midlines while they perform symmetrical upper-limb movements. The reflection generates the multisensory illusion that the paretic hand is functioning normally through a self-attribution of the reflection in the mirror, that is, the mirror illusion. Interestingly, mirror therapy has failed to exhibit the same efficacy in children with UCP [25] compared with adults after stroke [26]. While adults have a life of experienced HO before their stroke that may underpin the response to mirror therapy, it is possible that children with UCP who have developed from early life with atypical HO may not be as responsive to the mirror illusion and therapy. This hypothesis is supported by recent research suggesting that cross-modal visuo-tactile integration is dependent on body ownership [27]. Therefore, the effectiveness of cross-modal rehabilitative interventions might depend on the integrity of the patients' body ownership. The process of body ownership develops from infancy [28] and has already been strongly established based on visual–tactile integration by early childhood [10]. Therefore, early sensorimotor intervention, specifically geared at supporting multisensory integration as related to hand movement and agency, may support a more typical development of HO, thus supporting future hand function. Such an intervention could focus on driving the child's visual, tactile, and proprioceptive attention towards the affected hand, for example, by the activation of luminous and vibratory cues synchronised with guided or voluntary hand movement.

Our sample size may have underpowered our detection of potential differences between groups. Specifically, Figure 2 hints that PD for the non-paretic hand of teenagers with UCP may be higher than that for the dominant hand of TD teenagers. Despite not attaining statistical significance, this could be a sign of a more diffuse issue in the development of body ownership beyond the paretic body parts. Our sample size could have restricted our ability to demonstrate meaningful associations between body ownership and motor or sensory functions. Studies with larger sample sizes, a prospective observation of the development of HO throughout childhood, and the integration of additional co-factors, including brain imaging, are necessary to further define the extent and likely variability of HO issues in UCP, as well as their neurobiological underpinnings.

In conclusion, teenagers with UCP have an altered sense of HO with an excessive reliance on visual input, evocative of an abnormal maturation of visual–proprioceptive processes, and a distorted subjective and explicit experience of HO that most probably stems from the early dysfunction of complex sensory–motor integration related to their brain lesions. Abnormal HO most likely interacts with motor impairment and may prove a target for early sensorimotor intervention to improve the development of HO and, ultimately, hand function.

Author Contributions: Conceptualization, C.J.N.; methodology, C.N.G. and C.J.N.; formal analysis, C.N.G., D.L.G. and C.J.N.; investigation, D.L.G.; data curation, D.L.G.; writing—original draft preparation C.N.G. and C.J.N.; writing—review and editing, C.N.G., D.L.G., and C.J.N.; supervision, C.N.G. and C.J.N.; project administration, C.N.G. and C.J.N.; funding acquisition, C.N.G. and C.J.N. All authors have read and agreed to the published version of the manuscript.

Funding: This research was funded by la Fondation Paralysie Cérébrale (Paris, France) and the Anna Müller Grocholski Stiftung (Zürich, Switzerland).

Institutional Review Board Statement: The study was conducted in accordance with the Declaration of Helsinki, and approved by the Research Ethics Committee of Canton Vaud, Lausanne, Switzerland (CER-VD decision 2017-0208).

Informed Consent Statement: Informed consent was obtained from all subjects involved in the study.

Data Availability Statement: The data that support the findings of this study are available upon request from the corresponding author. The data are not publicly available due to privacy or ethical restrictions.

Acknowledgments: We thank Thomas Pavlik and Manon Burkhard for assisting in participant recruitment; Roselyne Bruchez, Diane Wellinger, and Caroline Carrasco for their advice on the methods and experimental set-up; and the participants and their families for their commitment.

Conflicts of Interest: The authors declare no conflict of interest. The funders had no role in the design of the study; in the collection, analyses, or interpretation of data; in the writing of the manuscript; or in the decision to publish the results.

References

1. Houwink, A.; Geerdink, Y.A.; Steenbergen, B.; Geurts, A.C.; Aarts, P.B. Assessment of upper-limb capacity, performance, and developmental disregard in children with cerebral palsy: Validity and reliability of the revised Video-Observation Aarts and Aarts module: Determine Developmental Disregard (VOAA-DDD-R). *Dev. Med. Child Neurol.* **2013**, *55*, 76–82. [CrossRef] [PubMed]
2. Liu, K.C.; Chen, H.L.; Wang, T.N.; Shieh, J.Y. Developing the Observatory Test of Capacity, Performance, and Developmental Disregard (OTCPDD) for Children with Cerebral Palsy. *PLoS ONE* **2016**, *11*, e0151798. [CrossRef] [PubMed]
3. Zielinski, I.M.; Jongsma, M.L.; Baas, C.M.; Aarts, P.B.; Steenbergen, B. Unravelling developmental disregard in children with unilateral cerebral palsy by measuring event-related potentials during a simple and complex task. *BMC Neurol.* **2014**, *14*, 6. [CrossRef]
4. Houwink, A.; Aarts, P.B.; Geurts, A.C.; Steenbergen, B. A neurocognitive perspective on developmental disregard in children with hemiplegic cerebral palsy. *Res. Dev. Disabil.* **2011**, *32*, 2157–2163. [CrossRef] [PubMed]
5. Brozzoli, C.; Ehrsson, H.H.; Farne, A. Multisensory representation of the space near the hand: From perception to action and interindividual interactions. *Neuroscientist* **2014**, *20*, 122–135. [CrossRef]
6. Blanke, O. Multisensory brain mechanisms of bodily self-consciousness. *Nat. Rev. Neurosci.* **2012**, *13*, 556–571. [CrossRef]
7. Tsakiris, M.; Haggard, P. The rubber hand illusion revisited: Visuotactile integration and self-attribution. *J. Exp. Psychol. Hum. Percept. Perform.* **2005**, *31*, 80–91. [CrossRef]
8. Makin, T.R.; Holmes, N.P.; Ehrsson, H.H. On the other hand: Dummy hands and peripersonal space. *Behav. Brain Res.* **2008**, *191*, 1–10. [CrossRef]
9. Botvinick, M.; Cohen, J. Rubber hands 'feel' touch that eyes see. *Nature* **1998**, *391*, 756. [CrossRef]
10. Cowie, D.; Makin, T.R.; Bremner, A.J. Children's responses to the rubber-hand illusion reveal dissociable pathways in body representation. *Psychol. Sci.* **2013**, *24*, 762–769. [CrossRef]
11. Cowie, D.; Sterling, S.; Bremner, A.J. The development of multisensory body representation and awareness continues to 10 years of age: Evidence from the rubber hand illusion. *J. Exp. Child Psychol.* **2016**, *142*, 230–238. [CrossRef]
12. Burin, D.; Livelli, A.; Garbarini, F.; Fossataro, C.; Folegatti, A.; Gindri, P.; Pia, L. Are movements necessary for the sense of body ownership? Evidence from the rubber hand illusion in pure hemiplegic patients. *PLoS ONE* **2015**, *10*, e0117155. [CrossRef]
13. Kammers, M.P.; de Vignemont, F.; Verhagen, L.; Dijkerman, H.C. The rubber hand illusion in action. *Neuropsychologia* **2009**, *47*, 204–211. [CrossRef]
14. Gerber, C.N.; Labruyere, R.; van Hedel, H.J. Reliability and Responsiveness of Upper Limb Motor Assessments for Children With Central Neuromotor Disorders: A Systematic Review. *Neurorehabil. Neural Repair* **2016**, *30*, 19–39. [CrossRef]
15. Holmefur, M.M.; Krumlinde-Sundholm, L. Psychometric properties of a revised version of the Assisting Hand Assessment (Kids-AHA 5.0). *Dev. Med. Child Neurol.* **2016**, *58*, 618–624. [CrossRef]
16. Louwers, A.; Krumlinde-Sundholm, L.; Boeschoten, K.; Beelen, A. Reliability of the Assisting Hand Assessment in adolescents. *Dev. Med. Child Neurol.* **2017**, *59*, 926–932. [CrossRef]
17. Cooper, J.; Majnemer, A.; Rosenblatt, B.; Birnbaum, R. The determination of sensory deficits in children with hemiplegic cerebral palsy. *J. Child Neurol.* **1995**, *10*, 300–309. [CrossRef]
18. Ehrsson, H.H.; Holmes, N.P.; Passingham, R.E. Touching a rubber hand: Feeling of body ownership is associated with activity in multisensory brain areas. *J. Neurosci.* **2005**, *25*, 10564–10573. [CrossRef]
19. Limanowski, J.; Blankenburg, F. Fronto-Parietal Brain Responses to Visuotactile Congruence in an Anatomical Reference Frame. *Front. Hum. Neurosci.* **2018**, *12*, 84. [CrossRef]
20. Olivé, I.; Tempelmann, C.; Berthoz, A.; Heinze, H.J. Increased functional connectivity between superior colliculus and brain regions implicated in bodily self-consciousness during the rubber hand illusion. *Hum. Brain Mapp.* **2015**, *36*, 717–730. [CrossRef]
21. Wawrzyniak, M.; Klingbeil, J.; Zeller, D.; Saur, D.; Classen, J. The neuronal network involved in self-attribution of an artificial hand: A lesion network-symptom-mapping study. *NeuroImage* **2018**, *166*, 317–324. [CrossRef]
22. Karabanov, A.N.; Ritterband-Rosenbaum, A.; Christensen, M.S.; Siebner, H.R.; Nielsen, J.B. Modulation of fronto-parietal connections during the rubber hand illusion. *Eur. J. Neurosci.* **2017**, *45*, 964–974. [CrossRef]
23. Tsakiris, M.; Prabhu, G.; Haggard, P. Having a body versus moving your body: How agency structures body-ownership. *Conscious. Cogn.* **2006**, *15*, 423–432. [CrossRef] [PubMed]
24. Garbarini, F.; Pia, L.; Piedimonte, A.; Rabuffetti, M.; Gindri, P.; Berti, A. Embodiment of an alien hand interferes with intact-hand movements. *Curr. Biol.* **2013**, *23*, R57–R58. [CrossRef] [PubMed]
25. Bruchez, R.; Jequier Gygax, M.; Roches, S.; Fluss, J.; Jacquier, D.; Ballabeni, P.; Grunt, S.; Newman, C.J. Mirror therapy in children with hemiparesis: A randomized observer-blinded trial. *Dev. Med. Child Neurol.* **2016**, *58*, 970–978. [CrossRef] [PubMed]
26. Thieme, H.; Morkisch, N.; Mehrholz, J.; Pohl, M.; Behrens, J.; Borgetto, B.; Dohle, C. Mirror therapy for improving motor function after stroke. *Cochrane Database Syst. Rev.* **2018**, *7*, CD008449. [CrossRef] [PubMed]
27. Fossataro, C.; Bruno, V.; Bosso, E.; Chiotti, V.; Gindri, P.; Farne, A.; Garbarini, F. The sense of body-ownership gates cross-modal improvement of tactile extinction in brain-damaged patients. *Cortex* **2020**, *127*, 94–107. [CrossRef] [PubMed]
28. Rochat, P. The innate sense of the body develops to become a public affair by 2–3 years. *Neuropsychologia* **2010**, *48*, 738–745. [CrossRef]

Journal of
Clinical Medicine

Article

Upper Body Physical Rehabilitation for Children with Ataxia through IMU-Based Exergame

Alberto Romano [1], Martina Favetta [1], Susanna Summa [1,*], Tommaso Schirinzi [2], Enrico Silvio Bertini [3], Enrico Castelli [1], Gessica Vasco [1,†] and Maurizio Petrarca [1,†]

1. Movement Analysis and Robotics Laboratory (MAR Lab), Intensive Neurorehabilitation and Robotics Department, "Bambino Gesù" Children's Hospital, IRCCS, 00050 Rome, Italy; alberto.romano01@ateneopv.it (A.R.); martina.favetta@opbg.net (M.F.); enrico.castelli@opbg.net (E.C.); gessica.vasco@opbg.net (G.V.); maurizio.petrarca@opbg.net (M.P.)
2. Department of Systems Medicine, University of Rome "Tor Vergata", 00133 Rome, Italy; t.schirinzi@yahoo.com
3. Unit of Neuromuscolar and Neurodegenerative Diseases, Department of Neurosciences, "Bambino Gesù" Children's Hospital, IRCCS, 00146 Rome, Italy; enricosilvio.bertini@opbg.net
* Correspondence: susanna.summa@opbg.net
† These authors contributed equally to this work.

Abstract: Background: Children with ataxia experience balance and movement coordination difficulties and needs intensive physical intervention to maintain functional abilities and counteract the disorder. Exergaming represents a valuable strategy to provide engaging physical intervention to children with ataxia, sustaining their motivation to perform the intervention. This paper aims to describe the effect of a home-conducted exergame-based exercise training for upper body movements control of children with ataxia on their ataxic symptoms, walking ability, and hand dexterity. Methods: Eighteen children with ataxia were randomly divided into intervention and control groups. Participants in the intervention group were asked to follow a 12-week motor activity program at home using the Niurion® exergame. Blind assessments of participants' ataxic symptoms, dominant and non-dominant hand dexterity, and walking ability were conducted. Results: On average, the participants performed the intervention for 61.5% of the expected time. At the end of the training, participants in the intervention group showed improved hand dexterity that worsened in the control group. Conclusion: The presented exergame enhanced the participants' hand dexterity. However, there is a need for exergames capable of maintaining a high level of players' motivation in playing. It is advisable to plan a mixed intervention to take care of the multiple aspects of the disorder.

Keywords: ataxia; exergaming; telerehabilitation; hand dexterity; treatment adherence and compliance

1. Introduction

Ataxia refers to a group of motor disorders associated with the cerebellum or its afferent and efferent projections dysfunction or damage [1]. People with ataxia experience a lack of balance and movement coordination that leads to difficulties in walking and standing, poor limbs and fine hand function control, muscle tone alterations, dysarthria, and altered ocular motor function [2,3]. Children with ataxia show similar sensorimotor impairment as adults [4]. A recent literature review estimated a prevalence of 26/100,000 different forms of ataxia in European children [5]. The impairments derived from ataxia are especially debilitating during childhood as motor development, and learning processes are still ongoing [4]. Moreover, age is likely to affect engagement and compliance with the chosen intervention modality and may impact the targeting and timing of rehabilitation efforts. Children have different information-processing capacities compared to adults and respond differently to motor learning and skill-acquisition paradigms, suggesting children may require more exercise practice time before learning is consolidated [6].

As no effective curative treatments are available, exercise and physical therapy represent the core interventions available to these children [7,8]. Physical treatment should start as soon as the diagnosis of ataxia is given, even if only mild symptoms are present. Although the effectiveness of physical therapy intervention for children with ataxia is still not established [9,10], the therapeutic scenario might rapidly change because of the upcoming disease-modifying treatments or other symptomatic and rehabilitative interventions [9–14]. Moreover, a growing body of literature emerged in the last decade regarding exergames usage to provide physical therapy interventions to young patients with ataxia. The term exergame refers to digital games that require bodily movements to play, stimulating an active gaming experience to function as a form of physical activity [15–17]. Ilg and colleagues used three Microsoft Xbox Kinect (MXK) videogames to improve the balance and gait quality of six children and four adults with several types of progressive spinocerebellar ataxia [18]. Similarly, Schatton et al. reported the use of Nintendo Wii and MXK games to increase the body balance of six children and four adults with different types of ataxia [19]. Both studies reported a reduction in the participants' ataxia symptoms, particularly related to gait and balance. Despite these preliminary positive results, the efficacy of exergame providing physical therapy to children with ataxia was, to date, only mildly tested. Moreover, the available studies focused on balance and gait, overlooking other key ataxia symptoms such as upper-limb function. A recent literature review [9] identified a sole case study proposing an elbow movements dexterity training for a 5-year old girl who had undergone surgical resection of a cerebellar tumor [20]. The patient was asked to track the movements of a pseudo-random target on a computer screen using elbow joint flexion and extension for two weeks, 10 min a day. The authors described an improvement in the participant's elbow and hand movement dexterity.

Exergames hold the potential to support the motivation of children with ataxia to perform therapeutic activities in an intensive way and in a meaningful context that was found fundamental to achieve improvements in ataxia symptoms [8,21].

This paper aims to describe the effect of a home-conducted exergame-based exercise training for upper body movements control of children with ataxia on their hand dexterity, ataxic symptoms, and walking ability.

2. Materials and Methods

2.1. Ethical Issues

The study was conducted according to the ethical principles of the Helsinki Declaration and local regulations. All details relating to the study procedure were discussed with the candidates' parents, and an informed consent document was signed for all participants. Enrolment was voluntary, with participants not receiving any incentives, financial or otherwise, for participation. The Ethical Committee of the Bambino Gesù Children's Hospital approved the study.

2.2. Participants

Eighteen children and adolescents (mean age: 11.6 ± 3.5 years; age range: 5.1–17.2 years) were enrolled in this study. The inclusion criteria for this study were the presence of a confirmed diagnosis of ataxia and the absence of any signs of inflammatory, vascular malformation, or tumor central nervous system disease. During the recruitment phase, all participants underwent a specialist medical examination that assessed their cognitive and motor aspects to ensure that they could carry out the tests provided in the study protocol. Patients presenting with intellectual disabilities were excluded from the current investigation. All the candidates met the inclusion criteria. Participants' age, sex, and ataxia characteristics are presented in Table 1. Two participants (11.1%) were diagnosed with non-genetic ataxia. All participants followed an individual physical therapy treatment for one 45-min session per week. These interventions concerned the development of activities aimed at improving the control of gross and fine motor movements, balance in sitting, standing, and walking, and dexterity in skills related to the activity of daily living (ADL).

Table 1. Participants' group, age at baseline (T0), diagnosis, and SARA items and total scores. The horizontal line separates the data obtained from participants in the IG and CG.

Group	Pt.	Age at T0 (Years)	Sex	Diagnosis	Gait	Stance	Sitting	Speech Disturbance	Finger Chase	Nose-Finger Test	Fast Alternating Hand Movements	Heel-Shin Slide	SARA Total Score
IG	1	14.9	F	Non-genetic ataxia	2	1	0	2	1	1	3	1	11
	2	10.2	M	Joubert's ataxia	3	1	0	1	1	0	1	1	8
	3	10	F	ARCA2	3	0	0	1	1	1	3	1	10
	4	8.6	M	ARCA2	1	0	0	0	0	1	1.5	0.5	4
	5	15.5	F	ARCA2	1	0	0	2	1	1	3	1	9
	6	9.5	F	Friedreich's ataxia *	2	2	1	0	1	1	3	2	11
	7	8.5	M	Friedreich's ataxia *	2	2	0	1	1	1	1	2	10
	8	16.9	F	Friedreich's ataxia *	2	2	0	2	0.5	1	0	1.5	9
	9	10.5	F	ARSACS *	2	1	0	1	1	1	2.5	2	10.5
CG	10	17.2	F	Non-genetic ataxia	1	1	0	1	1	1	1	2	8
	11	15.5	F	Joubert's ataxia	1	1	0	1	1	1	0	0	5
	12	11.2	M	Joubert's ataxia	1	1	0	0	1	1	1	1	6
	13	10.4	M	ARCA2	2	2	0	2	1	1	3	1.5	12.5
	14	7.7	M	ARCA2	2	2	0	2	1	1.5	3	3.5	15
	15	9	F	Friedreich's ataxia *	3	3	0	1	1	1.5	3	2.5	15
	16	12.6	F	Friedreich's ataxia *	1	2	0	1	0.5	1	0.5	1.5	7.5
	17	15.4	M	Friedreich's ataxia *	3	2	1	0	1	1	1	3	12
	18	5.1	F	Ataxia telangiectasia *	2	2	0	1	1	0	3	1	10

Abbreviation list: IG = Intervention Group; CG = Control Group; Pt. = Participants; M = Male; F = Female; ARCA2 = Autosomal Recessive Cerebellar Ataxia 2; ARSACS = Autosomal recessive spastic ataxia of Charlevoix-Saguenay; SARA = Scale for the Assessment and Rating of Ataxia. *: progressive ataxia.

2.3. Procedure

All participants' informed consents for participation were collected from their parents at the recruitment. Before starting the intervention (T0), all participants' outcome measures were collected by two independent assessors with previous experience in the rehabilitation of people with ataxia. After the evaluation, the participants were randomly and consecutively assigned to the Intervention Group (IG) and Control Group (CG). The assessors did not know which group the participants were assigned at any study stage. Then, participants in the IG were given the exergame for upper body rehabilitation (Niurion® kit—P2R, Bergamo, Italy). This inertial measurement unit (IMU) based rehabilitation device comprises five IMUs, a data receiver connected with a computer, an adherent shirt, and the software itself. The exergame included eight specific exercises aimed at improving the trunk and upper limbs movements control and muscle strength. Specific activities performed during each exercise were the following: elbows flexion, shoulders abduction at 90° and 180°, shoulders flexion at 90° and 180°, target reaching with the hand and arm in the ipsilateral and contralateral space, and anteroposterior trunk oscillation. Participants were asked to wear an adherent shirt and insert the IMUs in their designed pocket on the shirt (see Figure 1).

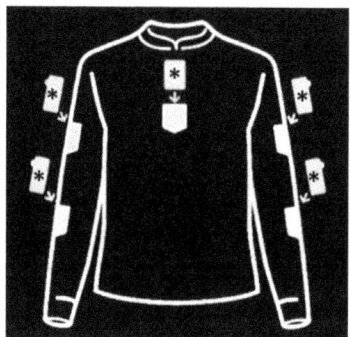

Figure 1. Visual description of IMU sensors (marked with asterisks) placement in the Niurion® shirt.

Then, a calibration occurs, and an avatar reproducing the upper body movements of the participant was constructed by the software, and the exercises began. During each exercise, the participant stood in front of the screen and saw the avatar moving accordingly with his movements in the virtual space (see Figure 2).

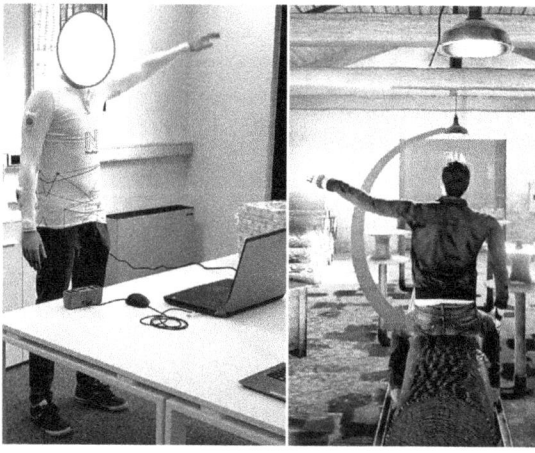

Figure 2. Example of shoulder 180° abduction exercise execution with related avatar movement.

Each exercise was performed in a different virtual space. The participant had to move his arms or body to interact with the environment and complete the game. The software was designed to recognize the trunk, the arm, and forearm movements allowing the interaction with the targets in the virtual environment. Moreover, the in-built algorithm of the software provides a real-time adaptation of the difficulty of the proposed tasks to avoid frustration due to continuous failures or motivation falling due to carrying out activities that are too simple for the subject. Each exercise lasted for seven minutes, and a 30 s recovery time was provided between the exercises (duration of the entire session: ~1 h). Each subject in the IG participated in two individual training sessions to be taught to use the system correctly. Participants' parents also participate in these meetings to better comprehend the system's functioning. At the end of the second training session, participants in the IG were asked to start the intervention at their home, performing the entire session (all the eight exercises) five days a week for 12 weeks (total of 60 sessions for each exercise). The time spent by each participant in the IG in the activities foreseen by the treatment was collected by the Niurion® software (version 1.2.0, P2R, Italy) and analyzed to establish the participant's adherence to the proposed intervention. Meanwhile, participants in the CG continued with the same therapeutic regimen conducted at a rehabilitation facility with their reference physiotherapist, without any change. None of the subjects in the IG changed their regimen of physical therapy sessions during the intervention period. Therefore, each participant received 12 physical therapy sessions within the duration of the current intervention.

At the end of the intervention (T1), the outcome measures were collected again for all participants, and obtained data were analyzed. Each participant's number of therapeutic sessions was collected from their reference therapists at the end of the protocol.

2.4. Outcome Measure

The 9-Hole Peg Test (9HPT) was administered to obtain a timed measure of the participants' pre- and post-intervention finger dexterity. This commonly used test requires placing and removing nine pegs in a pegboard as quickly as possible. The total time (seconds) to complete the task was recorded for both the dominant and non-dominant hands three times, and the mean of the three tests for each hand was calculated. This test has established intra- and inter-rater and test–retest reliability and normative reference values [22–25].

The Scale for the Assessment and Rating of Ataxia (SARA) was used to describe the ataxia severity level. Higher values reflect higher disease severity. This is a reliable and valid clinical scale measuring the severity of ataxia to be used in all cerebellar disorders [26–28]. SARA is "recommended" to assess cerebellar symptoms of different types of ataxia. It has been utilized by research groups other than the developer [3,29–32], and adequate psychometric proprieties support its use [33].

The Timed 25-Foot Walk test (T25FW) was used to assess the impact of the treatment on the participants' global mobility ability. The test required the participant to walk a 25-foot-long path as fast as possible. The test was performed twice. The time (seconds) to complete the path was recorded for each trial, and the mean score was then calculated. The T25FW was found highly representative of mobility function and disability stage in patients with Friedreich ataxia [34,35].

2.5. Statistical Analysis

Due to the small sample size, the non-parametric statistic was used to analyze the collected data. The Mann–Whitney U test was first used to evaluate the comparability of participants' age, sex, and the pre-intervention outcome measures scores among the IC and GC groups. The same test was conducted at the end of the intervention to compare the outcome measures variations between participants in the two groups. A delta was calculated with the difference between the scores obtained by each participant at T1 and T0 ($\Delta = T1 - T0$) to obtain the outcome measures variations. The Wilcoxon Signed-Rank test was used to evaluate the variation that occurred in the outcome measures of participants of each group separately. The threshold for significance for the analyses above was assumed to be α = 0.05. No correction was applied for multiple comparisons [36].

3. Results

No difference was found between IG and CG when comparing the participants' sex, age, and outcome measures scores at T0, proving the comparability of the two groups.

All the participants in the IG completed the protocol. The average adherence of each exercise is presented in Table 2. The average adherence was slightly varied among the exercises (range: 53.3–66.1%). All participants attended all the physical therapy sessions planned during the protocol (12 sessions). Individual participants' adherence data and related descriptive statistics are available as Supplementary Material (Table S1).

Table 2. Average adherence for each exercise and the whole treatment. The percentage represents the average portion of time spent by participants in the IG in each exercise compared to the time required by the protocol (60 1 h sessions).

Exercises	Adherence Avg (SD)
Elbow flexion	53.3 ± 0.4%
Shoulder 90° abduction	64.1 ± 0.2%
Shoulder 180° abduction	58.0 ± 0.3%
Shoulder 90° flexion	64.4 ± 0.3%
Shoulder 180° flexion	66.1 ± 0.3%
Ipsilateral target reaching	62.8 ± 0.3%
Controlateral target reaching	56.4 ± 0.3%
Trunk oscillation	63.9 ± 0.3%
General adherence	61.5 ± 3.9%

Abbreviation list: Avg = Average; SD = Standard Deviation.

The collected outcome measures scores and statistical analysis results are reported in Table 3. Participants' individual scores for each outcome measure are available as Supplementary Material (Table S2). A significant change occurred in both groups' dominant hand dexterity scores measured with the 9HPT at T1. Participants in the IG, on average, reduced the time needed to complete the task (representing an improvement—p: 0.05), while those in the CG increased it (representing a worsening—p: 0.03). In this test, the score changes that occurred in the IG and CG were statistically different (p: 0.01). The same trend was observable for the non-dominant hand. However, this difference did not reach the statistical significance between and within groups comparison analysis.

Participants' individual data collected at T0 and T1 for each outcome measure are available as Supplementary Materials. Looking at the 9HPT scores, among the IG, improvements in the 9HPT scores were found in eight participants (88.9%) for the dominant hand and in six of them (77.8%) for the non-dominant hand. Conversely, in the CG, one subject (11.1%) ameliorated his dominant hand score, and four (44.4%) improved their performance with the non-dominant hand. Participants' individual 9HPT scores are graphically represented in Figure 3.

Table 3. Descriptive statistics and statistical analysis of outcome measures scores for IC and CG at T0 and T1 and occurred scores variation (Δ). "IG" (T0 and T1), "CG" (T0 and T1), and "Δ Scores" (Δ IG and Δ CG) columns report the average score and standard deviation (in parenthesis) for each outcome measure. "p-value IG T0 vs. T1" and "p-value CG T0 vs. T1" columns report the results obtained from the Wilcoxon Signed-Rank test analyzing the scores difference between T0 and T1 for each group. "p-value Δ IG vs. Δ CG" column reports the results attained from the Mann–Whitney U test comparing the variation in the scores (Δ) of the IG and CG.

		IG		p-Value IG T0 vs. T1	CG		p-Value CG T0 vs. T1	Δ Scores		p-Value Δ IG vs. Δ CG
		T0	T1		T0	T1		Δ IG	Δ CG	
SARA Scores	Gait	2 (0.7)	2.1 (0.9)	0.65	1.8 (0.8)	2 (0.5)	0.48	−0.1 (0.8)	−0.2 (1)	0.60
	Stance	1 (0.9)	1.1 (0.8)	0.32	1.8 (0.7)	1.6 (0.7)	0.16	−0.1 (0.3)	0.2 (0.4)	0.09
	Sitting	0.1 (0.3)	0 (0)	0.32	0.1 (0.3)	0.3 (0.7)	0.16	0.1 (0.3)	−0.2 (0.4)	0.09
	Speech disturbance	1.1 (0.8)	1.2 (0.8)	1.00	1 (0.7)	1.4 (1)	0.18	0 (0.5)	−0.4 (1)	0.30
	Finger Chase	0.8 (0.4)	0.8 (0.4)	0.32	0.9 (0.2)	1.1 (0.8)	0.59	−0.1 (0.2)	−0.2 (0.8)	0.90
	Nose-finger test	0.9 (0.3)	1 (0)	1.00	1 (0.4)	1.2 (0.8)	0.71	0 (0)	−0.2 (0.8)	1.00
	Fast alternating hand movements	2 (1.1)	1.9 (0.9)	1.00	1.7 (1.3)	1.8 (1.2)	0.32	0.1 (0.8)	−0.1 (0.2)	0.90
	Heel-shin slide	1.3 (0.6)	1.4 (0.6)	0.16	1.8 (1.1)	1.7 (1)	1.00	−0.1 (0.2)	0.1 (0.8)	0.80
	SARA Total score	9.2 (2.2)	9.6 (2.4)	0.18	10.1 (3.7)	11.1 (3.9)	0.02 *↓	−0.4 (0.9)	−0.9 (1)	0.31
	T25FW	5.3 (1)	5.3 (0.5)	0.86	6.3 (1.4)	5.9 (1.2)	0.31	0.1 (0.8)	0.3 (0.7)	0.31
	9HPT Dominant hand	37.9 (8.4)	34.9 (6)	0.05 *↑	39.1 (8.9)	41.9 (11)	0.03 *↓	3 (3.9)	−2.6 (3.1)	0.01 *
	9HPT Non-dominant hand	40.2 (9)	38.3 (7.5)	0.17	45.2 (10.1)	46.6 (9.9)	0.37	1.9 (3.3)	−1.6 (3.9)	0.08

Abbreviation list: SARA = Scale for Assessment and Rating of Ataxia; T25FW = Timed 25-Foot Walk; 9HPT = 9-Hole Peg Test; IG = Intervention Group; CG = Control Group; T0 = pre-intervention evaluation; T1 = post-intervention evaluation. Δ: Delta; *: p-value ≤ 0.05; ↑: statistically significant change reflects an improvement; ↓: statistically significant change reflects a worsening.

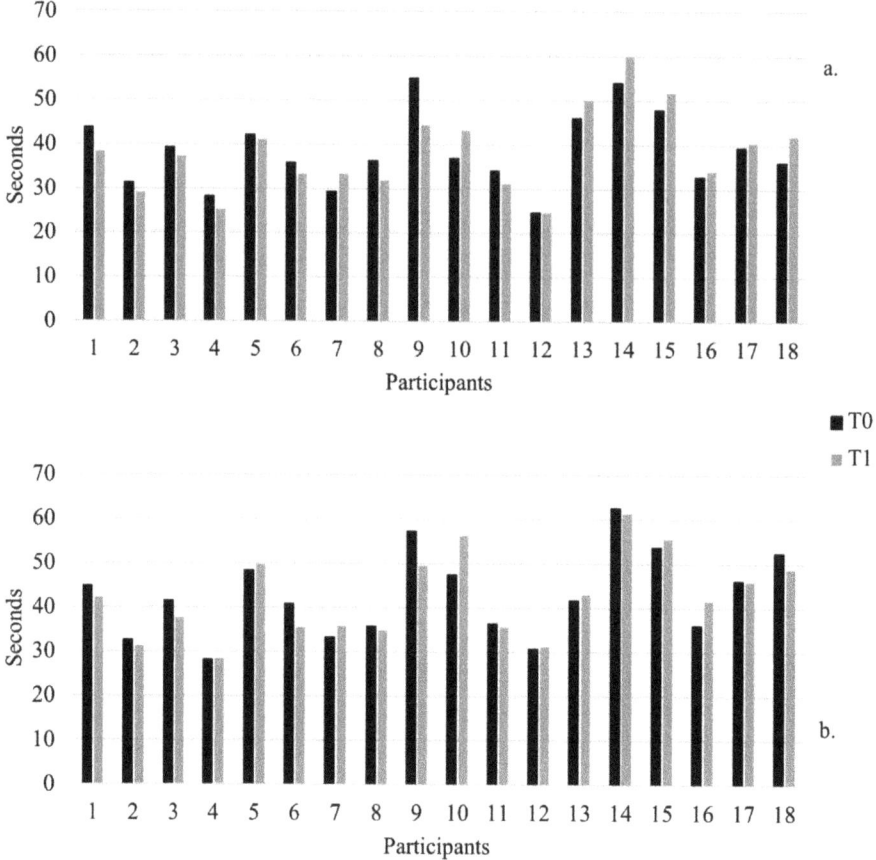

Figure 3. (**a**) Dominant and (**b**) non-dominant hands individual 9HPT scores for each participant at T0 and T1. Participants in the IG are numbered from one to nine; those in the CG are numbered from 10 to 18. Lower values represent better performance.

No statistically significant changes were identified in the SARA items and total scores collected from the IG at T0 and T1. Conversely, a significant increment of the SARA total score was found for the CG at T1. However, although a more substantial change occurred in the CG, no statistical difference emerged comparing the SARA items and total score variation between the two groups.

No significant change was recognized when analyzing the T25FW scores. A minor improvement can be found in both groups at this test, with the CG reducing its scores slightly more than the IG.

4. Discussion

The present article described the effects of exergame use for upper body physical rehabilitation training for children with ataxia on participants' hand dexterity, disease severity, and walking ability.

On average, the proposed intervention improved the hand dexterity of participants in the IG, while those in the CG worsened their performance. This result was confirmed when looking at the individual participants' 9HPT scores showing that most of the subjects in the IG reduced their scores, and most of those in the CG increased the time required to complete the test. The 9HPT test–retest error margin was identified as 5% for the dominant hand

and 2.4% for the non-dominant hand for the population with spinocerebellar ataxia [37]. Although minor changes occurred in the participants' scores, the 9HPT deltas exceeded the test's test–retest error margin in eight subjects for both the dominant and non-dominant hand in the IG. Of these, seven participants (77.8%) for the dominant hand and six (66.7%) for the non-dominant hand improved their score. Conversely, 9HPT deltas of six subjects for the dominant hand and five for the non-dominant hand surpass the test–retest error margin. Of them, five (55.6%) for the dominant hand and four (44.4%) for the non-dominant hand worsened their score. The authors believe that the conducted training strengthened the participants' body and arms muscles and increased their body segments control, improving the trunk, shoulders, and arms stabilization during the hand dexterity task performance. These findings echo those of Ada and colleagues [20], who reported that computer-based elbow dexterity training positively affected the ipsilateral hand dexterity.

The disease severity data show that no significant change occurred for participants in the IC while those in the CG showed a significant increment of their SARA scores. This result should be interpreted with caution due to the small sample size. Moreover, although the disease progression resulted in diminished IC, no statistical difference was found between SARA score deltas of subjects in the IC and CG. Previous research reported better outcomes of exergame training on children's ataxia symptoms assessed with the SARA [18,19]. However, these papers proposed treatments that focused more on balance and gait, while the one presented mainly involved arms movements. This discrepancy hints that a mixed intervention aimed at taking in charge different key aspects of the disorder may lead to more global improvements.

The walking ability changed accordingly in both groups showing no impact of the intervention on this skill. This result is not surprising as the implemented training was performed in a standing position and involved accurate upper limbs and trunk movements. Again, keeping in mind the globality of the motor impairment of children and adolescents with ataxia, it is advisable to combine interventions to take care of as many critical aspects of the pathology as possible. This finding is in line with a previous report suggesting that postural control can be enhanced using exergame as complementary training in adults with Ataxia [38]. The use of various exergames involving different body parts and skills across the week could also increase the child's interest, supporting the adherence to the program.

Adherence data suggest that the presented results can be attained even with a less intensive intervention than expected. The authors believe that the Niurion® exergame supported the participants' motivation to follow and adhere to the intervention, but it was insufficient to sustain the required adherence. These data align with previous statements reporting exergames' difficulties in maintaining the player's interest over long periods [17,39]. The literature recommends intensive, daily physical intervention for this population that could lead to even better results if reached [8,21,38]. Highly motivating virtual environments are needed to stimulate young users to adhere to long-lasting intensive practices and achieve ecologic and meaningful treatment [40]. The individuality of the motivational factors necessary to sustain prolonged treatments requires the possibility of pursuing the same therapeutic goal throughout multiple virtual environments and tasks, adapting to personal and age adequate preferences. Although previous studies suggested some factors supporting the children's motivation to play an exergame [41,42], the implementation of such elements remains technically challenging. However, exergaming is a relatively young and constantly developing technology, and its real potential in health promotion is far from being expressed [17].

Finally, considerations should be made on the fact that the present intervention was conducted at home, with minimal remote supervision of the health care professionals. These options represent a great advantage for monitoring and treating people with a rare pathology such as ataxia, which is widely distributed across the territory, sometimes with limited access to rehabilitation facilities. Moreover, as the proposed training acts as a supplementary intervention for the individuals in the IG, it could be speculated that the obtained improvement could be strictly related to the increased amount of time spent by participants in performing therapeutic activities, according to the existing literature [8,21,38]. Therefore, exergames could represent a cost-effective solution to increase the number of therapeutic sessions received by children with ataxia. The exergames cost-effectiveness is still limited by the hardware and software development price. However, more widely affordable solutions are emerging, such as the one used in this study and others [17,43–47].

This study presents some limitations. Although a robust experimental design was applied, a small number of participants was enrolled, limiting the generalization of the results. Enrolling large samples of patients with rare disorders in clinical rehabilitation research is difficult. Greater collaboration between scientists, clinicians, and the association of patients and families is needed to enhance the research quality in this field [11]. The external validity of our results is also challenged by the lack of a baseline and wash-out phases. Future studies should establish these phases to confirm the cause/effect relationship between the intervention and the occurred changes and their maintenance after the treatment interruption. In addition, there is a lack in the literature related to the expected change in the 9HPT score for the pediatric population with ataxia, challenging the possibility of comparing the presented results with the natural history of these patients. Finally, the effect of the intervention on the participants' activity of daily living was not assessed within the current project and could represent an interesting study of the efficacy of exergame.

5. Conclusions

The presented exergame effectively enhanced the hand dexterity of children with ataxia. However, there is a need for more engaging and fun exergames capable of maintaining a high level of players' interest and motivation in playing. Moreover, it is advisable to plan a mixed intervention (eventually with more than one exergame) to take care of the multiple aspects of the disorder.

Supplementary Materials: The following supporting information can be downloaded at: https://www.mdpi.com/article/10.3390/jcm11041065/s1, Table S1: Adherence individual data for each participant and related descriptive statistics; Table S2: Participants' individual scores for each outcome measure.

Author Contributions: Conceptualization, G.V. and M.P.; Data curation, A.R., M.F. and S.S.; Formal analysis, A.R., S.S. and T.S.; Funding acquisition, E.C. and M.P.; Investigation, A.R., M.F., T.S. and G.V.; Methodology, E.S.B., G.V. and M.P.; Project administration, E.S.B., E.C., G.V. and M.P.; Resources, E.C. and M.P.; Supervision, E.S.B., E.C., G.V. and M.P.; Validation, S.S., T.S., G.V. and M.P.; Visualization, A.R., M.F., E.S.B. and E.C.; Writing—original draft, A.R.; Writing—review and editing, A.R., S.S., T.S., G.V. and M.P. All authors have read and agreed to the published version of the manuscript.

Funding: This research was funded by the Italian Ministry of Health, within the grant "Progetto di Rete NET-2013-02356160-3".

Institutional Review Board Statement: The study was conducted in accordance with the Declaration of Helsinki and approved by the Ethics Committee of the Bambino Gesù Children's Hospital (NET-2013-02356160 WP3, nr. 1619-2018).

Informed Consent Statement: Informed consent was obtained from all subjects involved in the study.

Data Availability Statement: Data are available as Supplementary Materials (see Tables S1 and S2).

Acknowledgments: We thank the patients and their families for their collaboration and commitment.

Conflicts of Interest: The authors declare no conflict of interest.

References

1. Manto, M.-U. Clinical signs of cerebellar disorders. In *The Cerebellum and Its Disorders*; Cambridge University Press: Cambridge, UK, 2010; pp. 97–120. [CrossRef]
2. Mariotti, C.; Fancellu, R.; Di Donato, S. An overview of the patient with ataxia. *J. Neurol.* **2005**, *252*, 511–518. [CrossRef] [PubMed]

3. Summa, S.; Schirinzi, T.; Favetta, M.; Romano, A.; Minosse, S.; Diodato, D.; Olivieri, G.; Martinelli, D.; Sancesario, A.; Zanni, G.; et al. A wearable video-oculography based evaluation of saccades and respective clinical correlates in patients with early onset ataxia. *J. Neurosci. Methods* **2020**, *338*, 108697. [CrossRef] [PubMed]
4. Konczak, J.; Timmann, D. The effect of damage to the cerebellum on sensorimotor and cognitive function in children and adolescents. *Neurosci. Biobehav. Rev.* **2007**, *31*, 1101–1113. [CrossRef]
5. Musselman, K.E.; Stoyanov, C.T.; Marasigan, R.; Jenkins, M.E.; Konczak, J.; Morton, S.M.; Bastian, A.J. Prevalence of ataxia in children: A systematic review. *Neurology* **2014**, *82*, 80–89. [CrossRef] [PubMed]
6. Sullivan, K.J.; Kantak, S.S.; Burtner, P.A. Motor learning in children: Feedback effects on skill acquisition. *Phys. Ther.* **2008**, *88*, 720–732. [CrossRef] [PubMed]
7. Bodranghien, F.; Bastian, A.; Casali, C.; Hallett, M.; Louis, E.D.; Manto, M.; Mariën, P.; Nowak, D.A.; Schmahmann, J.D.; Serrao, M.; et al. Consensus paper: Revisiting the symptoms and signs of cerebellar syndrome. *Cerebellum* **2016**, *15*, 369–391. [CrossRef] [PubMed]
8. Lanza, G.; Casabona, J.A.; Bellomo, M.; Cantone, M.; Fisicaro, F.; Bella, R.; Pennisi, G.; Bramanti, P.; Pennisi, M.; Bramanti, A. Update on intensive motor training in spinocerebellar ataxia: Time to move a step forward? *J. Int. Med. Res.* **2019**, *48*, 300060519854626. [CrossRef] [PubMed]
9. Hartley, H.; Cassidy, E.; Bunn, L.; Kumar, R.; Pizer, B.; Lane, S.; Carter, B. Exercise and physical therapy interventions for children with ataxia: A systematic review. *Cerebellum* **2019**, *18*, 951–968. [CrossRef] [PubMed]
10. Marquer, A.; Barbieri, G.; Pérennou, D. The assessment and treatment of postural disorders in cerebellar ataxia: A systematic review. *Ann. Phys. Rehabil. Med.* **2014**, *57*, 67–78. [CrossRef] [PubMed]
11. Lacorte, E.; Bellomo, G.; Nuovo, S.; Corbo, M.; Vanacore, N.; Piscopo, P. The use of new mobile and gaming technologies for the assessment and rehabilitation of people with ataxia: A systematic review and meta-analysis. *Cerebellum* **2020**, *20*, 361–373. [CrossRef]
12. Bates, C.; Baxter, P.; Bonney, H.; Bremner, F.; Bunn, L.; Carrillo Perez-Tome, M.; Chung, M.; Cipolotti, L.; de Silva, R.; Duberley, K. *Management of the Ataxias towards Best Clinical Practice*, 3rd ed.; Ataxia UK: London, UK, 2016.
13. Sarva, H.; Shanker, V.L. Treatment options in degenerative cerebellar ataxia: A systematic review. *Mov. Disord. Clin. Pract.* **2014**, *1*, 291–298. [CrossRef] [PubMed]
14. Tartarisco, G.; Bruschetta, R.; Summa, S.; Ruta, L.; Favetta, M.; Busa, M.; Romano, A.; Castelli, E.; Marino, F.; Cerasa, A.; et al. Artificial intelligence for dysarthria assessment in children with ataxia: A hierarchical approach. *IEEE Access* **2021**, *9*, 166720–166735. [CrossRef]
15. Gao, Z.; Lee, J.E.; Pope, Z.; Zhang, D. Effect of active videogames on underserved children's classroom behaviors, effort, and fitness. *Games Health J.* **2016**, *5*, 318–324. [CrossRef] [PubMed]
16. Best, J.R. Exergaming in youth: Effects on physical and cognitive health. *Z. Psychol.* **2013**, *221*, 72–78. [CrossRef]
17. Benzing, V.; Schmidt, M. Exergaming for children and adolescents: Strengths, weaknesses, opportunities and threats. *J. Clin. Med.* **2018**, *7*, 422. [CrossRef] [PubMed]
18. Ilg, W.; Schatton, C.; Schicks, J.; Giese, M.A.; Schöls, L.; Synofzik, M. Video game-based coordinative training improves ataxia in children with degenerative ataxia. *Neurology* **2012**, *79*, 2056–2060. [CrossRef] [PubMed]
19. Schatton, C.; Synofzik, M.; Fleszar, Z.; Giese, M.A.; Schöls, L.; Ilg, W. Individualized exergame training improves postural control in advanced degenerative spinocerebellar ataxia: A rater-blinded, intra-individually controlled trial. *Park. Relat. Disord.* **2017**, *39*, 80–84. [CrossRef] [PubMed]
20. Ada, L.; Sherrington, C.; Canning, C.G.; Dean, C.M.; Scianni, A. Computerized tracking to train dexterity after cerebellar tumour: A single-case experimental study. *Brain Inj.* **2009**, *23*, 702–706. [CrossRef] [PubMed]
21. Milne, S.C.; Corben, L.A.; Roberts, M.; Szmulewicz, D.; Burns, J.; Grobler, A.C.; Williams, S.; Chua, J.; Liang, C.; Lamont, P.J.; et al. Rehabilitation for ataxia study: Protocol for a randomised controlled trial of an outpatient and supported home-based physiotherapy programme for people with hereditary cerebellar ataxia. *BMJ Open* **2020**, *10*, e040230. [CrossRef]
22. Corben, L.A.; Tai, G.; Wilson, C.; Collins, V.; Churchyard, A.J.; Delatycki, M.B. A comparison of three measures of upper limb function in Friedreich ataxia. *J. Neurol.* **2010**, *257*, 518–523. [CrossRef] [PubMed]
23. Gagnon, C.; Lessard, I.; Brais, B.; Côté, I.; Lavoie, C.; Synofzik, M.; Mathieu, J. Validity and reliability of outcome measures assessing dexterity, coordination, and upper limb strength in autosomal recessive spastic ataxia of charlevoix-saguenay. *Arch. Phys. Med. Rehabil.* **2018**, *99*, 1747–1754. [CrossRef]
24. Mathiowetz, V.; Weber, K.; Kashman, N.; Volland, G. Adult norms for the nine hole peg test of finger dexterity. *Occup. Ther. J. Res.* **1985**, *5*, 24–38. [CrossRef]
25. Lynch, D.R.; Farmer, J.M.; Tsou, A.Y.; Perlman, S.; Subramony, S.H.; Gomez, C.M.; Ashizawa, T.; Wilmot, G.R.; Wilson, R.B.; Balcer, L.J. Measuring Friedreich ataxia: Complementary features of examination and performance measures. *Neurology* **2006**, *66*, 1711–1716. [CrossRef]
26. Subramony, S.H. SARA—A new clinical scale for the assessment and rating of ataxia: Commentary. *Nat. Clin. Pract. Neurol.* **2007**, *3*, 136–137. [CrossRef]
27. Yabe, I.; Matsushima, M.; Soma, H.; Basri, R.; Sasaki, H. Usefulness of the scale for assessment and rating of ataxia (SARA). *J. Neurol. Sci.* **2008**, *266*, 164–166. [CrossRef]

28. Schmitz-Hübsch, T.; Du Montcel, S.T.; Baliko, L.; Berciano, J.; Boesch, S.; Depondt, C.; Giunti, P.; Globas, C.; Infante, J.; Kang, J.S.; et al. Scale for the assessment and rating of ataxia: Development of a new clinical scale. *Neurology* **2006**, *66*, 1717–1720. [CrossRef]
29. Summa, S.; Schirinzi, T.; Bernava, G.M.; Romano, A.; Favetta, M.; Valente, E.M.; Bertini, E.; Castelli, E.; Petrarca, M.; Pioggia, G.; et al. Development of SaraHome: A novel, well-accepted, technology-based assessment tool for patients with ataxia. *Comput. Methods Programs Biomed.* **2020**, *188*, 105257. [CrossRef]
30. Summa, S.; Tartarisco, G.; Favetta, M.; Buzachis, A.; Romano, A.; Bernava, G.M.; Vasco, G.; Pioggia, G.; Petrarca, M.; Castelli, E.; et al. Spatio-temporal parameters of ataxia gait dataset obtained with the Kinect. *Data Br.* **2020**, *32*, 106307. [CrossRef]
31. Schirinzi, T.; Favetta, M.; Romano, A.; Sancesario, A.; Summa, S.; Minosse, S.; Zanni, G.; Castelli, E.; Bertini, E.; Petrarca, M.; et al. One-year outcome of coenzyme Q10 supplementation in ADCK3 ataxia (ARCA2). *Cerebellum Ataxias* **2019**, *6*, 15. [CrossRef]
32. Summa, S.; Tartarisco, G.; Favetta, M.; Buzachis, A.; Romano, A.; Bernava, G.M.; Sancesario, A.; Vasco, G.; Pioggia, G.; Petrarca, M.; et al. Validation of low-cost system for gait assessment in children with ataxia. *Comput. Methods Programs Biomed.* **2020**, *196*, 105705. [CrossRef]
33. Perez-Lloret, S.; van de Warrenburg, B.; Rossi, M.; Rodríguez-Blázquez, C.; Zesiewicz, T.; Saute, J.A.M.; Durr, A.; Nishizawa, M.; Martinez-Martin, P.; Stebbins, G.T.; et al. Assessment of ataxia rating scales and cerebellar functional tests: Critique and recommendations. *Mov. Disord.* **2021**, *36*, 283–297. [CrossRef]
34. Fahey, M.C.; Corben, L.A.; Collins, V.; Churchyard, A.J.; Delatycki, M.B. The 25-foot walk velocity accurately measures real world ambulation in Friedreich ataxia. *Neurology* **2007**, *68*, 705–706. [CrossRef]
35. Lynch, D.R.; Farmer, J.M.; Wilson, R.L.; Balcer, L.J. Performance measures in Friedreich ataxia: Potential utility as clinical outcome tools. *Mov. Disord.* **2005**, *20*, 777–782. [CrossRef]
36. Armstrong, R.A. When to use the Bonferroni correction. *Ophthalmic Physiol. Opt.* **2014**, *34*, 502–508. [CrossRef]
37. Schmitz-Hübsch, T.; Giunti, P.; Stephenson, D.A.; Globas, C.; Baliko, L.; Saccà, F.; Mariotti, C.; Rakowicz, M.; Szymanski, S.; Infante, J.; et al. SCA functional index. *Neurology* **2008**, *71*, 486–492. [CrossRef]
38. Ayvat, E.; Onursal Kılınç, Ö.; Ayvat, F.; Savcun Demirci, C.; Aksu Yıldırım, S.; Kurşun, O.; Kılınç, M. The effects of exergame on postural control in individuals with ataxia: A rater-blinded, randomized controlled, cross-over study. *Cerebellum* **2021**, 1–9. [CrossRef]
39. Liang, Y.; Lau, P.W.C. Effects of active videogames on physical activity and related outcomes among healthy children: A systematic review. *Games Health J.* **2014**, *3*, 122–144. [CrossRef]
40. Vaz, D.V.; Silva, P.L.; Mancini, M.C.; Carello, C.; Kinsella-Shaw, J. Towards an ecologically grounded functional practice in rehabilitation. *Hum. Mov. Sci.* **2017**, *52*, 117–132. [CrossRef]
41. Chin A Paw, M.J.M.; Jacobs, W.M.; Vaessen, E.P.G.; Titze, S.; van Mechelen, W. The motivation of children to play an active video game. *J. Sci. Med. Sport* **2008**, *11*, 163–166. [CrossRef]
42. Baranowski, T.; Maddison, R.; Maloney, A.; Medina, E.; Simons, M. Building a better mousetrap (exergame) to increase youth physical activity. *Games Health J.* **2014**, *3*, 72–78. [CrossRef]
43. Arpaia, P.; Cimmino, P.; De Matteis, E.; D'Addio, G. A low-cost force sensor-based posturographic plate for home care telerehabilitation exergaming. *Measurement* **2014**, *51*, 400–410. [CrossRef]
44. Barry, G.; Galna, B.; Rochester, L. The role of exergaming in Parkinson's disease rehabilitation: A systematic review of the evidence. *J. Neuroeng. Rehabil.* **2014**, *11*, 33. [CrossRef] [PubMed]
45. Yoo, S.; Kay, J. VRun: Running-in-place virtual reality exergame. In Proceedings of the 28th Australian Conference on Computer-Human Interaction, Launceston, Australia, 29 November–2 December 2016; pp. 562–566.
46. de Souza, J.T. *"Free to Fly": Development and Evaluation of a Novel Exergame with a Low-Cost 3D Tracking Method for Post-Stroke Rehabilitation*; Universidade Federal de Uberlândia: Uberlândia, Brazil, 2021.
47. Sato, K.; Kuroki, K.; Saiki, S.; Nagatomi, R. Improving walking, muscle strength, and balance in the elderly with an exergame using Kinect: A randomized controlled trial. *Games Health J.* **2015**, *4*, 161–167. [CrossRef] [PubMed]

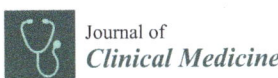

Article

Estimation of Gross Motor Functions in Children with Cerebral Palsy Using Zebris FDM-T Treadmill

Mariusz Bedla *, Paweł Pięta, Daniel Kaczmarski and Stanisław Deniziak

Faculty of Electrical Engineering, Automatic Control and Computer Science, Kielce University of Technology, al. Tysiąclecia Państwa Polskiego 7, 25-314 Kielce, Poland; p.pieta@tu.kielce.pl (P.P.); d.kaczmarski@tu.kielce.pl (D.K.); deniziak@tu.kielce.pl (S.D.)
* Correspondence: m.bedla@tu.kielce.pl

Abstract: A standardized observational instrument designed to measure change in gross motor function over time in children with cerebral palsy is the Gross Motor Function Measure (GMFM). The process of evaluating a value for the GMFM index can be time consuming. It typically takes 45 to 60 min for the patient to complete all tasks, sometimes in two or more sessions. The diagnostic procedure requires trained and specialized therapists. The paper presents the estimation of the GMFM measure for patients with cerebral palsy based on the results of the Zebris FDM-T treadmill. For this purpose, the regression analysis was used. Estimations based on the Generalized Linear Regression were assessed using different error metrics. The results obtained showed that the GMFM score can be estimated with acceptable accuracy. Because the Zebris FDM-T is a widely used device in gait rehabilitation, our method has the potential to be widely adopted for objective diagnostics of children with cerebral palsy.

Keywords: Gross Motor Function Measure; cerebral palsy; estimation; Zebris FDM-T; regression

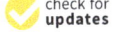

Citation: Bedla, M.; Pięta, P.; Kaczmarski, D.; Deniziak, S. Estimation of Gross Motor Functions in Children with Cerebral Palsy Using Zebris FDM-T Treadmill. *J. Clin. Med.* **2022**, *11*, 954. https://doi.org/10.3390/jcm11040954

Academic Editors: Hideki Nakano, Akiyoshi Matsugi, Naoki Yoshida and Yohei Okada

Received: 13 November 2021
Accepted: 8 February 2022
Published: 12 February 2022

Publisher's Note: MDPI stays neutral with regard to jurisdictional claims in published maps and institutional affiliations.

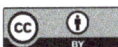

Copyright: © 2022 by the authors. Licensee MDPI, Basel, Switzerland. This article is an open access article distributed under the terms and conditions of the Creative Commons Attribution (CC BY) license (https:// creativecommons.org/licenses/by/ 4.0/).

1. Introduction

Cerebral palsy (CP) is a group of permanent disorders of the development of movement and posture that are considered one of the most frequent causes of non-progressive motor disability in children [1,2]. Symptoms of CP vary from person to person, ranging from mild to very severe movement difficulties [1,2]. CP is a very diverse problem accompanied by multiple comorbidities such as communication impairment, cognitive impairment, visual and hearing impairment, reduced alertness, epilepsy, seizures, musculoskeletal problems, feeding difficulties, behavioral disorders, mental retardation, and even sleep disorders [1–5]. Due to the complexity of this condition and the fact that there is no cure for CP, its treatment is also very complex: it includes botulinum toxin therapies, certain surgical techniques (such as orthopedic surgery and rhizotomy), and supportive treatments (such as physiotherapy or focal vibration (FV) on limb muscles)—these procedures help alleviate symptoms of the disease and improve motor skills of patients [1,6].

The volume of data that describe patients with CP is constantly expanding, and the diversity of these data is also increasing [3–5,7–9]. A significant problem associated with CP is the dispersion and inconsistency of data related to this condition, as well as the lack of dedicated information systems that would facilitate the observation of patients and help determine the most appropriate treatment process [2]. The Mobilize Center information system addresses the problem of data spread [10]. Moreover, in this work Ku et al. identified Big Data Analytics (BDA) and Machine Learning (ML) as potential methodologies that could revolutionize research on human mobility. Over the last few years, these approaches have been used extensively in numerous studies related to CP [11–20]. The growing amount of data obtained as a result of human biomechanical studies makes it imperative to develop advanced methods of multivariate analysis and ML. Current trends and future directions regarding Computer Vision (CV) and ML in CP research have been summarized in several works [9,21,22].

Because CP is a complex disorder, different morphological and functional Gait Classification Systems (GCSs) have been developed, many of whom express either gait pathology or functional impairment [23,24]. GCSs help categorize gait pathologies, allow for the assessment of patient health over time, provide a standardized way to compare gaits between different patients, simplify treatment recommendations and planning, and improve data exchange between clinicians and researchers [23,24]. To increase the efficiency of gait classification and quantify gait compared to the unimpaired gait of typically developing individuals (TD), data obtained with the use of three-dimensional Instrumented Gait Analysis (3DIGA) have been used to introduce gait indices such as the Gillette Gait Index (GGI), the Gait Deviation Index (GDI), and the Gait Profile Score (GPS) [24–26]. GGI has been proven to show an excellent correlation with Gross Motor Function Measure (GMFM), and GDI is strongly correlated with Gross Motor Function Classification System (GMFCS) [24]. Also, it should be noted that GDI and GPS were not developed exclusively for gait assessment in patients with CP, but as a more general measure of gait pathology [24,26]. Another test that is frequently used to evaluate functional exercise capacity of children with CP and is inexpensive to administer is the 6-minute Walk Test (6MWT) [27,28]. Furthermore, a work by Thomason et al. proposed a novel assessment of gait function in children with CP—the Gait Outcomes Assessment List (GOAL) [29]. This index tries to capture the complex nature of physical ability by taking into account contextual factors that contribute to functioning, as well as expectations of children and their parents.

Some of the GCSs are more efficient to administer, such as GGI and GDI, but require sophisticated and expensive equipment to measure certain kinematic and spatiotemporal parameters of a patient's gait [24]. Other indices like GMFM do not require the use of such equipment, but have other disadvantages. Because the GMFM score is evaluated using 88 (GMFM-88) or 66 (GMFM-66) items (measurements) grouped into 5 dimensions, the process of obtaining a value of this index can be time consuming—typically, it takes 45 to 60 min for the patient to complete all tasks, sometimes in two or more sessions [30,31]. Individual test items are scored from 0 to 3, and even though trained therapists reach a high level of agreement when administering and scoring GMFM [30,31], it may not be the case for young, inexperienced, untrained therapists, or those unfamiliar with the method of measurement. Moreover, if the child is tired or other factors related to the child are present, it is not always feasible to complete all the measurements [31]. To increase the efficiency of the evaluation of the GMFM index, its abbreviated forms were developed: GMFM-66-IS and GMFM-66 B&C [32]. GMFM-66-IS can be administered in approximately 20 to 30 min [31], so the time needed to evaluate the GMFM score can be reduced by two-thirds. A recent work proposed another reduced version of the GMFM-66 index named rGMFM-66 [31]. In this study Duran et al. used several artificial intelligence approaches to estimate the GMFM-66 value with the fewest possible measurements, e.g., by the means of Random Forest (RF), or Support Vector Machine (SVM).

An important direction of research on CP is the search for associations in patients health data, e.g., to find correlations with various classification systems and measures, such as: the Communication Function Classification System (CFCS) [33,34], the Five-Times-Sit-to-Stand Test (FTSST) [35], GDI [35–40], GMFCS [33,34,36,41,42], GMFM [43], the Manual Ability Classification System (MACS) [34], and also to identify other associations and correlations [39,40,44–50]. Strongly correlated data are essential for BDA and ML algorithms, e.g., to develop successful regression models.

Another direction of research is an attempt to predict the values of some of the previously mentioned classification systems and measures, as well as other health parameters of patients with CP, mainly by means of ML. In Ries et al. [51] developed a statistical orthosis selection model using RF. The goal of this model was to predict which of the five orthosis designs would provide the best gait outcome (defined as the change in GDI) for patients with diplegic CP. In Galarraga et al. [52] predicted postoperative lower limb kinematics utilizing multiple linear regressions. Another study by these authors [53] proposed a system that predicts postoperative kinematics considering a large number of surgical combinations and gait patterns in CP. In [54], Rosenberg and Steele used musculoskeletal models to simulate walking kinematics of children with CP, with and without passive ankle foot orthoses (AFOs). The work of Rajagopal et al. [55] built regression models to estimate the effect of single-event multilevel surgery (SEMLS) in improving gait in patients with CP. In [56], Duran et al. developed a method that predicts the expected changes in the GMFM-66 measure of individual children with CP between two points in time that are 6 months apart. Pitto et al. in their research [57] developed the SimCP—a novel framework that allows to evaluate the outcome of different simulated surgeries, enabling clinicians to predict gait performance after orthopedic intervention in children with CP. In Kidziński et al. [58], presented ML models to predict clinically relevant motion parameters such as walking speed, cadence, knee flexion angle at maximum extension, and GDI. The methods used by the researchers included the Convolutional Neural Network (CNN), RF, and Ridge Regression (RR)—they were trained using ordinary videos of patients with CP. Another similar work was conducted by Jalata et al. [59]. They proposed a Graph Convolutional Neural Network (GCNN) that predicts similar gait measures based on a video of a patient. The research by Azhand et al. [60] demonstrated a novel gait assessment model using CNNs that can extract 3D skeleton joints from videos of walking humans taken with monocular smartphone cameras. Other interesting work by Afifi [61] proposed a model using RF to predict CP in very preterm infants. The model provided a good level of discrimination between children with and without CP.

The purpose of this study was to develop a method to estimate the GMFM measure for patients with cerebral palsy based on the Zebris FDM-T treadmill results. The proposed model was trained using data collected from 23 patients with CP. The Zebris FDM-T is a device that is widely used in gait rehabilitation, so our method has the potential to be widely adopted. Section 2 briefly characterizes the GMFM measure and the Zebris FDM-T treadmill device, as well as discusses the study population and data analysis methods used to carry out this work. Section 3 presents the experimental results obtained with our method. Finally, Section 4 provides the interpretation of these results and concludes the article highlighting future research directions.

2. Materials and Methods

The Materials and Methods section has been divided into 5 subsections. The first subsection describes the GMFM, an observational tool for measuring changes in gross motor function over time in children with cerebral palsy. Then, the Zebris FMD-T treadmill device was characterized, from which the results for analysis were obtained. The third subsection covers the study population, which was based on the use of data from 23 patients. The next subsection discusses the Zebris FDM-T treadmill diagnostics scheme that was used to obtain patient measurements. The last subsection describes the data analysis methods that were used to carry out our research.

2.1. Gross Motor Function Measure (GMFM)

The GMFM is a precise observational tool for measuring changes in gross motor function over time in children with CP [47]. It is based on the principles of developmental neurophysiology [62,63]. It is a quantitative scale: it was designed to minimize variation by including the assessment of 'does do' rather than 'can do' (it consists of objectively defined test items and it has a standardized scoring system) [64]. The GMFM examines the functional behavior of children in terms of major motor activities from infancy to 16 years of age. It focuses on monitoring the number of gross motor activities that a 5-year-old child can perform [32]. It is an insightful and comprehensive tool that is used to assess the effectiveness of various treatments due to its high sensitivity and repeatability [38,62,65]. In addition, it can be utilized to set the functional goals of the current or planned treatment of the child. Also, it allows one to determine the functional state of the child at a given moment and compare it with the previous state. Lastly, it can be used to establish the type of functional process of the child.

There are two versions of GMFM: GMFM-66 and GMFM-88 [66]. The GMFM-88 scale was developed for children with CP, but it is also used in children with Down syndrome and brain injuries [62]. It provides a more detailed description of the limitations and abilities of children with varying levels of motor disabilities [66]. The GMFM-88 can be administered with shoes and outpatient aids and/or orthoses [62]. The GMFM measures a child's ability in five different dimensions:

1. lying and rolling (17 measurements),
2. sitting (20 measurements),
3. crawling and kneeling (14 measurements),
4. standing (13 measurements),
5. walking, running, and jumping (24 measurements) [32,47,65].

During the GMFM assessment, the child receives points from 0 to 3 for each motor task. The obtained number of points reflects the degree of execution of a given activity:

- 0 points—does not initiate movement,
- 1 point—activity performed in the range below 10% (initiates movement),
- 2 points—activity executed in the range between 10–100%,
- 3 points—activity performed in 100%,
- NT—not tested [66].

A child scores 0 points for omitting a measurement or for being unable to complete one [66]. The points obtained are then calculated by the computer program GMAE (Gross Motor Ability Estimator), which returns the result as a percentage with a 95% confidence area [66]. The GMFM scale is used in rehabilitation centers that treat children with CP, although it cannot be administered to patients with behavioral disorders and those who do not understand verbal commands or demonstrations [66,67]. The tool allows monitoring even the smallest progress in motor development of children with CP, especially those with spastic forms of the disease, which is an important step in improving their functional state [66]. All information about progress in child activity is also of key importance for parents of young patients. It is recommended to complete all test items, even by older children who may be able to perform more advanced tasks. The final report should also contain information in the event of difficulties arising from lack of cooperation with a child [66,67].

2.2. Zebris FDM-T Treadmill Device

The Zebris FDM-T treadmill [68] is a very universal rehabilitation and diagnostic device that supports various modes of operation. It can be used both for dynamic gait analysis and for static analysis while a patient is standing. The treadmill is used for the diagnosis and rehabilitation of lower limbs in patients with CP. In addition, a camera can be connected to the device, as well as an electromyography (EMG) set and a projector to display the footprints on a treadmill that a patient should follow, or a monitor that displays a customizable track with obstacles that a patient should avoid. Measurement results can be exported in the form of text, graphics, and video. Basic parameters that can be measured include values of forces and pressures of a feet, as well as time-space parameters of gait [69].

In this study, the results of the following measurements obtained with the use of the Zebris FDM-T device were analyzed: static analysis when standing with eyes open and closed, and gait analysis at a preferred speed determined for each patient at the first attempt. During the stance analysis, more than 20 parameters are recorded, such as forces, COP positions, 95% confidence ellipse area, etc. More than 100 parameters representing different aspects of gait are recorded during gait analysis, such as forces, pressures, gait phases, times, anterior/posterior position, foot rotations, lateral symmetry, cadence, velocity, step length, step width, etc.

2.3. Study Population

Data that were analyzed in this research came from a part of the TWEC project carried out by PHU Technomex Sp. z o.o. The TWEC project concerns the realization of an IT system with a mobile application that optimizes the indications, intensity, and training loads for integrated use during technologically assisted gait education in people with CP using selected rehabilitation devices. The study included 23 patients with CP (8–24 years of age): 12 women and 11 men. The analysis used 55 data samples about patients belonging to the GMFCS 2 group that were recorded during different stages of the project (there may be from 1 to 4 samples per patient). In the project GMFM-88 scale values were used, which were determined by physicians: the results are shown in Figure 1 as a box plot, with specific values represented as blue dots (they may overlap).

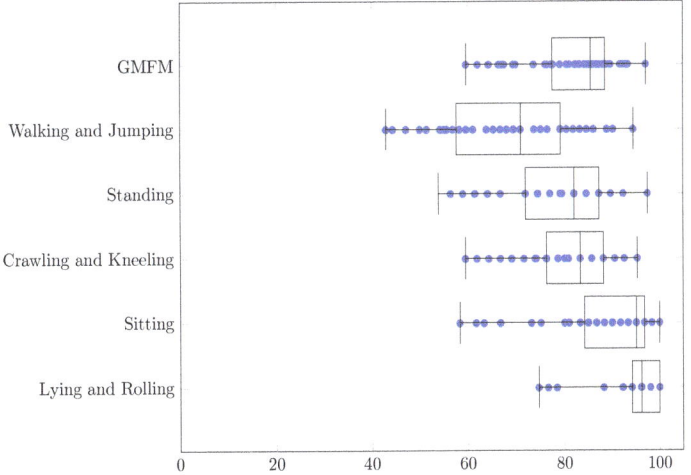

Figure 1. Patients' GMFM-88 values.

2.4. Zebris FDM-T Treadmill Diagnostics Scheme

This section describes the Zebris FDM-T treadmill diagnostics scheme that our partners (Department of Pediatric Orthopedics and Traumatology at Poznan University of Medical Sciences and PHU Technomex Sp. z o.o.) use in the TWEC project. Assessment on the treadmill is carried out in two ways: static (standing) and dynamic (walking). The first involves standing upright, while the second allows for the analysis of individual phases of gait and the assessment of many parameters describing gait that were mentioned in Section 2.2. The static measurement is performed at least twice for 30 s with eyes open and separately with eyes closed. When performing the test with eyes open, the screen should show a neutral image with no COP (center of pressure) feedback, or the screen should be obscured. In order to be able to perform a dynamic measurement, the examined person must get used to walking on moving ground. The period of acclimatization to walking on the treadmill lasts between 5 and 6 min, during which the patient's comfort speed is verified, trying to adjust the speed to obtain the natural locomotion speed of the ground (determined during the gait analysis in the optoelectronic system or the initial 6MWT fragment). If the patient does not feel comfortable after reaching the ground speed, the speed is gradually reduced every 30 s until the subject declares that the speed is appropriate. Then, a specific measurement is performed that lasts 60 s. After this period, the speed is gradually increased every 30 s until the maximum speed at which the patient is not afraid to move is achieved and another 60-s measurement is performed. On the treadmill, the patient walks barefoot and is allowed to hold the handrail if necessary. Patient diagnostics on the Zebris treadmill takes between 30 and 40 min.

2.5. Data Analysis

Many more parameters than data samples may lead to a problem with model fitting [70]. Therefore, direction of the learning process was performed. To improve the quality of the model, two types of operations were used. The first was the reduction of parameters to the ones most correlated with the target (GMFM dimensions). The second was based on an introduction of interaction features. At first, the parameters most correlated with the target were found. Then, they were multiplied by themselves and added to the original parameters. Lastly, the parameters that were most correlated with each other were removed. As a result, the remaining parameters were correlated with the target, but not with each other.

For data analysis, the Spark framework [71] was used. In particular, the MLlib library was utilized. The data were randomly divided into:

- training set—80% of the data,
- testing set—remaining 20% of the data.

Then, the Generalized Linear Regression using the Gaussian family. It allows flexible specification of a Generalized Linear Model (GLM) that can be applied to different types of predictive problems, including linear regression, Poisson regression, logistic regression, and more [71].

Finally, with the help of this tool, the following measures were calculated:

- Mean Squared Error (MSE),
- Root Mean Squared Error (RMSE),
- Mean Absolute Error (MAE),
- Mean Absolute Percentage Error (MAPE),
- Coefficient of Determination (R^2) [71].

The operations of dividing the data into training and testing were repeated 100 times. In the next section, errors are presented in two forms: plots and tables. The plots show the specific error values for each iteration as orange dots (they may overlap) and aggregated error values for all iterations in the form of a box plot. In the tables, the following symbols are used:

- min—minimal value,
- q1—first quartile,
- median—second quartile,
- q3—third quartile,
- max—maximal value,
- q3 − q1—difference between third and first quartile,
- range—difference between maximal and minimal value.

3. Results

In this section, experimental results concerning MSE, RMSE, MAPE, and R^2 are presented. Their description and interpretation are provided.

MSE is used to calculate the average squared difference between the observed and estimated values. RMSE is the square root of MSE. The smaller the values of these measures, the closer the model is to the actual data. The definitions used are as follows (https://spark.apache.org/docs/2.3.0/mllib-evaluation-metrics.html (accessed on 20 October 2021)):

$$\text{MSE} = \frac{1}{N} \sum_{i=0}^{N-1} (y_i - \hat{y}_i)^2, \ \text{RMSE} = \sqrt{\frac{1}{N} \sum_{i=0}^{N-1} (y_i - \hat{y}_i)^2} \quad (1)$$

Experimental results concerning MSE and RMSE are presented in the Tables 1 and 2 and in the Figures 2 and 3, respectively.

Table 1. The MSE values for the conducted experiments.

	Min	q1	Median	q3	Max	q3 − q1	Range
GMFM	9.4	33.7	47.5	58.7	89.5	25.0	80.1
Walking and Jumping	43.7	79.1	101.1	120.1	234.2	41.0	190.5
Standing	33.3	63.2	79.3	93.7	155.4	30.5	122.2
Crawling and Kneeling	12.2	31.8	41.2	59.0	109.9	27.3	97.7
Sitting	16.1	40.9	59.3	71.9	144.5	30.9	128.4
Lying and Rolling	2.8	8.0	13.1	18.2	38.5	10.2	35.7

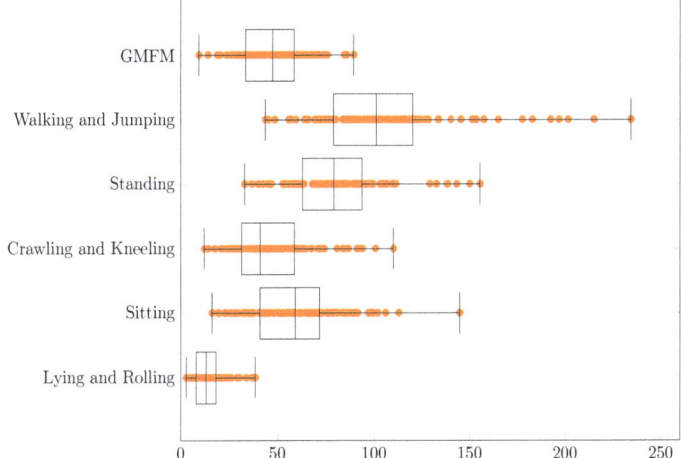

Figure 2. The MSE values for the conducted experiments.

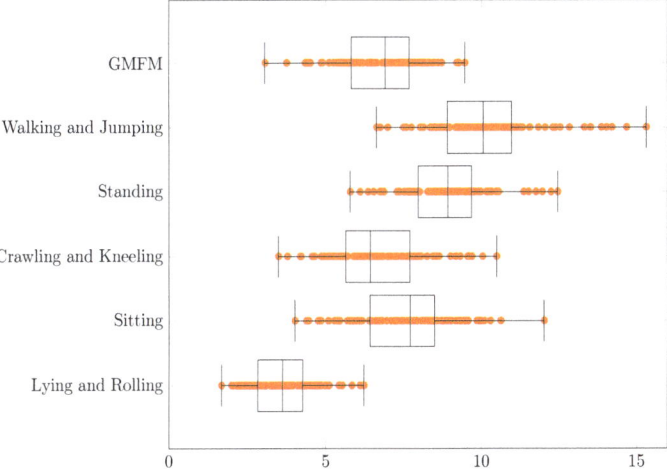

Figure 3. The RMSE values for the conducted experiments.

Table 2. The RMSE values for the conducted experiments.

	Min	q1	Median	q3	Max	q3 − q1	Range
GMFM	3.1	5.8	6.9	7.7	9.5	1.9	6.4
Walking and Jumping	6.6	8.9	10.1	11.0	15.3	2.1	8.7
Standing	5.8	7.9	8.9	9.7	12.5	1.7	6.7
Crawling and Kneeling	3.5	5.6	6.4	7.7	10.5	2.0	7.0
Sitting	4.0	6.4	7.7	8.5	12.0	2.1	8.0
Lying and Rolling	1.7	2.8	3.6	4.3	6.2	1.4	4.5

MAE is used to calculate the average absolute difference between the observed and estimated values. MAPE is the percentage version of MAE, where the absolute difference between the observed and estimated values is referred to the first one. Similarly to MSE and RMSE, the smaller the values of these measures, the closer the model is to the actual data. The MAE penalizes large errors more than MSE. The definitions used are as follows:

$$\text{MAE} = \frac{1}{N} \sum_{i=0}^{N-1} |y_i - \hat{y}_i|, \quad \text{MAPE} = \frac{100}{N} \sum_{i=0}^{N-1} \left| \frac{y_i - \hat{y}_i}{y_i} \right| \quad (2)$$

Experimental results concerning MAE and MAPE are presented in the Tables 3 and 4 and in the Figures 4 and 5, respectively.

Table 3. The MAE values for the conducted experiments.

	Min	q1	Median	q3	Max	q3 − q1	Range
GMFM	2.4	4.7	5.4	6.2	8.3	1.5	5.9
Walking and Jumping	5.4	7.7	8.6	9.4	13.3	1.7	7.9
Standing	4.4	6.7	7.5	8.1	11.0	1.5	6.6
Crawling and Kneeling	3.0	4.7	5.3	6.1	8.7	1.5	5.8
Sitting	3.4	4.9	5.8	6.7	9.7	1.8	6.4
Lying and Rolling	1.4	2.2	2.7	3.2	4.4	1.0	3.0

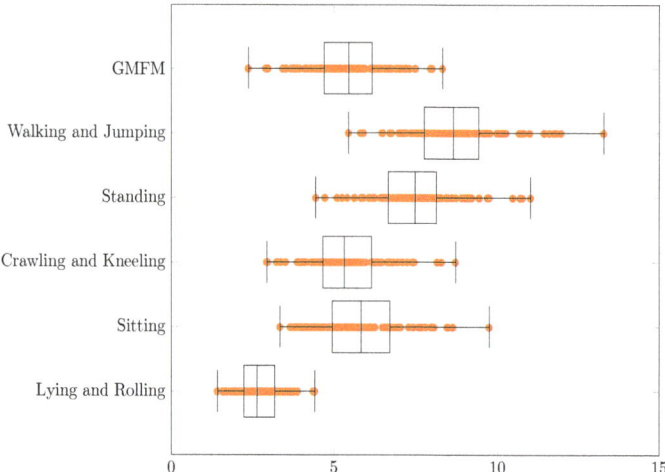

Figure 4. The MAE values for the conducted experiments.

Table 4. The MAPE [%] values for the conducted experiments.

	Min	q1	Median	q3	Max	q3 − q1	Range
GMFM	3.0%	5.9%	7.0%	8.0%	11.3%	2.2%	8.4%
Walking and Jumping	7.8%	11.4%	13.5%	15.5%	23.1%	4.2%	15.3%
Standing	6.0%	8.9%	10.1%	11.4%	16.0%	2.5%	10.0%
Crawling and Kneeling	3.5%	6.0%	6.9%	8.0%	11.9%	2.0%	8.3%
Sitting	3.6%	5.7%	6.9%	8.2%	14.5%	2.4%	11.0%
Lying and Rolling	1.6%	2.4%	2.8%	3.5%	5.5%	1.1%	3.9%

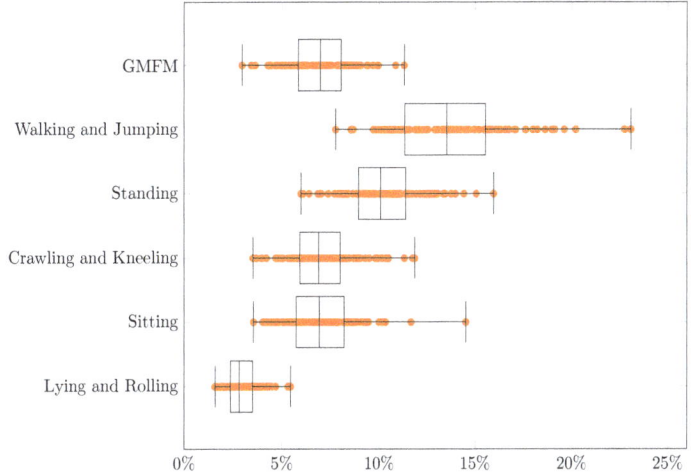

Figure 5. The MAPE [%] values for the conducted experiments.

For MSE, RMSE, MAE and MAPE the smallest errors can be observed for a dimension "Lying and Rolling" and the biggest errors for "Walking and Jumping". Significant similarities concerning MAPE between the dimensions "GMFM" (min = 3.0%, q1 = 5.9%, median = 7.0%, q3 = 8.0%, max = 11.3%, q3 − q1 = 2.2%, range = 8.4%) and "Crawling and Kneeling" (min = 3.5%, q1 = 6.0%, median = 6.9%, q3 = 8.0%, max = 11.9%, q3 − q1 = 2.0%, range = 8.3%) can be found in Table 4. This can also be noticed for various extents for MSE, RMSE and MAE (Tables 1–3, respectively). If the range (max–min) are taken into account, the smallest values always have "Lying and Rolling", and the largest have "Walking and Jumping". The results strongly depend on the selection of training and test data. In the best case, estimations for all dimensions can be made with a MAPE error $\leq 7.8\%$, and in the worst case $\leq 23.1\%$, which means an increase of almost 3 times. The error values in the dimensions probably follow to some extent from the actual results of the patients (Figure 1). They are also probably related to the different difficulties of the movements in the different dimensions.

R^2 is used to calculate the proportion of variance shared by the dependent variable and the independent variable(s). The higher the the value, the higher percentage of variation of dependent variable that is explained by the independent variable(s). The maximum value is 1 (100%). There are a few reason why R^2 may be negative [72], for example, the model is not good enough. According to [73] R^2 is more informative than other metrics in regression analysis evaluation. The definition used is as follows:

$$R^2 = 1 - \frac{\text{MSE}}{\text{VAR}(y)(N-1)} = 1 - \frac{\sum_{i=0}^{N-1}(y_i - \hat{y}_i)^2}{\sum_{i=0}^{N-1}(y_i - \bar{y}_i)^2} \quad (3)$$

Experimental results concerning R^2 are presented in the Table 5 and in the Figure 6.

Table 5. The R^2 values for the conducted experiments.

	Min	q1	Median	q3	Max	q3 − q1	Range
GMFM	−1.11	0.15	0.38	0.57	0.87	0.42	1.98
Walking and Jumping	−1.27	0.09	0.32	0.44	0.71	0.35	1.98
Standing	−0.82	0.11	0.30	0.40	0.65	0.29	1.47
Crawling and Kneeling	−0.72	0.19	0.37	0.55	0.80	0.36	1.53
Sitting	−3.70	0.11	0.43	0.65	0.84	0.54	4.54
Lying and Rolling	−1.58	0.41	0.65	0.75	0.95	0.35	2.53

For all dimensions, at least 75% of the cases (from q1 to max) have positive values of R^2. Median varies from about 0.30 for "Standing" to about 0.75 for "Lying and Rolling". Larger, non negative values would be desirable.

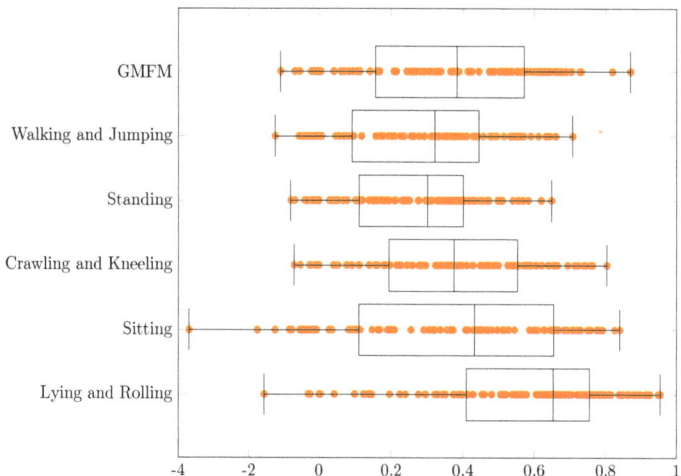

Figure 6. The R^2 values for the conducted experiments.

4. Discussion

Estimating the GMFM measure for patients with CP is a research topic that has not been extensively studied so far. Our experiments confirmed the hypothesis put forward in the introduction to the article: it is possible to estimate the value of this metric based on the Zebris FDM-T treadmill results, with the errors that were discussed in detail in the previous section. Some motor abilities (GMFM dimensions) are better estimated than others. The smallest errors can be observed for a dimension "Lying and Rolling" and the biggest errors for "Walking and Jumping". It may be related to the varying degree of difficulty of the tasks performed within each dimension. More complex exercises may lead to higher estimation errors because the patient may make more mistakes, e.g., as a result of greater fatigue or his/her impairment. Evidence that GMFM estimation is possible can also be found in the work by Duran et al. [56], who developed a method that predicts the expected changes in the GMFM-66 measure of individual children with CP between two points in time that are

6 months apart. In their work, the LMS (lambda-mu-sigma) method was used to generate age-related reference centile curves for the GMFM-66 score.

Because the Zebris FDM-T is a widely used device in gait rehabilitation, our proposition has the potential to be widely adopted. To the best of our knowledge, the approach presented in this paper has not been tried before, so our method can be considered novel. The main disadvantage regarding the GMFM index is related to the efficiency of its administration [30,31]. That is why its abbreviated forms were developed: GMFM-66-IS and GMFM-66 B&C [32]. In [31], Duran et al. proposed yet another reduced version of the GMFM-66 index named rGMFM-66, but its administration still requires some test items to be performed by the patient, although to a limited extent. Using our proposition, a value of GMFM can be estimated immediately when data from Zebris FDM-T are accessible, which can significantly shorten the time of a patient's examination.

Our method can be of great help for untrained therapists who are not familiar with the system of measurement. It can also be utilized by students during their didactic process. Furthermore, our proposition can be used to quickly assess the motor skills of a patient, and then, if a more thorough assessment is needed, a physician can administer the measure in a classic way.

There are many further research directions that can be investigated. It would be useful to estimate metrics with a larger sample of data from more patients. The impact of grouping patients with a similar disease type (e.g., CP type) on the estimation of the metric may also be examined. In projects that also include rehabilitation, estimation of changes in the patient's health may be researched. Furthermore, this approach can be extended to the estimation of changes in metrics as a consequence of surgeries that patients undergo, similarly to [52,53,55,57]. In addition, estimations can be based on patient data from different medical devices that may be used individually or together.

Author Contributions: Conceptualization, S.D., M.B., P.P. and D.K; methodology, M.B.; software, M.B.; validation, M.B. and S.D.; formal analysis, M.B., P.P. and D.K.; investigation, M.B., P.P. and D.K.; resources, S.D.; data curation, M.B. and D.K.; writing—original draft preparation, M.B., P.P. and D.K.; writing—review and editing, S.D., P.P. and M.B.; visualization, M.B.; supervision, S.D.; project administration, S.D.; funding acquisition, S.D. All authors have read and agreed to the published version of the manuscript.

Funding: This research was funded by The Polish National Centre for Research and Development grant number POIR.04.01.04-00-0035/19-00.

Data Availability Statement: Data sets used and analyzed in this research are available from the corresponding author on reasonable request.

Acknowledgments: We thank the staff of the Department of Pediatric Orthopedics and Traumatology at Poznan University of Medical Sciences and PHU Technomex Sp. z o.o. for providing the data used in our research.

Conflicts of Interest: The authors declare no conflict of interest.

Abbreviations

The following abbreviations are used in this manuscript:

CP	Cerebral palsy
BDS	Big Data Analytics
ML	Machine Learning
FV	Focal Vibration
CV	Computer Vision
GCSs	Gait Classification Systems
TD	Typically developing
3DIGA	Three-dimensional Instrumented Gait Analysis
GGI	Gillette Gait Index
GDI	Gait Deviation Index

GPS	Gait Profile Score
GMFM	Gross Motor Function Measure
GMFCS	Gross Motor Function Classification System
6MWT	6-m Walk Test
GOAL	Gait Outcomes Assessment List
RF	Random Forest
SVM	Support Vector Machine
CFCS	Communication Function Classification System
FTSST	Five-Times-Sit-to-Stand Test
MACS	Manual Ability Classification System
CNN	Convolutional Neural Network
RR	Ridge Regression
GCNN	Graph Convolutional Neural Network
GMAE	Gross Motor Ability Estimator
TWEC	Technologicznie Wspomagana Edukacja Chodu
COP	Center of Pressure
GLM	Generalized Linear Model
MSE	Mean Squared Error
RMSE	Root Mean Squared Error
MAE	Mean Absolute Error
MAPE	Mean Absolute Percentage Error
R^2	Coefficient of Determination

References

1. Sadowska, M.; Sarecka-Hujar, B.; Kopyta, I. Cerebral palsy: Current opinions on definition, epidemiology, risk factors, classification and treatment options. *Neuropsychiatr. Dis. Treat.* **2020**, *16*, 1505. [CrossRef] [PubMed]
2. Afzali, M.; Etemad, K.; Kazemi, A.; Rabiei, R. Cerebral palsy information system with an approach to information architecture: A systematic review. *BMJ Health Care Inform.* **2019**, *26*, e100055. [CrossRef] [PubMed]
3. Zhang, J.Y.; Oskoui, M.; Shevell, M. A population-based study of communication impairment in cerebral palsy. *J. Child Neurol.* **2015**, *30*, 277–284. [CrossRef] [PubMed]
4. Reid, S.M.; Meehan, E.M.; Arnup, S.J.; Reddihough, D.S. Intellectual disability in cerebral palsy: A population-based retrospective study. *Dev. Med. Child Neurol.* **2018**, *60*, 687–694. [CrossRef] [PubMed]
5. Whitney, D.G.; Warschausky, S.A.; Peterson, M.D. Mental health disorders and physical risk factors in children with cerebral palsy: A cross-sectional study. *Dev. Med. Child Neurol.* **2019**, *61*, 579–585. [CrossRef] [PubMed]
6. Lopez, S.; Bini, F.; Del Percio, C.; Marinozzi, F.; Celletti, C.; Suppa, A.; Ferri, R.; Staltari, E.; Camerota, F.; Babiloni, C. Electroencephalographic sensorimotor rhythms are modulated in the acute phase following focal vibration in healthy subjects. *Neuroscience* **2017**, *352*, 236–248. [CrossRef]
7. Coker-Bolt, P.; Downey, R.J.; Connolly, J.; Hoover, R.; Shelton, D.; Seo, N.J. Exploring the feasibility and use of accelerometers before, during, and after a camp-based CIMT program for children with cerebral palsy. *J. Pediatr. Rehabil. Med.* **2017**, *10*, 27–36. [CrossRef]
8. Sartori, M.; Fernandez, J.; Modenese, L.; Carty, C.; Barber, L.; Oberhofer, K.; Zhang, J.; Handsfield, G.; Stott, N.; Besier, T.; et al. Toward modeling locomotion using electromyography-informed 3D models: Application to cerebral palsy. *Wiley Interdiscip. Rev. Syst. Biol. Med.* **2017**, *9*, e1368. [CrossRef]
9. Zhang, J. Multivariate analysis and machine learning in cerebral palsy research. *Front. Neurol.* **2017**, *8*, 715. [CrossRef]
10. Ku, J.P.; Hicks, J.L.; Hastie, T.; Leskovec, J.; Ré, C.; Delp, S.L. The mobilize center: An NIH big data to knowledge center to advance human movement research and improve mobility. *J. Am. Med. Inform. Assoc.* **2015**, *22*, 1120–1125. [CrossRef]
11. Bergamini, L.; Calderara, S.; Bicocchi, N.; Ferrari, A.; Vitetta, G. Signal Processing and Machine Learning for Diplegia Classification. In Proceedings of the International Conference on Image Analysis and Processing, Catania, Italy, 11–15 September 2017; Springer: Berlin/Heidelberg, Germany, 2017; pp. 97–108.
12. Kuntze, G.; Nettel-Aguirre, A.; Ursulak, G.; Robu, I.; Bowal, N.; Goldstein, S.; Emery, C.A. Multi-joint gait clustering for children and youth with diplegic cerebral palsy. *PLoS ONE* **2018**, *13*, e0205174. [CrossRef] [PubMed]
13. Ferrari, A.; Bergamini, L.; Guerzoni, G.; Calderara, S.; Bicocchi, N.; Vitetta, G.; Borghi, C.; Neviani, R.; Ferrari, A. Gait-based diplegia classification using lsmt networks. *J. Healthc. Eng.* **2019**, *2019*, 3796898. [CrossRef] [PubMed]
14. Zhang, Y.; Ma, Y. Application of supervised machine learning algorithms in the classification of sagittal gait patterns of cerebral palsy children with spastic diplegia. *Comput. Biol. Med.* **2019**, *106*, 33–39. [CrossRef] [PubMed]
15. Ihlen, E.A.; Støen, R.; Boswell, L.; de Regnier, R.A.; Fjørtoft, T.; Gaebler-Spira, D.; Labori, C.; Loennecken, M.C.; Msall, M.E.; Möinichen, U.I.; et al. Machine learning of infant spontaneous movements for the early prediction of cerebral palsy: A multi-site cohort study. *J. Clin. Med.* **2020**, *9*, 5. [CrossRef]

16. Choisne, J.; Fourrier, N.; Handsfield, G.; Signal, N.; Taylor, D.; Wilson, N.; Stott, S.; Besier, T.F. An unsupervised data-driven model to classify gait patterns in children with cerebral palsy. *J. Clin. Med.* **2020**, *9*, 1432. [CrossRef]
17. Sukhadia, N.; Kamboj, P. Detection of Spastic Cerebral Palsy Using Different Techniques in Infants. In *ICT Analysis and Applications*; Springer: Berlin/Heidelberg, Germany, 2021; pp. 57–71.
18. Kurowski, B.G.; Greve, K.; Bailes, A.F.; Zahner, J.; Vargus-Adams, J.; Mcmahon, M.A.; Aronow, B.J.; Mitelpunkt, A. Electronic health record and patterns of care for children with cerebral palsy. *Dev. Med. Child Neurol.* **2021**, *63*, 1337–1343. [CrossRef]
19. Harris, C.M.; Wright, S.M. Malnutrition in hospitalized adults with cerebral palsy. *J. Parenter. Enter. Nutr.* **2021**, *45*, 1749–1754. [CrossRef]
20. Sakkos, D.; Mccay, K.D.; Marcroft, C.; Embleton, N.D.; Chattopadhyay, S.; Ho, E.S. Identification of Abnormal Movements in Infants: A Deep Neural Network for Body Part-Based Prediction of Cerebral Palsy. *IEEE Access* **2021**, *9*, 94281–94292. [CrossRef]
21. Phinyomark, A.; Petri, G.; Ibáñez-Marcelo, E.; Osis, S.T.; Ferber, R. Analysis of big data in gait biomechanics: Current trends and future directions. *J. Med. Biol. Eng.* **2018**, *38*, 244–260. [CrossRef]
22. Silva, N.; Zhang, D.; Kulvicius, T.; Gail, A.; Barreiros, C.; Lindstaedt, S.; Kraft, M.; Bölte, S.; Poustka, L.; Nielsen-Saines, K.; et al. The future of General Movement Assessment: The role of computer vision and machine learning–A scoping review. *Res. Dev. Disabil.* **2021**, *110*, 103854. [CrossRef]
23. Papageorgiou, E.; Nieuwenhuys, A.; Vandekerckhove, I.; Van Campenhout, A.; Ortibus, E.; Desloovere, K. Systematic review on gait classifications in children with cerebral palsy: An update. *Gait Posture* **2019**, *69*, 209–223. [CrossRef] [PubMed]
24. Tsitlakidis, S.; Schwarze, M.; Westhauser, F.; Heubisch, K.; Horsch, A.; Hagmann, S.; Wolf, S.I.; Götze, M. Gait Indices for Characterization of Patients with Unilateral Cerebral Palsy. *J. Clin. Med.* **2020**, *9*, 3888. [CrossRef] [PubMed]
25. Rasmussen, H.M.; Nielsen, D.B.; Pedersen, N.W.; Overgaard, S.; Holsgaard-Larsen, A. Gait Deviation Index, Gait Profile Score and Gait Variable Score in children with spastic cerebral palsy: Intra-rater reliability and agreement across two repeated sessions. *Gait Posture* **2015**, *42*, 133–137. [CrossRef] [PubMed]
26. Baker, R.; McGinley, J.L.; Schwartz, M.H.; Beynon, S.; Rozumalski, A.; Graham, H.K.; Tirosh, O. The gait profile score and movement analysis profile. *Gait Posture* **2009**, *30*, 265–269. [CrossRef] [PubMed]
27. Fitzgerald, D.; Hickey, C.; Delahunt, E.; Walsh, M.; O'Brien, T. Six-minute walk test in children with spastic cerebral palsy and children developing typically. *Pediatr. Phys. Ther.* **2016**, *28*, 192–199. [CrossRef]
28. Guinet, A.; Desailly, E. Six-minute walk test (6MWT) in children with cerebral palsy. Systematic review and proposal of an adapted version. *Ann. Phys. Rehabil. Med.* **2018**, *61*, e304. [CrossRef]
29. Thomason, P.; Tan, A.; Donnan, A.; Rodda, J.; Graham, H.K.; Narayanan, U. The Gait Outcomes Assessment List (GOAL): Validation of a new assessment of gait function for children with cerebral palsy. *Dev. Med. Child Neurol.* **2018**, *60*, 618–623. [CrossRef]
30. Palisano, R.J.; Hanna, S.E.; Rosenbaum, P.L.; Russell, D.J.; Walter, S.D.; Wood, E.P.; Raina, P.S.; Galuppi, B.E. Validation of a model of gross motor function for children with cerebral palsy. *Phys. Ther.* **2000**, *80*, 974–985. [CrossRef]
31. Duran, I.; Stark, C.; Saglam, A.; Semmelweis, A.; Lioba Wunram, H.; Spiess, K.; Schoenau, E. Artificial intelligence to improve efficiency of administration of gross motor function assessment in children with cerebral palsy. *Dev. Med. Child Neurol.* **2021**, *64*, 228–234. [CrossRef]
32. Brunton, L.K.; Bartlett, D.J. Validity and reliability of two abbreviated versions of the Gross Motor Function Measure. *Phys. Ther.* **2011**, *91*, 577–588. [CrossRef]
33. Margaretha, V.; Prananta, M.S.; Alam, A. Correlation between gross motor function classification system and communication function classification system in children with cerebral palsy. *Althea Med. J.* **2017**, *4*, 221–227. [CrossRef]
34. Mutlu, A.; Kara, Ö.K.; Livanelioğlu, A.; Karahan, S.; Alkan, H.; Yardımcı, B.N.; Hidecker, M.J.C. Agreement between parents and clinicians on the communication function levels and relationship of classification systems of children with cerebral palsy. *Disabil. Health J.* **2018**, *11*, 281–286. [CrossRef] [PubMed]
35. Ito, T.; Noritake, K.; Sugiura, H.; Kamiya, Y.; Tomita, H.; Ito, Y.; Sugiura, H.; Ochi, N.; Yoshihashi, Y. Association between gait deviation index and physical function in children with bilateral spastic cerebral palsy: A cross-sectional study. *J. Clin. Med.* **2020**, *9*, 28. [CrossRef] [PubMed]
36. Malt, M.A.; Aarli, Å.; Bogen, B.; Fevang, J.M. Correlation between the Gait Deviation Index and gross motor function (GMFCS level) in children with cerebral palsy. *J. Child. Orthop.* **2016**, *10*, 261–266. [CrossRef]
37. Matsunaga, N.; Ito, T.; Noritake, K.; Sugiura, H.; Kamiya, Y.; Ito, Y.; Mizusawa, J.; Sugiura, H. Correlation between the Gait Deviation Index and skeletal muscle mass in children with spastic cerebral palsy. *J. Phys. Ther. Sci.* **2018**, *30*, 1176–1179. [CrossRef]
38. Nicholson, K.; Lennon, N.; Church, C.; Miller, F. Gait analysis parameters and walking activity pre-and postoperatively in children with cerebral palsy. *Pediatr. Phys. Ther.* **2018**, *30*, 203–207. [CrossRef]
39. Goudriaan, M.; Nieuwenhuys, A.; Schless, S.H.; Goemans, N.; Molenaers, G.; Desloovere, K. A new strength assessment to evaluate the association between muscle weakness and gait pathology in children with cerebral palsy. *PLoS ONE* **2018**, *13*, e0191097. [CrossRef]
40. Guinet, A.L.; Néjib, K.; Eric, D. Clinical gait analysis and physical examination don't correlate with physical activity of children with cerebral palsy. Cross-sectional study. *Int. Biomech.* **2020**, *7*, 88–96. [CrossRef]
41. Shevell, M.I.; Dagenais, L.; Hall, N.; Consortium, R. The relationship of cerebral palsy subtype and functional motor impairment: A population-based study. *Dev. Med. Child Neurol.* **2009**, *51*, 872–877. [CrossRef]

42. Jeon, H.; Jung, J.H.; Yoon, J.A.; Choi, H. Strabismus is correlated with gross motor function in children with spastic cerebral palsy. *Curr. Eye Res.* **2019**, *44*, 1258–1263. [CrossRef]
43. Al-Nemr, A.; Abdelazeim, F. Relationship of cognitive functions and gross motor abilities in children with spastic diplegic cerebral palsy. *Appl. Neuropsychol. Child* **2018**, *7*, 268–276. [CrossRef] [PubMed]
44. Kim, H.Y.; Cha, Y.H.; Chun, Y.S.; Shin, H.S. Correlation of the torsion values measured by rotational profile, kinematics, and CT study in CP patients. *Gait Posture* **2017**, *57*, 241–245. [CrossRef] [PubMed]
45. Panibatla, S.; Kumar, V.; Narayan, A. Relationship between trunk control and balance in children with spastic cerebral palsy: A cross-sectional study. *J. Clin. Diagn. Res. JCDR* **2017**, *11*, YC05. [CrossRef] [PubMed]
46. Li, H.; Wang, X.L.; Wu, Y.Q.; Liu, X.M.; Li, A.M. Correlation of the predisposition of Chinese children to cerebral palsy with nucleotide variation in pri-miR-124 that alters the non-canonical apoptosis pathway. *Acta Pharmacol. Sin.* **2018**, *39*, 1453–1462. [CrossRef]
47. Kallem Seyyar, G.; Aras, B.; Aras, O. Trunk control and functionality in children with spastic cerebral palsy. *Dev. Neurorehabilit.* **2019**, *22*, 120–125. [CrossRef]
48. van Gorp, M.; Dallmeijer, A.J.; van Wely, L.; de Groot, V.; Terwee, C.B.; Flens, G.; Stam, H.J.; van der Slot, W.; Roebroeck, M.E.; on behalf of the PERRIN DECADE Study Group. Pain, fatigue, depressive symptoms and sleep disturbance in young adults with cerebral palsy. *Disabil. Rehabil.* **2021**, *43*, 2164–2171. [CrossRef]
49. Monica, S.; Nayak, A.; Joshua, A.M.; Mithra, P.; Amaravadi, S.K.; Misri, Z.; Unnikrishnan, B. Relationship between Trunk Position Sense and Trunk Control in Children with Spastic Cerebral Palsy: A Cross-Sectional Study. *Rehabil. Res. Pract.* **2021**, *2021*, 9758640. [CrossRef]
50. O'Sullivan, R.; French, H.P.; Van Rossom, S.; Jonkers, I.; Horgan, F. The association between gait analysis measures associated with crouch gait, functional health status and daily activity levels in cerebral palsy. *J. Pediatr. Rehabil. Med.* **2021**, *14*, 227–235. [CrossRef]
51. Ries, A.J.; Novacheck, T.F.; Schwartz, M.H. A data driven model for optimal orthosis selection in children with cerebral palsy. *Gait Posture* **2014**, *40*, 539–544. [CrossRef]
52. Galarraga, C.O.A.; Vigneron, V.; Dorizzi, B.; Khouri, N.; Desailly, E. Predicting postoperative gait in cerebral palsy. *Gait Posture* **2017**, *52*, 45–51. [CrossRef]
53. Galarraga, O.; Vigneron, V.; Khouri, N.; Dorizzi, B.; Desailly, E. Predictive simulation of surgery effect on cerebral palsy gait. *Comput. Methods Biomech. Biomed. Eng.* **2017**, *20*, S85–S86. [CrossRef] [PubMed]
54. Rosenberg, M.; Steele, K.M. Simulated impacts of ankle foot orthoses on muscle demand and recruitment in typically-developing children and children with cerebral palsy and crouch gait. *PLoS ONE* **2017**, *12*, e0180219. [CrossRef] [PubMed]
55. Rajagopal, A.; Kidziński, Ł.; McGlaughlin, A.S.; Hicks, J.L.; Delp, S.L.; Schwartz, M.H. Estimating the effect size of surgery to improve walking in children with cerebral palsy from retrospective observational clinical data. *Sci. Rep.* **2018**, *8*, 16344. [CrossRef] [PubMed]
56. Duran, I.; Stark, C.; Martakis, K.; Hamacher, S.; Semler, O.; Schoenau, E. Reference centiles for the gross motor function measure and identification of therapeutic effects in children with cerebral palsy. *J. Eval. Clin. Pract.* **2019**, *25*, 78–87. [CrossRef]
57. Pitto, L.; Kainz, H.; Falisse, A.; Wesseling, M.; Van Rossom, S.; Hoang, H.; Papageorgiou, E.; Hallemans, A.; Desloovere, K.; Molenaers, G.; et al. SimCP: A simulation platform to predict gait performance following orthopedic intervention in children with cerebral palsy. *Front. Neurorobot.* **2019**, *13*, 54. [CrossRef]
58. Kidziński, Ł.; Yang, B.; Hicks, J.L.; Rajagopal, A.; Delp, S.L.; Schwartz, M.H. Deep neural networks enable quantitative movement analysis using single-camera videos. *Nat. Commun.* **2020**, *11*, 4054. [CrossRef]
59. Jalata, I.K.; Truong, T.D.; Allen, J.L.; Seo, H.S.; Luu, K. Movement Analysis for Neurological and Musculoskeletal Disorders Using Graph Convolutional Neural Network. *Future Internet* **2021**, *13*, 194. [CrossRef]
60. Azhand, A.; Rabe, S.; Müller, S.; Sattler, I.; Heimann-Steinert, A. Algorithm based on one monocular video delivers highly valid and reliable gait parameters. *Sci. Rep.* **2021**, *11*, 14065. [CrossRef]
61. Afifi, J. Prediction of Cerebral Palsy in Very Preterm Infants. Ph.D. Thesis, Dalhousie University Halifax, Halifax, NS, Canada, 2021.
62. Russell, D.J.; Avery, L.M.; Rosenbaum, P.L.; Raina, P.S.; Walter, S.D.; Palisano, R.J. Improved scaling of the gross motor function measure for children with cerebral palsy: Evidence of reliability and validity. *Phys. Ther.* **2000**, *80*, 873–885. [CrossRef]
63. Pietrzak, S.; Jóźwiak, M. Subjective and objective scales to assess the development of children cerebral palsy. *Ortop. Traumatol. Rehabil.* **2001**, *3*, 487–489.
64. Russell, D.J.; Rosenbaum, P.L.; Cadman, D.T.; Gowland, C.; Hardy, S.; Jarvis, S. The gross motor function measure: A means to evaluate the effects of physical therapy. *Dev. Med. Child Neurol.* **1989**, *31*, 341–352. [CrossRef] [PubMed]
65. Ko, J.; Kim, M. Reliability and responsiveness of the gross motor function measure-88 in children with cerebral palsy. *Phys. Ther.* **2013**, *93*, 393–400. [CrossRef] [PubMed]
66. Alotaibi, M.; Long, T.; Kennedy, E.; Bavishi, S. The efficacy of GMFM-88 and GMFM-66 to detect changes in gross motor function in children with cerebral palsy (CP): A literature review. *Disabil. Rehabil.* **2014**, *36*, 617–627. [CrossRef] [PubMed]
67. Engelen, V.; Ketelaar, M.; Gorter, J.W. Selecting the appropriate outcome in paediatric physical therapy: How individual treatment goals for children with cerebral palsy are reflected in GMFM-88 and PEDI. *J. Rehabil. Med.* **2007**, *39*, 225–231. [CrossRef] [PubMed]

68. Zebris Medical GmbH. Zebris FDM-T System Specifications and Operating Instructions. Available online: https://www.zebris.de/fileadmin/Editoren/zebris-PDF-Manuals/Medizin/Hardware/Alte_Versionen/FDM-T_Hardware-Manual_160119_en.pdf (accessed on 19 October 2021).
69. Zebris Medical GmbH. *The Zebris FDM-T System for Stance and Gait Analysis*. Available online: https://www.zebris.de/fileadmin/Editoren/zebris-PDF/zebris-Prospekte-EN/FDM-T_Prospekt_en_120901_72dpi.pdf (accessed on 20 October 2021).
70. James, G.; Witten, D.; Hastie, T.; Tibshirani, R. *An Introduction to Statistical Learning with Applications in R*, 2nd ed.; Springer: Berlin/Heidelberg, Germany, 2021.
71. MLlib: Main Guide. Classification and Regression, Version 3.2.0. Available online: https://spark.apache.org/docs/3.2.0/ml-guide.html (accessed on 20 October 2021).
72. Barten, A.P. The coefficient of determination for regression without a constant term. In *The Practice of Econometrics: Studies on Demand, Forecasting, Money and Income*; Springer: Dordrecht, The Netherlands, 1987; pp. 181–189. [CrossRef]
73. Chicco, D.; Warrens, M.J.; Jurman, G. The coefficient of determination R-squared is more informative than SMAPE, MAE, MAPE, MSE and RMSE in regression analysis evaluation. *PeerJ Comput. Sci.* **2021**, *7*, e623. [CrossRef] [PubMed]

Article

Effectiveness of Radial Extracorporeal Shock Wave Therapy and Visual Feedback Balance Training on Lower Limb Post-Stroke Spasticity, Trunk Performance, and Balance: A Randomized Controlled Trial

Emanuela Elena Mihai [1], Ilie Valentin Mihai [2,*] and Mihai Berteanu [1,3]

1. Physical and Rehabilitation Medicine Department, Carol Davila University of Medicine and Pharmacy Bucharest, 050451 Bucharest, Romania; emanuela-elena.mihai@drd.umfcd.ro (E.E.M.); mihai.berteanu@umfcd.ro (M.B.)
2. Department of Telecommunications, University Politehnica of Bucharest, 060042 Bucharest, Romania
3. Physical and Rehabilitation Medicine Department, Elias University Emergency Hospital, 011461 Bucharest, Romania
* Correspondence: valentin.mihai.syl@gmail.com

Citation: Mihai, E.E.; Mihai, I.V.; Berteanu, M. Effectiveness of Radial Extracorporeal Shock Wave Therapy and Visual Feedback Balance Training on Lower Limb Post-Stroke Spasticity, Trunk Performance, and Balance: A Randomized Controlled Trial. *J. Clin. Med.* 2022, 11, 147. https://doi.org/10.3390/jcm11010147

Academic Editors: Akiyoshi Matsugi, Naoki Yoshida, Hideki Nakano and Yohei Okada

Received: 24 November 2021
Accepted: 24 December 2021
Published: 28 December 2021

Publisher's Note: MDPI stays neutral with regard to jurisdictional claims in published maps and institutional affiliations.

Copyright: © 2021 by the authors. Licensee MDPI, Basel, Switzerland. This article is an open access article distributed under the terms and conditions of the Creative Commons Attribution (CC BY) license (https://creativecommons.org/licenses/by/4.0/).

Abstract: Stroke remains one of the leading causes of disability in adults, and lower limb spasticity, affected stance, and balance impact everyday life and activities of such patients. Robotic therapy and assessment are becoming important tools to clinical evaluation for post-stroke rehabilitation. The aim of this study was to determine in a more objective manner the effects of visual feedback balance training through a balance trainer system and radial extracorporeal shock wave therapy (rESWT), along with conventional physiotherapy, on lower limb post-stroke spasticity, trunk control, and static and dynamic balance through clinical and stabilometric assessment. The study was designed as a randomized controlled trial. The experimental group underwent conventional physiotherapy, visual feedback balance training, and rESWT. The control group underwent conventional physiotherapy, visual feedback training and sham rESWT. The statistical analysis was performed using GraphPad Software and MATLAB. Primary clinical outcome measures were The Modified Ashworth Scale (MAS), passive range of motion (PROM), Visual Analogue Scale (VAS), and Clonus score. Secondary outcome measures were trunk performance, sensorimotor, and lower limb function. Stabilometric outcome measures were trunk control, static balance, and dynamic balance. Visual feedback training using the Prokin system and rESWT intervention, along with conventional physiotherapy, yielded statistically significant improvement both on clinical and stabilometric outcome measures, enhancing static and dynamic balance, trunk performance, sensorimotor outcome, and limb function and considerably diminishing lower limb spasticity, pain intensity, and clonus score in the experimental group.

Keywords: radial extracorporeal shock wave therapy; stroke; spasticity; balance trainer; stabilometric assessment; neurological rehabilitation

1. Introduction

Stroke remains one of the leading causes of death and disability all over the world [1–3]. Trunk control and sitting balance are commonly affected in post-stroke patients and are considered important features to predict functional outcome and hospital stay [4–9]. Moreover, balance and gait impairments are known to highly interfere within the recovery process of standing and walking ability in post-stroke patients [10–12]. Another important characteristic in many post-stroke patients is spasticity, along with muscle weakness, sensorimotor deficits, and cognitive impairments [13–15]. In addition, trunk impairment, spasticity grade, poor balance, and altered stance in post-stroke patients are increasing the risk for falls and impaired mobility [14].

Trunk deviations may also imply balance deficit, gait impairment, and diminished functional ability, but core stability exercises may also provide more efficient use of the lower limbs for static and dynamic balance, as well as for gait [7,15–18]. Given that, in the acute phase of stroke, trunk function is a major indicator for functional independence outcome, clinical assessments for trunk deviations and lower extremity tests are both used, predicting independent walking at six months [19,20]. To ensure an adapted rehabilitation program and assess the main determinant, it is important to differentiate the intrinsic trunk control deficiency from underlying lower extremity deficits. Nevertheless, to our knowledge, it has not yet been evaluated, nor determined, to what extent trunk deficits and lower limb post-stroke spasticity may correlate and impact stance and balance in post-stroke patients. Therefore, the aim of our study was to assess, in a more objective, global manner, both clinically and through stabilometric system Prokin, the relationship between stance, balance, trunk deviations, and lower limb post-stroke spasticity. Moreover, the trial aimed to determine whether conventional physical therapy in conjunction with visual feedback balance training and two radial extracorporeal shock wave therapy (rESWT) sessions might have a positive impact on stance, balance, and spasticity grade, and we assessed their relationship with trunk performance in post-stroke patients. Additional primary and secondary outcome measures were also evaluated. Core stability exercises and visual feedback training were used, with promising results [4,10,16,21,22]. The stabilometric computerized system is both an assessment tool and a training system for static, dynamic balance, and trunk. To date, it was used in various clinical trials as a training tool for promoting stance and balance improvement in several neurorehabilitation programs [10,23,24].

For spasticity management, along with physical therapy programs, anti-spastic medications or botulinum toxin type A injections, selective neurotomy, chemical neurolysis, and orthopedic surgery, techniques, such as whole body vibration, local muscle vibration, neuromuscular electrical stimulation (NMES), and therapeutic ultrasound, were also used, but there is no clear consensus yet regarding their long-term effects, number or sessions, or duration of treatment [25]. The whole body vibration seemed to reduce lower limb spasticity in cerebral palsy patients, and local muscle vibration therapy granted effectiveness in the management of chronic post-stroke patients [26,27]. In addition, NMES alone or combined with other interventions showed beneficial effects on lower limb motor function in chronic stroke patients [28]. Therapeutic ultrasound seemed to have good efficacy when also compared to extracorporeal shock wave therapy (ESWT) [29]. During the last few years, extracorporeal shock wave therapy, a novel, non-invasive intervention has become a potential therapy in the non-invasive management of post-stroke spasticity, with promising results also on the long-term [29–32]. The principle of this therapeutic intervention involves a sequence of an acoustic pulse producing high peak pressure, fast rise in pressure, and short time cycle targeting the wanted area and providing effective outcomes [29,33]. The mechanism of propagation of the shock wave refers either to radial extracorporeal shock wave therapy (rESWT) or focused extracorporeal shock wave therapy (fESWT). rESWT actions on a larger interventional area and delivers the high energy in the superficial tissue, modifying globally the mechanical properties of the muscle, in comparison to fESWT, where the shock wave action is delivered to a selected, deeper intervention area [29–31].

Considering the rESWT mechanism of action and its positive results from the literature with regard to spasticity, we aimed to assess rESWT effects in conjunction with conventional physiotherapy and balance training for post-stroke patients affected by lower limb spasticity. Therefore, we conducted a randomized controlled trial to further investigate and assess the relationship between lower limb spasticity and trunk deficits during static and dynamic balance in post-stroke patients who underwent either rESWT or sham rESWT intervention, visual feedback balance training using the Prokin system, and conventional physical therapy. The stabilometric assessment complemented the clinical evaluation and also provided an objective evaluation of combined therapeutic effect of the used therapies. Additional outcomes focused on the effectiveness of rESWT delivery on pain intensity, clonus, passive range of motion, lower limb sensorimotor function, and functionality. The adverse events were also attentively monitored during the trial.

2. Materials and Methods

2.1. Ethical Approval

The present study was conducted according to the Declaration of Helsinki, the guidelines for Consolidated Standards of Reporting Trials (CONSORT) and the CONSORT Statement [34]. The study protocol was approved by the Ethics Committee of the Elias University Emergency Hospital, Bucharest, Romania, Prot. No. 2090/C.E. Written informed consent was received from all participants taking part in the study, as well as from their relatives, when necessary.

2.2. Study Design

The study is designed as a prospective, double-blind randomized controlled trial, single-center, with an intention-to-treat analysis, and two groups with 1:1 allocation ratio. Patients were recruited between January 2021 and August 2021 during the pandemic COVID-19 period and were randomly allocated either to a control or an experimental group. The allocation method was concealed in numbered, opaque, sealed envelopes. The recruitment of patients, conventional rehabilitation program, intervention delivery, and data collection were performed at the Physical and Rehabilitation Medicine Department, Elias University Emergency Hospital, Bucharest, Romania.

2.3. Study Participants

A total of 273 patients admitted to the Physical and Rehabilitation Medicine Department, Elias University Emergency Hospital, Bucharest, Romania, between January 2021 and August 2021, were evaluated for eligibility, and 39 patients met the eligibility criteria. Seven participants declined to take part in the study ($n = 7$), and four participants were not able to initiate the rehabilitation program because of interfering acute diseases ($n = 4$), other complications ($n = 4$). One patient was not able to complete the rehabilitation program due to early discharge related to personal and family matters ($n = 1$). The final analysis and results are based on 23 patients with post-stroke lower limb spasticity who were enrolled and completed the study. No significant differences were found at the baseline comparison. Post-treatment data for the patients not completing the study were not available.

Patients with stroke were included if they stated the following inclusion criteria: (1) a hemorrhagic or ischemic stroke in acute, subacute, or chronic phase; (2) no history of previous stroke; (3) lower limb post-stroke spasticity and spasticity grade ≥ 1 on the Modified Ashworth Scale (MAS); (4) pain intensity measured on Visual Analogue Scale (VAS) ≥ 1; (5) ability to stand unassisted in upright position for 30 s; (6) no change in anti-spastic drug dose or treatment, and no changes in analgesic medication, as it could affect the results on the Modified Ashworth Scale and the Visual Analogue Scale; and (7) adult patients (>18 years old). Exclusion criteria consisted of: (1) other neurological and orthopedic disorders or lower limb deformities that could interfere with motor performance and balance; (2) myopathies; (3) severe cognitive impairment, severe aphasia or inability to understand instructions; (4) severe spasticity; (5) visual field conditions or hemineglect; (6) patients unable to undergo follow-up evaluation and excluded from the final analysis; and (7) anti-coagulant medication or any contraindication to receive rESWT, or any contraindication to physical therapy. Informed consent was obtained from all the patients prior to their participation, and the study was approved by the hospital's Ethics Committee according to the Declaration of Helsinki.

In the study and final analysis, there were enrolled 13 male patients and 10 female patients, with an average age of 68.18 ± 11.51 years old in the control group and 60.33 ± 11.5 in the experimental group. The average duration of disease was of 24.97 ± 34.17 months in the control group and 25.02 ± 39.23 in the experimental group. There were 17 cases diagnosed with ischemic stroke based on cerebral MRI or cerebral CT scan, and 6 cases diagnosed with hemorrhagic stroke.

2.4. Radial Extracorporeal Shock Wave Therapy (rESWT) Intervention

Conventional physiotherapy could be defined as the therapeutic interventions and techniques carried out in accordance to each rehabilitation department. In our study, we referred to it as a treatment involving any of the following practices and therapies for post-stroke patients (range of motion exercises, stretching, stance and balance training, core stability exercises, gait training, functional training, physical agents and other therapies, orthoses, braces, etc.). Both groups had the same conventional physical therapy program, consisting of techniques of verticalization, passive and active movements, stretching exercises, stance and balance techniques, gait training, functional training, therapeutic massage, local heat, or cryotherapy. The conventional physiotherapy program lasted 1 h/day, 5 days/week, for 2 weeks. A summary of the parameters for the control group and the experimental group is presented in Table 1.

Table 1. Therapeutic interventions and parameters for the control group and the experimental group.

	Control Group	Experimental Group
Treatment type	CP+sham rESWT+Prokin	CP+rESWT+Prokin
CP session length	1 h/day; 5 days/week; 2 weeks	1 h/day; 5 days/week; 2 weeks
rESWT session length	7 min/session; 1 session/week; 2 weeks	7 min/session; 1 session/week; 2 weeks
Visual feedback session length	20 min/day; 5 times/week; 2 weeks	20 min/day; 5 times/week; 2 weeks

Abbreviations: CP: conventional physiotherapy; rESWT: radial extracorporeal shock wave therapy; sham rESWT: sham radial extracorporeal shock wave therapy.

After performing the baseline screening and assessment, random allocation was used to generate allocation sequence and assign the patients to one of the two groups. Patients considered eligible were assigned to an experimental group (receiving conventional physiotherapy, visual feedback balance training using the Prokin and rESWT) or a control group (receiving conventional physiotherapy, visual feedback balance training using the Prokin and sham rESWT). Treatment allocation was concealed from all the participants and the outcome assessors during the trial.

After choosing the intervention site, rESWT (Endopuls 811; Enraf Nonius B.V. Vareseweg 127, 3047 AT Rotterdam MedTech, The Netherlands) was applied at the myotendinous junction of both the gastrocnemius and the soleus muscles in post-stroke spasticity patients. No ultrasonography was used to detect the intervention site. All the patients completed two rESWT sessions once a week for two weeks. Participants were comfortably placed during the rESWT intervention, and 2000 shots were applied on the gastrocnemius and soleus myotendinous junction with a frequency of 10 Hz and energy density of 60 mJ (1 bar), within tolerable pain limits. The control group received sound over the myotendinous junction of gastrocnemius and soleus with transducer-like contact. Treatment sessions lasted for approximately 7 min each, 2 sessions in total, 1 session/week, for 2 weeks, for sham rESWT and rESWT. The rESWT and sham rESWT sessions were delivered during the hospital stay, 15 min after the conventional rehabilitation program and the visual feedback balance training. Figure 1 presents the rESWT delivery.

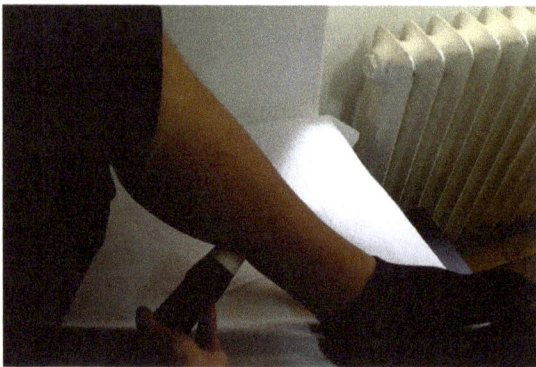

Figure 1. Radial extracorporeal shock wave therapy delivery on a patient from the clinical trial; original picture taken by the author EE Mihai in the Department of Physical and Rehabilitation Medicine, Elias University Emergency Hospital, Bucharest, using a digital camera (Nikon D3300; Nikon Corporation, Tokyo, Japan).

Clinical and stabilometric assessments were performed before the first rESWT session and the beginning of physical therapy program. The second evaluation was performed at the end of the rehabilitation program, after the last session of treatment by the same assessor, who also performed the first assessment. Adverse events were attentively monitored during the study.

2.5. Visual Feedback Balance Training Using the Prokin

All the patients in the experimental and the control group performed visual feedback balance training using Prokin, in addition to the conventional rehabilitation program, rESWT intervention, and sham rESWT, respectively. They were given precise information, and they were asked to wear normal clothing in order to create a more friendly environment during the session. Each training session lasted for 20 min/day, 5 times/week, for 2 weeks, and was delivered 15 min after the conventional physiotherapy program, as post-stroke patients are usually becoming easily fatigued. Through real-time visual feedback, patients were asked to move their Center of Pressure (CoP) in different directions, maintaining the specified area on the screen. They had to move forward, backward, sideways, and to perform a circular motion. For trunk training, they had to perform the same movements while they were seated on the specific Prokin trunk sensor. The patients were also given the possibility to play one game of their choice at the end of the training. Figure 2 shows one of the patients on the stabilometric system, Prokin balance trainer, and assessment tool.

2.6. Clinical Outcome Measures and Methods of Clinical Evaluation

The primary clinical outcome measures were spasticity grade assessed using the Modified Ashworth Scale (MAS), knee and ankle passive range of motion (PROM), pain intensity evaluated through Visual Analogue Scale (VAS), and Clonus score. For the MAS evaluation for gastrocnemius and soleus muscles, patients were laying in supine position with the knee fully extended and the joint stabilized. The MAS measures muscle resistance during passive muscle stretching. The MAS score ranges from 0 (no increase in muscle tone) to 4 (rigid) and includes a rating of 1+. For a suitable statistical analysis, a MAS grade 1+ was matched to 2 points and grade 2, 3, and 4 were matched to 3, 4, and 5 points, respectively. Knee and ankle passive mobility were assessed by PROM, using a hand-held goniometer, and summing the angles of maximum plantar flexion and dorsiflexion. Pain intensity was evaluated by the VAS using a vertical 10-cm line (starting pain-free to the worst imaginable pain). The Clonus score evaluated the beats' number up to sustained clonus.

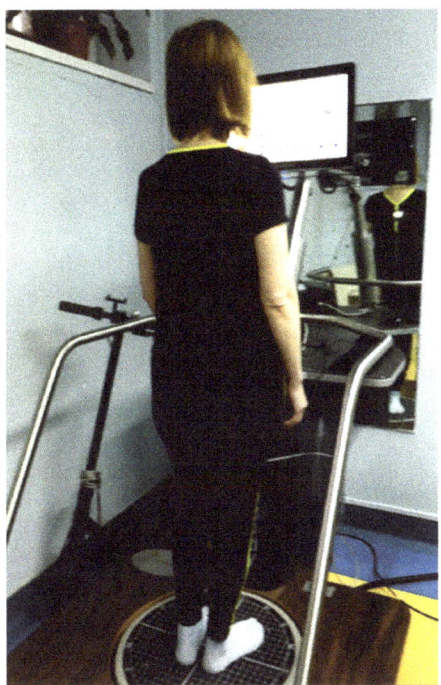

Figure 2. Patient from the clinical trial during a session of visual feedback balance training and stabilometric assessment using the Prokin system; original picture taken by the author EE Mihai in the Department of Physical and Rehabilitation Medicine, Elias University Emergency Hospital, Bucharest, using a digital camera (Nikon D3300; Nikon Corporation, Tokyo, Japan).

The secondary outcomes were gait and balance assessed by Tinetti Assessment Tool, Functional Ambulation Categories (FAC), and Fugl-Meyer Assessment for Lower Extremity (FMA-LE). FMA-LE assessed lower limb sensorimotor impairment, and Trunk Impairment Scale (TIS) evaluated static and dynamic sitting balance and trunk coordination in a sitting position. The functional impairments were assessed through Tinetti Assessment Tool and FAC. The outcomes were classified in relation to the baseline (T0) and the follow-up period after two sessions of rESWT intervention or sham rESWT intervention(T1), and between the control and the experimental group. ESWT was applied once a week for two weeks, and the assessment was performed pre-treatment and after the second session. The assessment was conducted at baseline and follow-up by the same blind assessor, who did not know which patients underwent rESWT or sham rESWT.

2.7. Stabilometric Assessment

The stabilometric assessment was performed by a blind assessor using the Prokin system (PK 252, TecnoBody, Bergamo, Italy), and the assessor did not know which patients underwent rESWT or sham rESWT. Prokin system consists of a force-sensitive stabilometric platform which assists with the assessment of trunk, stance, and static and dynamic balance. Additionally to clinical measures, we aimed to evaluate stance and balance in an objective manner, while correlating the clinical assessment with the data obtained using the Prokin system. Focusing on an objective approach and trying to recreate a daily life environment, the patients were asked to wear comfortable clothing. They were given precise instructions and were reminded of them when needed; they were positioned in a standardized way on the stabilometric platform (barefoot or wearing socks, but no footwear), and the feet position was adapted by using a Y shaped frame (called yova) with a 3-cm distance between the internal malleoli. In addition, the medial border of the feet was rotated 12 degrees in correlation with the anteroposterior axis. Patients were instructed to stand still, keep their arms by their sides, and look ahead at the screen positioned in front of them focusing on a stationary or moving target. Each participant performed various tests in standing position and also in seated position, allowing the evaluation of stance, balance, and trunk. In addition, the tests were performed either with eyes open (EO) or eyes closed (EC), and a skilled physiotherapist stood behind the patient to prevent any risk of falls. The perimeter and the ellipse area for static balance, dynamic balance, and trunk parameters were measured, and results were evaluated accordingly.

Clinical evaluation and stabilometric assessment using the Prokin system at baseline and follow-up were both performed in two sessions. Conventional rehabilitation program, visual feedback balance training using the Prokin, and rESWT or sham rESWT intervention, clinical evaluation, and instrumental assessment were performed, and patients were asked to use the same comfortable clothing, the same conditions were recreated and instructions were once again given to all the participants. For both the control group and experimental group, none of the patients experienced loss of balance during stabilometric assessment in any of the sensory conditions. None of the patients suffered any accident or fall during the assessments and study duration, physiotherapy program, nor during hospitalization. In addition, no adverse events related to rESWT intervention were reported during or after sessions. The stabilometric assessment using the Prokin platform was carried out by the same experienced physiotherapist, who was not involved in the screening, randomization sequence, baseline evaluation, and follow-up.

2.8. Statistical Analysis

The assessment of all the patients was conducted before and after the intervention. Patient characteristics were described as the mean and standard deviation for the control and the experimental group for the continuous data. The Pearson's Chi-square test was used when analyzing differences in categorical variables, and the Mann–Whitney U test and Independent t-test were used for continuous variables. The change score was also used to show the difference between the pre- and post-treatment, both for clinical outcome measures and stabilometric outcome measures. The change in outcome measures was compared between the control and the experimental group by means of the Mann–Whitney U test and Independent t-test.

All the statistical analyses were performed using GraphPad Software (San Diego, CA, USA) and MATLAB (R2016a, The MathWorks, Inc., Natick, MA, USA) to determine the variables of interest. The null hypothesis was rejected when the critical test statistical value α was exceeded by the F value/t value. A p-value < 0.05 was considered to be statistically significant.

3. Results

Figure 3 shows the study flow diagram and patient allocation. Out of the 273 participants screened, 24 patients were randomly assigned, with 12 patients either in the control group or the experimental group. One patient in the control group was discharged earlier due to personal matters and was excluded from the analysis. Therefore, the patients were randomized into two groups: a control group ($n = 11$) and an experimental group ($n = 12$).

Table 2 presents the characteristics of control and experimental group at baseline. No differences were identified among the groups related to the demographic variables, stroke type, affected side of the body, time since stroke onset, nor clinical and stabilometric outcomes. Comparisons between the groups showed homogeneity at baseline for all the parameters.

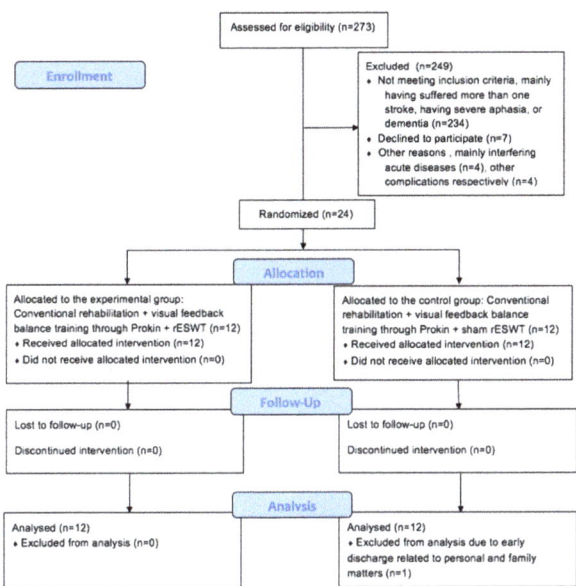

Figure 3. CONSORT 2010 Flow Diagram and patient allocation. Abbreviation: rESWT: radial extracorporeal shock wave therapy.

Table 2. Characteristics of participants at baseline, clinical, and stabilometric outcome measures.

	CG (Mean, SD)	EG (Mean, SD)	p-Value
Variables	n, 11	n, 12	
Age (years)	68.18 (11.51)	60.33 (11.5)	0.11 [a]
Weight (kg)	77.50 (11.53)	75.32 (17.88)	0.72 [a]
Height (cm)	174.09 (8.08)	171.16 (10.77)	0.46 [a]
Time since stroke onset (months)	24.97 (34.17)	25.02 (39.23)	0.99 [a]
Gender (M/F)	7/4	6/6	
Stroke type (Ischemic/Hemorrhagic)	8/3	9/3	0.5 [c]
Affected side of the body (Right/Left)	6/5	4/8	0.87 [c]
Clinical outcome measures			
MAS	2.54 (0.52)	2.58 (0.51)	0.86 [a]
Knee PROM (degrees)	116.90 (5.16)	116 (4.78)	0.66 [a]
Ankle PROM (degrees)	39.27 (3.16)	39.91 (4.1)	0.65 [a]
VAS	3.09 (1.13)	3 (1.12)	0.84 [a]
Clonus Score	2.36 (1.28)	2.25 (1.23)	0.82 [a]
TIS	14.63 (2.33)	14.58 (2.71)	0.85 [b]
Tinetti Assessment Tool	15.81 (4.33)	14.83 (5.62)	0.53 [b]
FAC	4.72 (0.9)	4.58 (1.37)	1.00 [b]
FMA-LE	19.27 (1.95)	19.66 (2.1)	0.60 [b]
Stabilometric outcome measures			
Dynamic	4.74 (1.04)	5.27 (3.01)	0.57 [a]
Trunk	202.54 (112.36)	193.21 (114.75)	0.84 [a]
Limits of stability	46.82 (9.17)	52.23 (20.44)	0.41 [a]
Static perimeter, mm (EO)	660.09 (289.16)	626.52 (244.94)	0.76 [a]
Static ellipse area, mm^2 (EO)	537.60 (95.62)	539.98 (276.06)	0.98 [a]
Static perimeter, mm (EC)	1079.28 (558.89)	1147.16 (492.65)	0.76 [a]
Static ellipse area, mm^2 (EC)	1092.48 (661.60)	1111.07 (467.81)	0.93 [a]

Abbreviations: CG: control group; EC: eyes closed; EG: experimental group; EO: eyes open; FAC: Functional Ambulation Categories; FMA-LE: Fugl-Meyer Assessment for Lower Extremity; MAS: Modified Ashworth Scale; M/F: Male/Female ratio; PROM: passive range of motion; SD: standard deviation; TIS: Trunk Impairment Scale; VAS: Visual Analogue Scale. Differences between groups were calculated by Independent t-test [a], Mann–Whitney U test [b] or Pearson's Chi-square test [c] depending on the data. p-value < 0.05.

3.1. Clinical Outcome Measures

Table 3 presents the comparison of the intervention effect among control and experimental group for primary and secondary clinical outcome measures. *p*-value shows the inter-group differences of the change score. For the primary and secondary clinical outcome measures, patients from the experimental group showed significant improvement compared to the control group in all the outcome measures except for knee PROM, TIS, and FAC.

Table 3. Comparison of change score of clinical outcome measures between CG and EG post-treatment.

Clinical Outcome Measures	CG (Mean, SD) n = 11 Post-Treatment	Change Score	EG (Mean, SD) n = 12 Post-Treatment	Change Score	Diff.	*p*-Value
MAS	2.18 (0.75)	0.36	1.50 (0.52)	1.08	0.72	0.02 [a]
Knee PROM (degrees)	122.63 (5.4)	5.73	126.33 (3.96)	10.33	4.6	0.07 [a]
Ankle PROM (degrees)	44.09 (3.47)	4.82	48.33 (2.26)	8.17	3.35	0.03 [a]
VAS	2.09 (1.22)	1	1 (0.85)	2	1	0.02 [a]
Clonus score	1.90 (1.13)	0.46	0.83 (0.83)	1.42	0.96	0.01 [a]
TIS	17.54 (2.06)	2.91	18.66 (2.38)	4.08	1.17	0.2 [a]
Tinetti Assessment Tool	21.09 (3.50)	5.28	24.66 (2.83)	9.83	4.55	0.02 [b]
FAC	5.45 (0.82)	0.73	5.5 (0.79)	0.92	0.19	0.92 [b]
FMA-LE	22.36 (2.06)	3.09	24.75 (2.01)	5.09	2	0.01 [b]

Abbreviations: CG: control group; Diff: Difference of the change score; EG: experimental group; FAC: Functional Ambulation Categories; FMA-LE: Fugl-Meyer Assessment for Lower Extremity; MAS: Modified Ashworth Scale; PROM: passive range of motion; SD: standard deviation; TIS: Trunk Impairment Scale; VAS: Visual Analogue Scale. Differences between groups were calculated by Independent *t*-test [a] and Mann–Whitney U test [b] depending on the data. *p*-value < 0.05.

The change score for the MAS was 1.08 in the experimental group, while, in the control group, it was 0.36, (*p*-value < 0.02). For ankle PROM, a statistically significant improvement was also stated, with a change score of 8.17 in the experimental group and 4.82 in the control group, (*p*-value < 0.03).

For the pain intensity assessment through VAS, the change score was 2 points in the experimental group, while the change score in the control group was 1 point, showing a statistically significant difference between the two groups after the intervention, (*p*-value of 0.02). Regarding the Clonus score, the score in the control group was 0.46 points, while, in the experimental group, it was 1.42 points (*p*-value < 0.01).

As for the other parameters, such as Tinetti Assessment Tool, the experimental group showed a change score of 9.83 points compared to the control group, which showed a change of 5.28 points (*p*-value < 0.02). With regard to the FMA-LE, the experimental group scored 5.09 points in the change score, and the control group registered 3.09 points (*p*-value < 0.01).

3.2. Stabilometric Outcome Measures

The stabilometric outcome measures evaluated using the Prokin system after the intervention are presented in Table 4. All the parameters showed statistically significant improvement, except for perimeter with eyes closed (EC). However, before the intervention, there were no differences between the control and the experimental group. Regarding the dynamic balance, the experimental group showed a change score of 2.17 compared to the control group, which registered a change score of 0.35 (*p*-value < 0.03). As for limits of stability testing, there was a score change of 265.64 points in the experimental group compared to the control group, where the change score was 109.04 points (*p*-value < 0.02).

Table 4. Comparison of change score of stabilometric outcome measures between CG and EG post-treatment.

Stabilometric Outcome Measures	CG (Mean, SD) n = 11 Post-Treatment	Change Score	EG (Mean, SD) n = 12 Post-Treatment	Change Score	Diff.	p-Value
Dynamic	4.39 (0.86)	0.35	3.10 (1.66)	2.17	1.82	0.03
Trunk	311.58 (128.28)	109.04	458.85 (166.33)	265.64	156.6	0.02
Limits of stability	51.92 (7.76)	5.1	68.37 (19.12)	16.14	11.04	0.01
Static-perimeter, mm (EO)	624.52 (201.91)	35.57	424.48 (108.40)	202.04	166.47	0.01
Static-ellipse area, mm^2 (EO)	482.81 (147.31)	54.79	328.59 (182.17)	211.39	156.60	0.03
Static-perimeter, mm (EC)	943.53 (412.42)	135.75	734.02 (332.75)	413.14	277.39	0.1
Static-ellipse area, mm^2 (EC)	1021.83 (583.39)	70.65	609.77 (128.26)	501.30	430.65	0.04

Abbreviations: CG: control group; Diff: Difference of the change score; EC: eyes closed; EG: experimental group; EO: eyes open; SD: standard deviation. Differences between groups were calculated by means of the Independent t-test. p-value < 0.05.

Concerning the trunk analysis, a statistically significant improvement was found (p-value < 0.02) in the experimental group, with a change score of 156.6. Regarding the static balance, the assessment of perimeter with eyes open (EO), ellipse area with EO, and ellipse area with EC showed that scores were significantly decreased after conventional physical therapy, Prokin visual feedback balance training, and rESWT intervention (p-value < 0.05) in the experimental group, compared to the control group.

Figures 4–6 present the data processed through MATLAB for one representative patient from the control and the experimental group pre- and post-treatment. Figure 4 showed that the experimental group gained a more pronounced improvement regarding the path recorded by the CoP for 30 s, which became more stable after the application of rESWT, visual feedback balance training, and conventional physiotherapy for the static stabilometric assessment. Regarding the dynamic stabilometric assessment, Figure 5 showed a smoother CoP path and a reduction of CoP path length for the experimental group after the intervention and, therefore, improvements for stance and dynamic balance. Figure 6 showed the processed data from trunk stabilometric assessment for trunk stability in the experimental group compared to the control group.

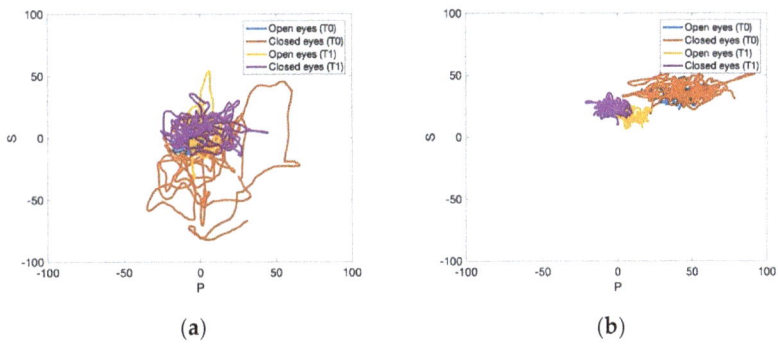

Figure 4. Static stabilometric assessment with eyes open and eyes closed for one representative patient in the control group (a) and experimental group (b) pre- and post-treatment. Abbreviations: T0: pre-treatment; T1: post-treatment.

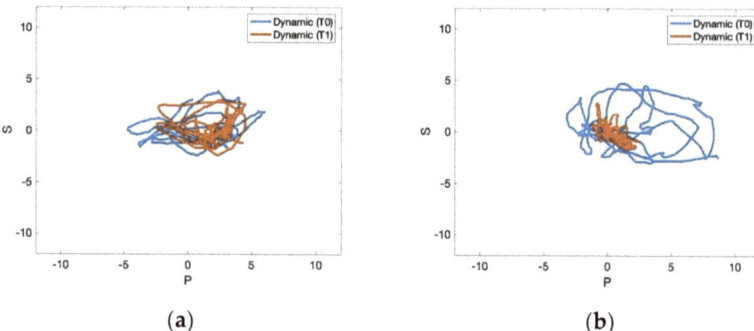

Figure 5. Dynamic stabilometric assessment for one representative patient in the control group (**a**) and experimental group (**b**) pre- and post-treatment. Abbreviations: T0: pre-treatment; T1: post-treatment.

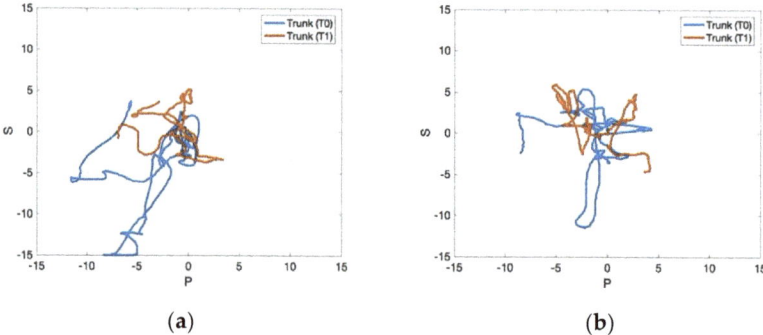

Figure 6. Trunk stabilometric assessment for one representative patient in the control group (**a**) and experimental group (**b**) pre- and post-treatment. Abbreviations: T0: pre-treatment; T1: post-treatment.

No adverse events, such as muscle hematoma, focal edema, pain, or skin petechiae, were reported during the study. No falls were registered, either, and all patients were assessed according to the study protocol.

4. Discussion

Post-stroke patients are often affected by limb spasticity, strength deficits, loss of function, loss of balance, and trunk deficits. Accordingly, novel interventions could complement conventional rehabilitation and common medications used in neurorehabilitation with satisfying results. This study's results showed that additional visual feedback training using the Prokin and rESWT intervention improved not only clinical parameters, but also stabilometric parameters in the experimental group. Since the control group received sham rESWT, and the results were less significant than in the experimental group, rESWT was considered the main determinant, especially for the clinical parameters. An important feature of the study is the objective, global assessment of post-stroke patients through clinical and stabilometric parameters. In our trial, Prokin was used as a training tool, as well as an assessment instrument.

To our knowledge, this is the first trial to assess, clinically and through stabilometric parameters, the effects of both visual feedback training using the Prokin system and rESWT intervention added to conventional physiotherapy for post-stroke survivors. In addition, we expanded the trial on correlating trunk deficits with lower limb spasticity and the cumulative effects of combined therapies on clinical and stabilometric outcome measures.

The visual feedback balance training and rESWT intervention added to conventional physiotherapy were implemented aiming to improve stance, balance, trunk deficits, and to decrease lower limb spasticity grade. The results are consistent with previous studies in which the main focus was either on core stability exercises, trunk training, or visual feedback training [4,10,14]. Virtual reality added to conventional rehabilitation also showed efficacy on improving balance and gait in neurologic patients [35,36]. As an additional treatment technique to the conventional physiotherapy, visual feedback balance training using the Prokin system has gained more interest since it enables patients to adjust their stance, balance, and overall performance in real-time through visual dynamic feedback. Therefore, patients were able to adapt the movement of the CoP and redress an abnormal stance, consequently improving balance function. This training system offers a novel, interactive tool as an alternative to sole conventional therapy. The training using the Prokin system ensures the projection of a more accurate proprioceptive sensing map, which helps the patient focus on regaining proprioceptive function, as well as to adjust more easily to sensorimotor perturbations, and this could also explain the beneficial effects on static and dynamic balance that we obtained in our study.

In our study, the experimental group showed a statistically significant change of the stabilometric outcome measures compared to the control group. Both static and dynamic balance were improved, which could also be correlated to the Tinetti Assessment Tool score through Pearson correlation analysis, obtaining clinical and stabilometric enhancement (p-value < 0.02). The dynamic module allowed the assessment and management of instability by the patient, offering real-time insights into adjusting mechanisms, thus allowing the patient to redress the stance, and, consequently, the balance, as well. The static module assessed the patients through the oscillation of the CoP, area, and the parameter of the CoP. For the experimental group, in the EO situation, area, as well as perimeter, decreased dramatically. A possible explanation could be that, after rESWT intervention the spasticity grade affecting the lower limb decreased, and the proprioceptive training was also performed more easily, leading to the smoothness of oscillation and a more stable CoP path. Moreover, these improvements may offer more information regarding the relationship between lower limb spasticity, trunk deficits, and balance. Another possible explanation could be related to the visual compensation, which can overcome the shortcomings of proprioceptive and vestibular function deficiency, enhancing neuroplasticity and, therefore, treatment efficacy. The only stabilometric parameter which showed no statistically significant change was perimeter in the EC situation.

The limits of stability assessed the participants' ability to voluntarily sway to various locations in space, as shown on the screen while tested. The measured parameters were maximum CoP excursion, endpoint CoP excursion, and directional control. After the intervention, both groups showed enhanced results, but the experimental group showed three times better results compared to the control group, showing that the rESWT component determined the more enhanced effect. The trunk module allowed the assessment of the pelvic area in the sitting position, and the trunk sensor detected oscillations of the torso in every direction. It offered information on peripheral control of the patient and possible compensation for poor stance. Compensation strategies are factors which are usually seen in post-stroke patients and sometimes interfere within the rehabilitation programs. Balance control is a key feature associated with gait recovery and the probability of suffering a fall in stroke patients, but adapted strategies and individualized rehabilitation programs augment therapeutic efficacy in the long-term [10,37–39]. Regarding trunk control, the stabilometric assessment showed a more pronounced effectiveness on this parameter in the experimental group compared to the control group. The clinical parameters, such as spasticity grade, clonus score, and passive range of motion, were also significantly enhanced for the group receiving rESWT, compared to the group receiving sham rESWT. These results may explain how adequate trunk control could lead to a smoother, more stable center of pressure path and, therefore, better static and dynamic balance. In addition, improved lower limb function could also enhance a more correct stance and balance.

Concerning spasticity grade assessed by the MAS, in one study, significant differences were found between the control and the experimental group, but a change score of one point was required for considering a detectable clinical change in stroke participants [15]. However, it was also observed that there was a pronounced tendency for the patients experiencing a more severe lower limb impairment to have more important trunk movement deviations, which could be related to the stability ensured by lower extremity [15]. Although, in our study, we found a change score of 0.68 points between the control and the experimental group, the change score in the experimental group post-treatment was 1.08 points and 0.36 points, respectively, in the control group. In our trial, patients with a higher spasticity grade also experienced more trunk deficits, and the intervention effect showed significant improvement of these parameters, both on clinical and stabilometric evaluations. In contrast to what was observed in another study, the lower limb spasticity grade improvements could not only be associated with transitory factors, since improvement in lower limbs spasticity had a significantly positive impact on stance and balance at the clinical and stabilometric evaluations and performance [4]. Accordingly, the relationship between lower limb spasticity grade and trunk deficits cannot be excluded and should be further analyzed.

The clinical improvement of MAS grade was three times greater in the experimental group compared to the control group showing the effectiveness of the rESWT component on spasticity management and also the dynamic real-time feedback through balance training. These results are consist with those from other clinical trials [10,29,40]. Although knee PROM showed no statistically significant improvement after the interventions, ankle PROM showed statistically significant improvement, which could be explained by the site of rESWT application and its effects on plantar flexor muscles and thus, on augmented ankle PROM. Another explanation for more significant improvement of ankle PROM may be related to the effects of rESWT on the entire muscle and the superficial tissue area. These results are in accordance with other studies [30,40]. In a previous study, rESWT seemed to provide greater improvement in ankle PROM than fESWT [29]. The difference between rESWT and fESWT lies in the penetration depth and physical properties, but the clinical difference is not yet determined [29]. However, to assess the effect on the muscle, reliable measurements of muscle thickness on ultrasonography are correlated with the time frame, as well as the side of the body [41]. Several studies have already showed that both rESWT and fESWT were effective as novel, non-invasive therapies for spasticity management in post-stroke patients [29,31,40]. In terms of lower limb pain intensity, the VAS showed better scores in the experimental group, twice as ameliorated than in the control group which received sham rESWT and Prokin visual feedback training, the results being consistent with another trial which also showed the beneficial effects of rESWT on this endpoint [42]. The effects on pain intensity could be explained through the properties of extracorporeal shock waves on the muscles and tendons, which was found to produce a long-term tissue regeneration effect, as well as a prompt antalgic and anti-inflammatory result [31,43,44]. No improvement was found for the TIS and FAC, although TIS was significantly improved in the experimental group. An explanation could be that many patients were already in the chronic phase of stroke, and, although the clinical improvement was registered, it was not found as statistically significant. Both Tinetti Assessment Tool and FMA-LE showed amelioration, demonstrating statistically and clinically significant sensorimotor and functional improvement. These parameters were also correlated with the stabilometric outcome measures.

The present study also has some limitations. Firstly, the small sample size could augment the overall effect of the intervention. However, correlations were performed, and all the clinical and stabilometric parameters were cautiously evaluated and measured. Secondly, study data might be limited since this is a single center trial. Nonetheless, this could provide more accurate data from groups assessed by the same team in the same medical unit and under the same circumstances. Thirdly, patients who could not tolerate the upright position for at least 30 s could not be eligible to take part in our trial, which limited the number of participants. Therefore, future research and larger samples of participants are highly needed to assess the efficacy of visual feedback balance training using the Prokin system combined with rESWT and conventional physiotherapy program in treating post-stroke patients, lower limb spasticity, and its relationship with trunk deficits and static and dynamic balance.

Despite these limitations, the present study has proved that combined rESWT intervention and visual feedback training, along with conventional physiotherapy, yielded statistically significant improvement, both on clinical and stabilometric outcome measures, enhancing static and dynamic balance, trunk performance, sensorimotor outcome, and limb function and considerably diminishing lower limb spasticity, pain intensity, and clonus score in the experimental group. Our results could also explain the relationship between spasticity, trunk deficits, and poor balance, as well as the way they influence each other.

5. Conclusions

In conclusion, rESWT intervention and visual feedback balance training using the Prokin system, along with conventional physiotherapy, improved trunk control and lower limb spasticity, and static and dynamic balance, decreased pain intensity and clonus score, and ameliorated the sensorimotor outcome and functionality in post-stroke patients. These results need to be further confirmed by larger clinical trials, and future research should further assess the effects of additional therapies as a complement to the conventional physiotherapy, to establish protocols and guidelines and to provide the best insight into the neurorehabilitation programs. Due to the COVID-19 pandemic, the hospitalization rate was reduced, as well as the rehabilitation program and hospital stay. For future research, we aim to recreate the study with a larger sample size, and a longer rehabilitation program during hospital stay, perhaps in correlation with a tele-rehabilitation strategy after discharge, as well. This would allow us track the progress and ensure continuity of the rehabilitation program for post-stroke patients with benefits in both the short and the long-term.

Author Contributions: Conceptualization, E.E.M., I.V.M. and M.B.; methodology, E.E.M. and M.B.; software, E.E.M. and I.V.M.; project administration, E.E.M.; validation, E.E.M., I.V.M. and M.B.; data curation, E.E.M. and I.V.M.; writing–original draft preparation, E.E.M.; writing–review and editing, E.E.M. and I.V.M.; visualization, E.E.M., I.V.M. and M.B.; supervision, E.E.M., I.V.M. and M.B. All authors have read and agreed to the published version of the manuscript.

Funding: This research received no external funding.

Institutional Review Board Statement: The study was conducted in accordance with the Declaration of Helsinki, and approved by the Ethics Committee of the Elias University Emergency Hospital, Bucharest, Romania, Prot. No. 2090/C.E.

Informed Consent Statement: Informed consent was obtained from all subjects involved in the study.

Data Availability Statement: Datasets used and analyzed during the clinical trial are available from the corresponding author on reasonable request.

Acknowledgments: Special thanks to Luca Gheorghe, Luminita Dumitru, Ruxandra Badea, Simona Savulescu, Horatiu Dinu, Marius Popescu, and Matei Teodorescu.

Conflicts of Interest: The authors declare no conflict of interest.

References

1. Guzik, A.; Bushnell, C. Stroke Epidemiology and Risk Factor Management. *Contin. Lifelong Learn. Neurol.* **2017**, *23*, 15–39. [CrossRef]
2. Donkor, E.S. Stroke in the 21st Century: A Snapshot of the Burden, Epidemiology, and Quality of Life. *Stroke Res. Treat.* **2018**, *2018*, 3238165. [PubMed]
3. Johnson, W.; Onuma, O.; Owolabi, M.; Sachdev, S. Stroke: A global response is needed. *Bull. World Health Organ.* **2016**, *94*, 634. [CrossRef]
4. Van Criekinge, T.; Hallemans, A.; Herssens, N.; Lafosse, C.; Claes, D.; De Hertogh, W.; Truijen, S.; Saeys, W. SWEAT2 Study: Effectiveness of Trunk Training on Gait and Trunk Kinematics After Stroke: A Randomized Controlled Trial. *Phys. Ther.* **2020**, *100*, 1568–1581. [CrossRef]

5. Van Criekinge, T.; Saeys, W.; Hallemans, A. Trunk biomechanics during hemiplegic gait after stroke: A systematic review. *Gait Posture* **2017**, *54*, 133–143. [CrossRef] [PubMed]
6. Verheyden, G.; Nieuwboer, A.; De Wit, L. Trunk performance after stroke: An eye catching predictor of functional outcome. *J. Neurol. Neurosurg. Psychiatry* **2007**, *78*, 694–698. [CrossRef] [PubMed]
7. Verheyden, G.; Vereeck, L.; Truijen, S.; Troch, M.; Herregodts, I.; Lafosse, C.; Nieuwboer, A.; De Weerdt, W. Trunk performance after stroke and the relationship with balance, gait and functional ability. *Clin. Rehabil.* **2006**, *20*, 451–458. [CrossRef] [PubMed]
8. Di Monaco, M.; Trucco, M.; Di Monaco, R.; Tappero, R.; Cavanna, A. The relationship between initial trunk control or postural balance and inpatient rehabilitation outcome after stroke: A prospective comparative study. *Clin. Rehabil.* **2010**, *24*, 543–554. [CrossRef]
9. Nitz, J.; Gage, A. Post stroke recovery of balanced sitting and ambulation ability. *Aust. J. Physiother.* **1995**, *41*, 263–267. [CrossRef]
10. Zhang, M.; You, H.; Zhang, H.; Zhao, W.; Han, T.; Liu, J.; Jiang, S.; Feng, X. Effects of visual feedback balance training with the Pro-kin system on walking and self-care abilities in stroke patients. *Medicine* **2020**, *99*, e22425. [CrossRef] [PubMed]
11. Lamb, S.E.; Ferrucci, L.; Volapto, S. Risk factors for falling in home- dwelling older women with stroke: The Women's Health and Aging Study. *Stroke* **2003**, *34*, 494–501. [CrossRef]
12. Lofgren, B.; Osterlind, O.; Gustafson, Y. In-patient rehabilitation after stroke: Outcome and factors associated with improvement. *Disabil. Rehabil.* **1998**, *20*, 55–61. [CrossRef]
13. Saleh, M.A.; Gaverth, J.; Yeung, E.; Marilyn, M.L. Assessment of spasticity after stroke using clinical measures: A systematic review. *Disabil. Rehabil.* **2015**, *37*, 2313–2323. [CrossRef]
14. Cabanas-Valdés, R.; Cuchi, G.U.; Bagur-Calafat, C. Trunk training exercises approaches for improving trunk performance and functional sitting balance in patients with stroke: A systematic review. *NeuroRehabilitation* **2013**, *33*, 575–592. [CrossRef] [PubMed]
15. Tamaya, V.C.; Wim, S.; Herssens, N.; Van de Walle, P.; Willem, H.; Steven, T.; Ann, H. Trunk biomechanics during walking after sub-acute stroke and its relation to lower limb impairments. *Clin. Biomech.* **2020**, *75*, 105013. [CrossRef] [PubMed]
16. Cabanas-Valdés, R.; Bagur-Calafat, C.; Girabent-Farrés, M.; Caballero-Gómez, F.M.; Hernández-Valiño, M.; Urrútia, C.G. The effect of additional core stability exercises on improving dynamic sitting balance and trunk control for subacute stroke patients: A randomized controlled trial. *Clin. Rehabil.* **2016**, *30*, 1024–1033. [CrossRef]
17. Willson, J.D.; Dougherty, C.P.; Ireland, M.L.; Davis, I.M.C. Core stability and its relationship to lower extremity function and injury. *J. Am. Acad. Orthop. Surg.* **2005**, *13*, 316–325. [CrossRef]
18. Fujita, T.; Sato, A.; Togashi, Y.; Kasahara, R.; Ohashi, T.; Tsuchiya, K.; Yamamoto, Y.; Otsuki, K. Identification of the affected lower limb and unaffected side motor functions as determinants of activities of daily living performance in stroke patients using partial correlation analysis. *J. Phys. Ther. Sci.* **2015**, *27*, 2217–2220. [CrossRef]
19. Veerbeek, J.M.; Van Wegen, E.E.; Harmeling-Van der Wel, B.C.; Kwakkel, G. EPOS, Investigators. Is accurate prediction of gait in nonambulatory stroke patients possible within 72 hours poststroke? The EPOS study. *Neurorehabil. Neural Repair* **2011**, *25*, 268–274. [CrossRef]
20. Smith, M.C.; Barber, P.A.; Stinear, C.M. The TWIST Algorithm Predicts Time to Walking Independently after Stroke. *Neurorehabilit. Neural Repair* **2017**, *3*, 955–964. [CrossRef]
21. Chung, E.; Lee, B.H.; Hwang, S. Core stabilization exercise with real-time feedback for chronic hemiparetic stroke: A pilot randomized controlled trials. *Restor. Neurol. Neurosci.* **2014**, *32*, 313–321. [CrossRef] [PubMed]
22. Yavuzer, G.; Eser, F.; Karakus, D. The effects of balance training on gait late after stroke: A randomized controlled trial. *Clin. Rehabil.* **2006**, *20*, 960–969. [CrossRef] [PubMed]
23. You, H.; Zhang, H.; Liu, J. Effect of balance training with Pro-kin System on balance in patients with white matter lesions. *Medicine* **2017**, *96*, e9057. [CrossRef] [PubMed]
24. Zhao, W.; You, H.; Jiang, S.; Zhang, H.; Yang, Y.; Zhang, M. Effect of Pro-kin visual feedback balance training system on gait stability in patients with cerebral small vessel disease. *Medicine* **2019**, *98*, e14503. [CrossRef] [PubMed]
25. Khan, F.; Amatya, B.; Bensmail, D.; Yelnik, A. Non-pharmacological interventions for spasticity in adults: An overview of systematic reviews. *Ann. Phys. Rehabil. Med.* **2019**, *62*, 265–273. [CrossRef] [PubMed]
26. Costantino, C.; Galuppo, L.; Romiti, D. Short-term effect of local muscle vibration treatment versus sham therapy on upper limb in chronic post-stroke patients: A randomized controlled trial. *Eur. J. Phys. Rehabil. Med.* **2017**, *53*, 32–40. [CrossRef] [PubMed]
27. Huang, M.; Liao, L.R.; Pang, M.Y. Effects of whole body vibration on muscle spasticity for people with central nervous system disorders: A systematic review. *Clin. Rehabil.* **2017**, *31*, 23–33. [CrossRef]
28. Hong, Z.; Sui, M.; Zhuang, Z.; Liu, H.; Zheng, X.; Cai, C.; Jin, D. Effectiveness of Neuromuscular Electrical Stimulation on Lower Limbs of Patients With Hemiplegia After Chronic Stroke: A Systematic Review. *Arch. Phys. Med. Rehabil.* **2018**, *99*, 1011–1022.e1. [CrossRef]
29. Radinmehr, H.; Ansari, N.N.; Naghdi, S.; Tabatabaei, A.; Moghimi, E. Comparison of Therapeutic Ultrasound and Radial Shock Wave Therapy in the Treatment of Plantar Flexor Spasticity After Stroke: A Prospective, Single-blind, Randomized Clinical Trial. *J. Stroke Cerebrovasc. Dis.* **2019**, *28*, 1546–1554. [CrossRef]
30. Wu, Y.T.; Chang, C.N.; Chen, Y.M.; Hu, G.C. Comparison of the effect of focused and radial extracorporeal shock waves on spastic equinus in patients with stroke: A randomized controlled trial. *Eur. J. Phys. Rehabil. Med.* **2018**, *54*, 518–525. [CrossRef]

31. Mihai, E.E.; Dumitru, L.; Mihai, I.V.; Berteanu, M. Long-Term Efficacy of Extracorporeal Shock Wave Therapy on Lower Limb Post-Stroke Spasticity: A Systematic Review and Meta-Analysis of Randomized Controlled Trials. *J. Clin. Med.* **2020**, *10*, 86. [CrossRef]
32. Martínez, I.M.; Sempere-Rubio, N.; Navarro, O.; Faubel, R. Effectiveness of Shock Wave Therapy as a Treatment for Spasticity: A Systematic Review. *Brain Sci.* **2020**, *11*, 15. [CrossRef]
33. Ogden, J.A.; Toth-Kischkat, A.; Schultheiss, R. Principles of shock wave therapy. *Clin. Orthop. Relat. Res.* **2001**, *387*, 8–17. [CrossRef]
34. Rennie, D. CONSORT revised—improving the reporting of randomized trials. *JAMA* **2001**, *285*, 2006–2007. [CrossRef] [PubMed]
35. Cano Porras, D.; Siemonsma, P.; Inzelberg, R.; Zeilig, G.; Plotnik, M. Advantages of virtual reality in the rehabilitation of balance and gait: Systematic review. *Neurology* **2018**, *90*, 1017–1025. [CrossRef] [PubMed]
36. Cano Porras, D.; Sharon, H.; Inzelberg, R.; Ziv-Ner, Y.; Zeilig, G.; Plotnik, M. Advanced virtual reality-based rehabilitation of balance and gait in clinical practice. *Ther. Adv. Chronic Dis.* **2019**, *10*, 2040622319868379. [CrossRef]
37. Mackintosh, S.F.; Hill, K.D.; Dodd, K.J. Balance score and a history of falls in hospital predict recurrent falls in the 6 months following stroke rehabilitation. *Arch. Phys. Med. Rehabil.* **2006**, *87*, 1583–1589. [CrossRef]
38. Pollock, A.; Baer, G.; Pomeroy, V. Physiotherapy treatment approaches for the recovery of postural control and lower limb function following stroke. *Cochrane Database Syst. Rev.* **2003**, *2*, CD001920.
39. Stucki, G.; Bickenbach, J.; Gutenbrunner, C.; Melvin, J. Rehabilitation: The health strategy of the 21st century. *J. Rehabil. Med.* **2018**, *50*, 309–316. [CrossRef]
40. Mihai, E.E.; Popescu, M.N.; Beiu, C.; Gheorghe, L.; Berteanu, M. Tele-Rehabilitation Strategies for a Patient With Post-stroke Spasticity: A Powerful Tool Amid the COVID-19 Pandemic. *Cureus* **2021**, *13*, e19201. [CrossRef]
41. Barotsis, N.; Tsiganos, P.; Kokkalis, Z.; Panayiotakis, G.; Panagiotopoulos, E. Reliability of muscle thickness measurements in ultrasonography. *Int. J. Rehabil. Res.* **2020**, *43*, 123–128. [CrossRef] [PubMed]
42. Ilieva, E.M. Radial shock wave therapy for plantar fasciitis: A one year follow-up study. *Folia Med.* **2013**, *55*, 42–48. [CrossRef] [PubMed]
43. Moon, S.W.; Kim, J.H.; Jung, M.J.; Son, S.; Lee, J.H.; Shin, H. The effect of extracorporeal shock wave therapy on lower limb spasticity in subacute stroke patients. *Ann. Rehabil. Med.* **2013**, *37*, 461–470. [CrossRef] [PubMed]
44. Mariotto, S.; Prati, A.C.; Cavalieri, E.; Amelio, E.; Marlinghaus, E.; Suzuki, H. Extracorporeal shock wave therapy in inflammatory diseases: Molecular mechanism that triggers anti-inflammatory action. *Curr. Med. Chem.* **2009**, *16*, 2366–2372. [CrossRef]

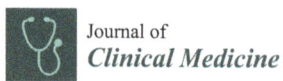

Article

Effectiveness of a New 3D-Printed Dynamic Hand–Wrist Splint on Hand Motor Function and Spasticity in Chronic Stroke Patients

Yu-Sheng Yang [1], Chi-Hsiang Tseng [2], Wei-Chien Fang [3], Ia-Wen Han [4] and Shyh-Chour Huang [2,*]

[1] Department of Occupational Therapy, College of Health Science, Kaohsiung Medical University, Kaohsiung 80708, Taiwan; yusheng@kmu.edu.tw
[2] Mechanical Engineering Department, National Kaohsiung University of Science and Technology, Kaohsiung 807618, Taiwan; jason012125@gmail.com
[3] Department of Physical Medicine and Rehabilitation, Kaohsiung Municipal United Hospital, Kaohsiung 80457, Taiwan; takako0703118@yahoo.com.tw
[4] Department of Physical Medicine and Rehabilitation, Kaohsiung Medical University Hospital, Kaohsiung 80756, Taiwan; yatwen1114@gmail.com
* Correspondence: shuang@nkust.edu.tw

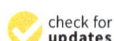

Citation: Yang, Y.-S.; Tseng, C.-H.; Fang, W.-C.; Han, I.-W.; Huang, S.-C. Effectiveness of a New 3D-Printed Dynamic Hand–Wrist Splint on Hand Motor Function and Spasticity in Chronic Stroke Patients. *J. Clin. Med.* **2021**, *10*, 4549. https://doi.org/10.3390/jcm10194549

Academic Editors: Naoki Yoshida, Hideki Nakano, Yohei Okada and Akiyoshi Matsugi

Received: 31 August 2021
Accepted: 27 September 2021
Published: 30 September 2021

Publisher's Note: MDPI stays neutral with regard to jurisdictional claims in published maps and institutional affiliations.

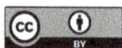

Copyright: © 2021 by the authors. Licensee MDPI, Basel, Switzerland. This article is an open access article distributed under the terms and conditions of the Creative Commons Attribution (CC BY) license (https://creativecommons.org/licenses/by/4.0/).

Abstract: Spasticity, a common stroke complication, can result in impairments and limitations in the performance of activities and participation. In this study, we investigated the effectiveness of a new dynamic splint on wrist and finger flexor muscle spasticity in chronic stroke survivors, using a randomized controlled trial. Thirty chronic stroke survivors were recruited and randomly allocated to either an experimental or control group; 25 completed the 6-week intervention program. The participants in the experimental group were asked to wear the dynamic splint at least 6 h/day at home, for the entire intervention. The participants in the control group did not wear any splint. All the participants were evaluated 1 week before, immediately, and after 3 and 6 weeks of splint use, with the modified Ashworth scale and the Fugl−Meyer assessment for upper extremity. User experience was evaluated by a self-reported questionnaire after the 6-week intervention. The timed within-group assessments showed a significant reduction in spasticity and improvements in functional movements in the experimental group. We found differences, in favor of the experimental group, between the groups after the intervention. The splint users indicated a very good satisfaction rating for muscle tone reduction, comfort, and ease of use. Therefore, this new splint can be used for at-home rehabilitation in chronic stroke patients with hemiparesis.

Keywords: stroke; spasticity; assistive technology

1. Introduction

Post-stroke spasticity is a common complication associated with other signs and symptoms of upper motor neuron syndrome, including agonist and antagonist co-contraction, weakness, and lack of coordination. Stroke survivors with more severe paresis in the upper-limb muscles have a higher risk for developing spasticity in the arm, and contractures of the wrist and finger flexor muscles [1,2]. These problems often develop 6–8 weeks after a stroke [3,4].

Spasticity limits muscle lengthening, which can lead to two consequences. First, spastic muscles have a tendency to stay in a shortened position for longer periods, and second, voluntary activities of antagonist muscles are frequently restricted [5]. An implicit assumption exists that states that spasticity results in muscle fibers and connective tissue changes that can lead to contractures [6,7]. Spasticity and contractures in the upperlimb can significantly affect many activities of daily living or sleep, or can lead to a lesser ability to function [8–10]. Without appropriate attention, stroke survivors with spasticity are at risk for developing a clenched fist, a hand that is deformed into a fist by permanent shortening of the flexor muscles of the fingers and soft tissue [11].

When left in the immobilized state with the flexor synergy pattern after stroke, the condition of the upper limbs progresses to a fibrotic state, which triggers changes in the muscle fiber and sarcomere properties, and the development of early contractures [12]. In such conditions, prolonged muscle stretching is one of the most used treatments to manage spasticity and improve the viscoelastic properties of the muscle–tendon units [13,14]. Static stretching is a widely used type of prolonged muscle stretching, and may be applied in different ways, including by self-stretching, clinical therapist's hands, splints, orthoses, or other physical modalities [13–18].

Splints can provide a safe low-load force to the spastic muscles, which facilitates muscle relaxation, maintains muscle length, and prevents contractures [19], thereby having widespread uses in many clinic settings. However, some previous studies did not support the effectiveness of hand splinting [20,21]. Systematic review research, conducted by Lannin and Herbert, concluded that there was insufficient evidence to either support or refute the effectiveness of hand splinting for adults, following stroke [22]. The effects of splinting may not be long lasting because of a failure to comply with the recommended procedures, and a lack of understanding of the effective dose of stretching within the rehabilitation process. A clear definition of "prolonged", with regard to the duration of stretch, is not yet clear, and further research is required to determine the most appropriate technique and duration to produce the desired effect. Moreover, some studies were conducted with a static splint, an immobilization or supportive splint [20,21]. It has no moving components, and only provides support and immobilization. The position of the static splint sets the wrist/hand in a fixed position. However, the level of spasticity varies during daytime, resulting in different positions of the wrist/hand. The chosen position of the static splint might not be adequate to manage these varying levels of spasticity. By contrast, compared with static splints, a dynamic splint has a static base onto which levels, springs, or pulleys can be attached. It can deliver various stretching options, such as a prolonged or short duration with a high or low intensity of force to counteract the different levels of spasticity. As a result, a dynamic splint is superior, offering more benefits, such as reducing spasticity, allowing comfortable stretch, repositioning fingers in extension positions, and increasing hand performance [23].

In many of the cases we have observed, patients did not like to wear such splints or orthoses. About 33–50% of stroke patients did not wear static splints or orthoses daily for >8 has advised because of discomfort [24]. They complained about an increase in pain and spasticity, which makes it difficult to endure the splints or orthoses for a longer period each day [24]. This discomfort can be a result of the static characteristics of the splints. During moments with high levels of spasticity, the wrist tries to flex against the splints, which can cause pain, pressure sores over the bony prominences (e.g., radial or ulna styloid process), and even wrist or finger flexor hypertonicity, as a result of the pain stimulus. However, without an appropriate splint design to keep the wrist and fingers firmly in the stretched state, both will try to shorten, leading to a lack of stretch.

In recent years, the introduction of 3D-printing techniques in orthopedic and rehabilitation practices has been extensively discussed, because the use of such techniques renders it possible to customize splints or orthoses as well as enhance patient treatment satisfaction levels [25,26]. Varieties of 3D-printed splints have been reported to address deficiencies of the post-stroke spastic hand [16,27–29]. Most of them employed finger caps with elastic cords to stretch the fingers apart in an extension. However, when the degree of finger flexor spasticity is large, it becomes difficult to wear the splint with finger caps against the tension in stretching elastic cords simultaneously. Moreover, these 3D-printed splints had finger enclosures that did not allow the user to have any proprioceptive feedback when picking up the objects. Accordingly, proprioceptive feedback is essential for planning and controlling the limb postures and movements needed for the successful accomplishment of most common motor tasks [30,31]. Finger enclosures may hinder paretic limb detection ability, potentially leading to decreased finger movements.

To overcome the problems, we developed a dynamic splint based on a pulley rotation design. The results demonstrated the beneficial effects of this dynamic splint in eight chronic stroke patients, during a 4-week intervention [32]. However, the dynamic splint was found to have some limitations in some chronic stroke survivors. First, it was difficult to maintain the fingers firmly in the stretched state because the string tended to lose its tension when encountering cases of severe spasticity. In addition, chronic hemiparetic stroke patients were required to put each string of the finger cap on each finger, respectively, so that each finger could be stretched; they found it somehow difficult to handle these strings alone. To resolve these issues, we improved the design and simplified its operations. As a result, we developed a new dynamic splint using a four-bar linkage mechanism as a hand joint exoskeleton to fit the range of finger trajectories. This dynamic splint was intended to be effective in reducing spasticity, easy to fabricate, convenient to operate, and comfortable to wear. Moreover, based on our previous research, we observed that chronic stroke patients who wore the dynamic splints for longer than scheduled showed tremendous improvement, as compared to the group who had a schedule of wearing the splints 3 h a day [32]. A previous study had also indicated that the use of a dynamic splint for at least 6 h per day significantly reduced wrist contractures, causing less pain [17]. Therefore, the primary aim of this study was to evaluate the effect of this new dynamic splint on hand motor function and spasticity in chronic hemiparetic stroke survivors. The secondary aim was to describe the self-reported experiences after the use of this new dynamic splint. We hypothesized that these stroke survivors would be able to relieve their wrist and finger flexors hypertonia, thereby enhancing hand motor function after wearing this dynamic splint. They were able to endure this splint for the prescribed 6 h a day without discomfort.

2. Materials and Methods

2.1. Participants

Thirty participants were recruited from outpatients visiting in the Kaohsiung Medical University Hospital. Participants were included if they met the following criteria: (1) were >18 years of age, (2) had a first-ever stroke resulting in upper-limb spastic hemiplegia >1year before admission to the study, and (3) had upper-limb spasticity (modified Ashworth scale (MAS) scores of 1–3 at the wrist and/or finger flexors). Participants were excluded if they (1) had deficits in language or cognitive impairments that were likely to interfere with their cooperation in the study, (2) presented with severe upper-limb contractures, and (3) had received botulinum toxin injections <6 months prior to study admission. Participants taking oral anti-spastic drugs were only included in the study if the dosage had not been changed during the month before joining. All participants provided informed written consent. The study was conducted in accordance with the Declaration of Helsinki Ethical Principles and Good Clinical Practices and was approved by the Institutional Review Board of Kaohsiung Medical University Chung-Ho Memorial Hospital (KMHIRB-F(I)-20200017).

2.2. Intervention

We randomly assigned participants following a simple randomization procedure (computerized random numbers) to an experimental or a control group. Both groups received the conventional rehabilitation therapy by experienced therapists, including putting patient's limbs in a normal position, the stretching technique of the wrist/finger flexor muscles, proprioceptive neuromuscular facilitation (PNF), neurodevelopmental technique (NDT), and task-oriented training to enhance the motor function and sensory function of the wrist and hand, and activities of daily living training for upper limb. Conventional rehabilitation therapy was performed 3 times per week, for 40 min per time during the 6-week intervention. Participants in the experimental group were asked to wear a custom-made, dynamic 3D-printed hand–wrist splint for at least 6 h per day at home for the 6-week intervention. Participants or caregivers who helped apply the splint self-recorded their actual daily splint wearing time in a diary. Participants in the control group did not wear a hand splint for the study period and were advised to stretch their wrist or finger flexors in a home exercise program.

The study flowchart is illustrated in Figure 1. We assessed the participants in both groups four times. All participants were assessed twice before wearing the dynamic splint within an interval of 1 week and assessed within a 3-week interval for 6 weeks after wearing the splint (first assessment: Pre-1; second assessment: Pre-0; third assessment: Pos-3; fourth assessment: Pos-6). The multiple-baseline design (Pre-1, Pre-0) used in this study enabled us to map improvements on the basis of changes in outcome measures.

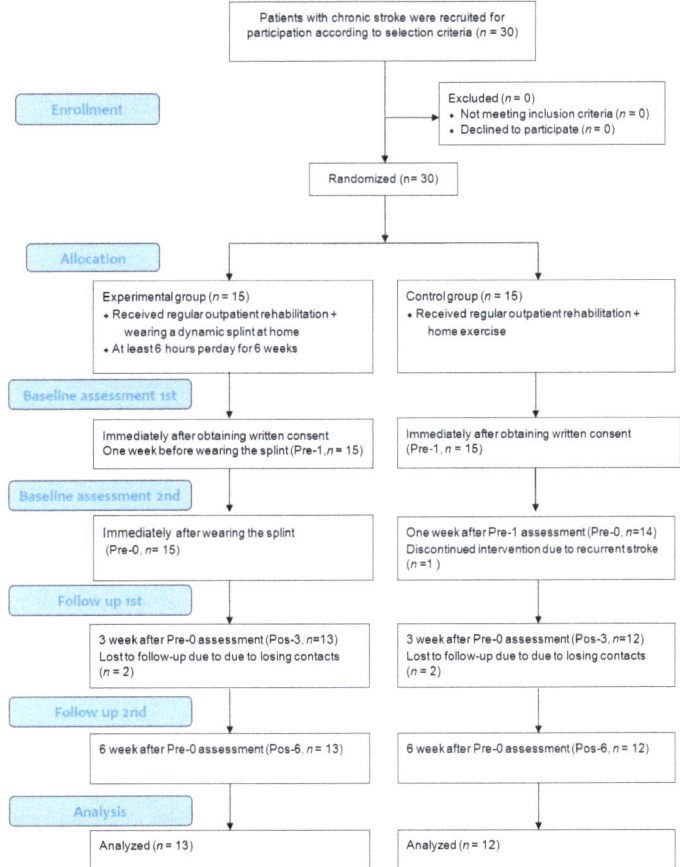

Figure 1. Experiment flowchart.

2.3. D-Printed Dynamic Splint

The 3D-printed dynamic splint consisted of a modified dorsal wrist splint, link bars, and finger caps (Figure 2). This splint held the wrist extended to a 45-degree position. To address the many practical and anatomical challenges of the hand exoskeleton design, we used a four-bar linkage mechanism as a hand joint exoskeleton to fit the range of finger trajectories [33]. The linkage was located at the dorsal wrist and attached to the medial phalanx of the finger just above the distal interphalangeal joint with a finger cap.

We designed the mechanism so that it did not interfere with the finger motion, and the user's fingertips and palm were free to touch real objects and experience tactile feedback. In addition, the fingers could be stretched in extension with the wrist, extended by a simple locking mechanism for a prolonged time. Our previous study had shown that stretching three fingers (thumb, index, and middle fingers) reduced the finger flexors' spasticity, and the splint was easy to self-use at home [32]. Therefore, we used a 3D-printed dynamic splint with a novel three-finger design in the current study.

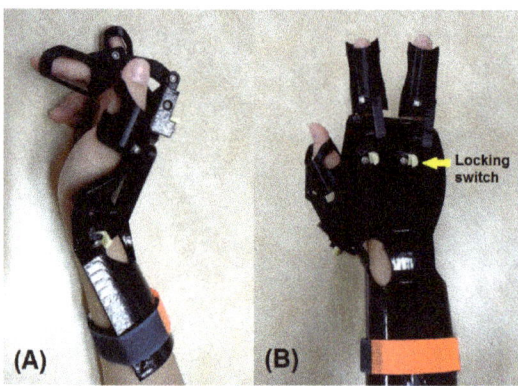

Figure 2. (**A**) Lateral view and (**B**) dorsal view of a 3D-printed dynamic hand–wrist splint.

This study used a fused deposition modeling (FDM)-based 3D printer (UP Box, Go Hot Technologies Co., Ltd., Taiwan) to print all components of this dynamic splint. Each individual part was printed with acrylonitrile–butadiene–styrene (ABS) filament, which has excellent mechanical strength and durability properties. The printing parameters were set as follows: layer thickness of 0.2 mm, 20% filling level, printing temperature of 230 °C, and printing speed of 60 mm/s. Our dynamic splint was customized and manufactured solely on the basis of participant's anthropometric measurements, such as the width of forearm, wrist and fingers; the length of middle finger, index, and thumb. The customized dynamic splint can be manufactured in only 10 h once all the parameters of the participants are measured. The total estimated cost of this dynamic splint is roughly USD 80. This includes the price of all components needed to fabricate the splints, with the exception of the 3D printer. However, considering that the amount of filament required for each splint is estimated to be between 100 and 150 g, depending on its size, the estimated price is expected to decrease further.

2.4. Outcome Measures

The primary outcome measure was the MAS for evaluation of the severity of wrist and finger flexor spasticity. The MAS, a six-category ordinal scale used to assess the resistance encountered during a passive muscle quickly stretching, not requiring instrumentation [34], is the most commonly used tool for evaluating the efficacy of pharmacological and rehabilitation interventions for spasticity among patients with stroke. To allow for the analysis by the statistical software, we modified the MAS scores 1+ to 4, to 2–5 for our analysis [15,18,35]. A smaller score indicated better improvement of spasticity release. Inter- and intra-rater agreement for the MAS measuring upper extremities was 0.78 and 0.84, respectively [36].

Another primary outcome measure was the Fugl–Meyer assessment for upper extremity (FMA-UE), which is the "gold standard" for assessing the motor recovery of post-stroke hemiparesis in clinical trials [37,38]. The FMA-UE consists of 30 items assessing motor function and 3 items assessing reflex function with total scores ranging between 0 and 66. Higher FMA-UE scores mean better motor function. Inter- and intra-rater agreement for the FMA-UE was 0.95 and 0.98, respectively [39–41].

A secondary outcome measure was a subjective self-reported questionnaire regarding pain, spasticity, satisfaction, and ease of self-wear. We measured each item as well with a 10cm visual analog scale(VAS), with 0 cm representing "no pain", "no spasticity", "extremely dissatisfied", or "extremely hard" and 10 cm representing "worst pain", "worst spasticity", "very satisfied", or "very easy". A senior therapist in stroke rehabilitation who was blinded to the group identities conducted all the outcome measures.

2.5. Statistical Analysis

The sample size was calculated based on G power software version 3.1.1 with expected differences between experimental and control groups on the MAS scale from a previous study [15]. The sample size calculation indicated that 15 patients per group should have been enrolled for $\alpha = 0.05$ and $1-\beta = 0.95$, with the effect size of 1.282. Therefore, the indicated overall number of 30 participants was achieved in this study. To summarize the results of the duration of wearing time, pain, subjective spasticity, level of satisfaction, and the easy self-wear descriptive statistics were used. Quantitative variables were compared using independent t-test/Mann–Whitney U test (when the data sets were not normally distributed) between the two groups. Categorical variables were compared using chi-square test. Analysis of covariance (ANCOVA) was used to compare MAS and FMA-UE scores at multiple time points between two groups after adjusting for the baseline values. Repeated measures analysis of variance (ANOVA) with Bonferroni adjustment was used for comparison of MAS and FMA–UE scores within each group between multiple time points. All statistical analyses were performed using the SPSS software (version 20 for Windows, IBM, Armonk, NY, USA), and the level of significance was set to 0.05.

3. Results

3.1. Participant Characteristics

Thirty stroke survivors were recruited in this study, but only 25 completed the 6-week intervention. One participant in the control group dropped out because of recurrent stroke, and four participants (three in the experimental group, one in the control group) were lost during follow-up. The participants' demographic and clinical characteristics are presented in Table 1. No significant demographic differences occurred between the groups, including age, gender, stroke history, and affected side.

Table 1. Participant demographic characteristics and clinical features between the groups.

Characteristic/Feature	Group		p-Value
	Experimental (n =13)	Control (n =12)	
Mean age, years	44.4 (10.2)	47.1 (9.2)	0.55
Gender (male/female)	11/2	10/2	0.93
History of stroke, months	22.5 (11.9)	20.0 (10.4)	0.48
Affected side (right/left)	7/6	6/6	0.86

Values are presented as means (standard deviations).

3.2. Clinical Assessments

The average MAS scores of the wrist and finger flexors at different assessments in the study groups are shown in Table 2. Within the experimental group, we found no significant differences in the wrist and finger flexors between Pre-1 and Pre-0. However, there was a significant decrease in the finger flexors at Pos-3 ($p = 0.03$) and at Pos-6 ($p < 0.01$ on wrist flexors, $p < 0.01$ on finger flexors), respectively, when compared to Pre-0. Within the control group, we found no significant serial MAS changes in either the wrist or finger flexors at Pre-1, Pre-2, Pos-3, and Pos-6, although we observed a slow decreasing tendency (Figure 3). Moreover, after 3 weeks of the wearing intervention, the average MAS of the finger flexors showed a significant decrease ($p = 0.05$); after 6 weeks, the average MAS of the wrist ($p < 0.01$) and finger ($p < 0.01$) flexors in the experimental group were significantly decreased compared with those in the control group.

Table 2. Average MAS scores of the wrist and finger flexors in the study groups.

Group	Pre-1	Pre-0	*p*-Value [a]	Pos-3	*p*-Value [a]	Pos-6	*p*-Value [a]
E-wrist	3.0 (0.6)	2.8 (0.7)	0.99	2.4 (0.8)	0.57	1.8 (0.7)	<0.01 *
C-wrist	2.5 (0.8)	2.3 (0.8)	0.99	2.4 (0.8)	0.9	2.2 (0.9)	0.99
p-value [b]	0.92	0.92	-	0.57	-	<0.01 *	-
Partial EtaSquared	<0.01	<0.01		0.02		0.28	
E-finger	3.3 (0.6)	3.2 (0.6)	0.99	2.4 (0.9)	0.03 *	2.0 (0.6)	<0.01 *
C-finger	2.8 (0.4)	2.9 (0.3)	0.99	2.8 (0.4)	0.99	2.8 (0.5)	0.99
p-value [b]	0.22	0.22	-	0.05 *	-	<0.01 *	-
Partial Eta Squared	0.07	0.07		0.17		0.61	

Values are presented as means (standard deviations); * $p < 0.05$. E-wrist: wrist flexors in the experimental group; C-wrist: wrist flexors in the control group; E-finger: finger flexors in the experimental group; C-finger: finger flexors in the control group. [a] *p*-value was determined by ANOVA using Bonferroni adjustment; [b] *p*-value after adjusting for multiple baseline using ANCOVA between experimental group and control group at each assessment.

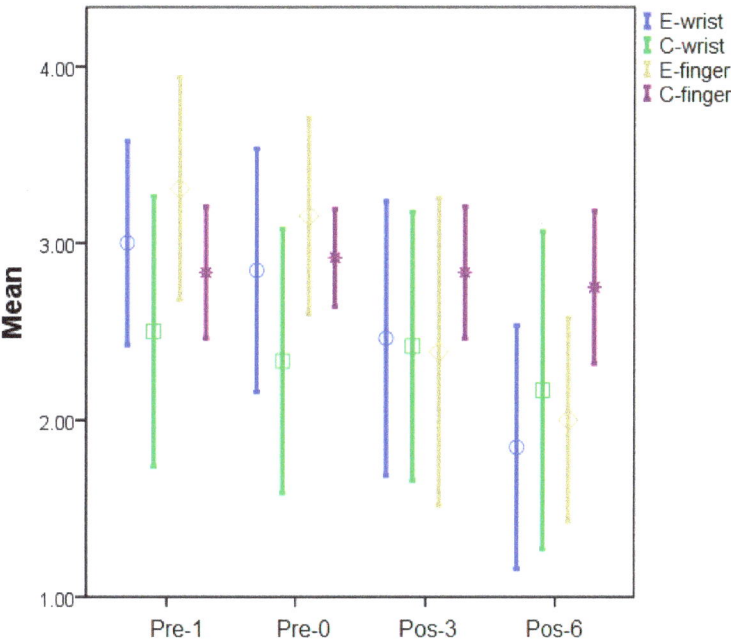

Figure 3. Sequential changes in mean MAS scores for the wrist and finger flexors in the study. Mean values and ±1 standard error were displayed. E-wrist: wrist flexors in the experimental group; C-wrist: wrist flexors in the control group; E-finger: finger flexors in the experimental group; C-finger: finger flexors in the control group.

The average FMA-UE scores at different assessments in the study groups are shown in Table 3. Similarly, for the experimental group, the average FMA–UE scoreat Pre-1 and Pre-0 showed no significant differences. We observed a significant improvement in Pos-3 ($p = 0.02$) and Pos-6 ($p < 0.01$), when compared to Pre-0. For the control group, we found no significant differences in the FMA-UE scores between Pre-1 and Pre-0. However, we noted a slight improvement in Pos-3 (Figure 4). Thereafter, we found a significant increase until Pos-6 ($p = 0.01$). Moreover, we found no significant differences in the FMA-UE scores in the experimental group, when compared to the control group, at Pre-1, Pre-0, and Pos-3. We did find a significant difference until Pos-6 ($p = 0.05$).

Table 3. Average FMA-UE scores in the study groups.

Group	Pre-1	Pre-0	p-value [a]	Pos-3	p-Value [a]	Pos-6	p-Value [a]
Exp	27.2 (11.4)	27.8 (11.7)	0.07	30.5 (12.0)	0.02 *	36.8 (11.2)	<0.01 *
Ctrl	21.1 (11.6)	21.6 (11.5)	0.13	23.0 (12.7)	0.06	26.0 (14.7)	0.01 *
p-value [b]	0.89	0.89		0.39		0.05 *	-
Partial EtaSquared	<0.01	<0.01		0.03		0.17	

Values are presented as means (standard deviations); * $p < 0.05$. [a] p-value was determined by ANOVA using Bonferroni adjustment; [b] p-value after adjusting for multiple baseline using ANCOVA between experimental group and control group at each assessment.

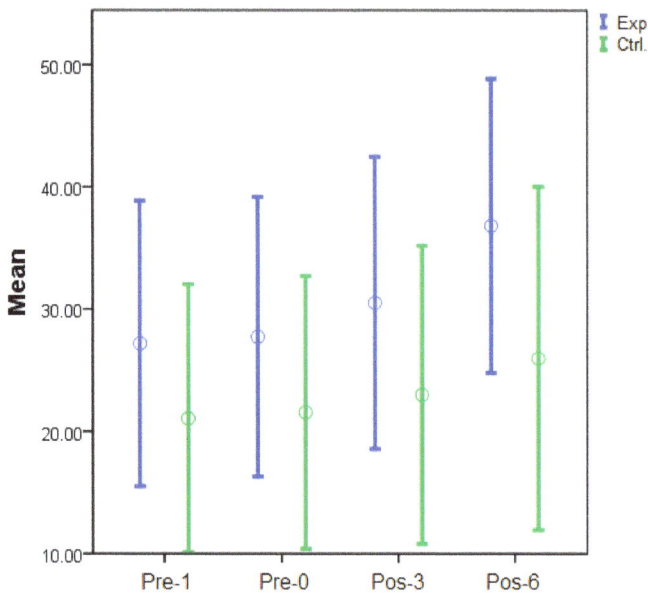

Figure 4. Sequential changes in mean FMA-UE scores in the study groups. Mean values and ±1 standard error were displayed. Exp.: experimental group; Ctrl.: control group.

3.3. Subjective Self-Reported Findings

The participants in the experimental group, at 6 weeks, showed significant differences in their attitudes towards splint wearing time ($p < 0.01$), reduced spasticity ($p < 0.01$), level of satisfaction ($p < 0.01$), and ease of use ($p < 0.01$) (Table 4). However, the pain ratings showed no statistical differences between Pos-3 and Pos-6 ($p = 0.89$). The participants reported that they had still experienced mild, annoying pain after wearing the splint for 6 weeks.

Table 4. Subjective reported wearing time, pain, spasticity, level of satisfaction, and ease of self-wear in the experimental group.

Time (n =13)	Wearing Time (h)	Pain (0–10)	Spasticity (0–10)	Satisfaction (0–10)	Easy to Use (0–10)
Pos-3	7.2	2.6	7.4	7.7	8.0
Pos-6	7.9	2.5	5.6	8.4	8.8
p-value	<0.01 *	0.89	<0.01 *	<0.01 *	<0.01 *

Values are presented as means; * $p < 0.05$.

4. Discussion

The results from this study indicated that our new 3D-printed dynamic hand–wrist splint was effective in significantly reducing wrist and finger flexor spasticity after 3 weeks of intervention. Furthermore, we observed a further effect on reducing spasticity after wearing the splint for 6 weeks. We also found significant alleviation in self-reported spasticity after 6 weeks of intervention.

Several previous studies have described a variety of dynamic splints that effectively improved motor function and relieved spasticity in stroke patients [16,17,32,42]. In comparison to a static splint, a dynamic splint consists of a static base that forms the foundation of the splint, and an outrigger, the mobile part consisting of levers, springs, or pulleys. It also included a dynamic component to facilitate splint mobility with the associated structures, such as finger springs and caps, an adjustable tensioner, and wrist mount areas. This dynamic component offers energy-storing properties and provides various resistance grades against spasticity. Therefore, as flexor tone increases in the patient's hand, the fingers remain within the splint instead of pulling out. The dynamic hand piece then repositions the fingers into extension, as tone increases.

Thus, a dynamic splint is far superior to a static splint because it provides more benefits, such as reducing spasticity, allowing for comfortable stretch, and repositioning fingers into extension positions. Many dynamic splints for reducing hand spasticity have been developed; however, most of these were too complicated to wear, involving a glove or hook-and-loop fasteners strapping each finger in firmly. Often, it is technically difficult for a stroke patient with spasticity to wear these types of splints alone at home.

The new dynamic hand–wrist splint presented in this study has a simple device configuration and low-cost fabrication. The finger cap has a similar design to the finger sleeve, for easy and quick wearing or removing. Furthermore, this splint uses a four-bar linkage mechanism to fit finger trajectories and caps to reposition the fingers. Therefore, it allows for a comfortable prolonged stretch and maintains the fingers in an extended position to decrease wrist and finger flexor spasticity.

The motor function of the affected wrist and hand (measured with the FMA-UE) showed statistically significant improvements after 3 weeks of intervention and had sustained improvement at 6 weeks. The average difference in improvement between Pre-0 and Pos-6, using the FMA-UE, was 9.1, which we believed to be clinically meaningful because the minimal clinically important difference of the FMA-UE has been established to be between 4.25 and 7.25 for patients with chronic stroke [43]. Moreover, 76.9% of the participants in the experimental group exceeded the MCID of 4.25. The increase in the FMA-UE score demonstrated the voluntary motor improvements achieved by the participants.

Historically, traditional rehabilitation approaches have focused on reducing spasticity as a prerequisite for improving motor function [44]. In stroke survivors with functionally useful voluntary limb movement, inappropriate co-activation of agonist and antagonist muscles can cause spastic co-contraction, thereby impeding normal limb movement [45,46]. One possible reason for the better performance in the FMA-UE score with decreased MAS in the experimental group was that the participants could be able to exert more voluntary effort in the reach-to-grasp tasks. People with stroke often have difficulty generating force in the finger extensor to open their hands, due to stronger wrist and finger flexor spasticity. The suppression of wrist and finger flexor spasticity, by prolonged stretching with a dynamic hand–wrist splint, can decrease the ability to counteract the agonist wrist and finger extensor muscles, thereby increasing the ability to voluntarily control hand opening. Furthermore, maximized involvement of voluntary effort in post-stroke limb practice has been found to be an important factor related to the significant release of muscle tone, with long-term effects [47]. When the affected hand was able to start performing the tasks they could not achieve (e.g., hand open) by themselves, they would be promoted to practice reach-to-grasp tasks. Our findings are also consistent with other robot-assisted therapy in upper extremity hemiparesis studies, suggesting that decreased muscle tone occurs in chronic stroke individuals with better voluntary motor functions [47–49].

Both groups received approximately 2 h of upper-limb therapies per week, as conventional stroke rehabilitation programs. The conventional program is patient-specific, task-specific, and consists of PNF and NDT. Presumably, those conventional treatments had a relevant influence on the patients' improvement. Consequently, the FMA–UE scores of the control group gradually increased by 4.5 points, from the baseline to Pos-6, but these scores were not superior to those in the experimental group. The use of a 3D-printed dynamic hand–wrist splint at home, combined with a conventional rehabilitation program, could provide additional long-term benefits in terms of upper extremity motor recovery and motor functioning.

The participants in this study reported a significant difference in reducing spasticity and in increasing wearing time before and since the use of this splint. The participants were willing to wear the splint from 6 h, as advised, to 7.9 h/day after the 6 weeks of intervention. The participants reported high levels of satisfaction and ease of use, finding it easy to wear this dynamic splint on their affected hand independently, without any problems.

The self-reported pain did not show a significant difference, although the spasticity complaints tended to decrease. Therefore, our new dynamic splint, using prolonged stretching principles to guard against increased spasticity, muscle stiffness, and shortening in the wrist and finger flexors, certainly caused some pain. Yet, after wearing the splint for 6 weeks, not one of the participants ceased wearing it because of a painful experience. On the contrary, the participants wore this splint for longer than the advised hours. One possible reason for this might be that these stroke patients experienced improvement in their hand function and thus were willing to keep wearing the splint.

The strength of our study is that it used a randomized controlled trial design. We selected the FMA–UE and MAS to measure primary outcomes and a self-reported questionnaire to measure secondary outcomes. However, there were limitations that need to be addressed in this study. First, this study was limited in that we surveyed the experimental group using a self-reported questionnaire, which is not a standardized questionnaire. This survey may simply lack sufficient validity and reliability. However, the self-reported data collected by this survey used VAS, which is a simple and frequently used method to evaluate variations in satisfaction or discomfort rating questionnaires. These self-reported outcomes may still give useful insights into the user's perspective on this dynamic splint. Another limitation was that the included participants were stroke patients; they often have a certain degree of cognitive impairment. We did not assess their cognitive abilities for both groups; however, we ensured that the participants in the experimental group understood how to wear this dynamic splint properly.

One more limitation was the choice of MAS as the spasticity assessment scale. The MAS is a muscle tone assessment scale used to assess the resistance experienced during a passive range of motion. It is the most commonly used tool to evaluate the efficacy of pharmacologic and rehabilitation interventions for the treatment; therefore, it can be easily compared with the results obtained in other studies. However, recent studies raised questions about the moderate inter- and intra-rater reliability [50,51] and validity of the MAS assessment of spasticity [51,52]. Spasticity, defined as hyper-resistance measured during passive rotation of a joint, is related to neural and non-neural factors. MAS does not address the velocity-dependent aspect of spasticity [51,52], and it has been described as a grading of muscle stiffness to solely assess resistance to passive movement [51]. Despite its popularity, MAS has been subject to criticism; the modified Tardieu scale (MTS) has been suggested as an alternative and suitable measure for use in the assessment of spasticity [52,53]. MTS could address the intensity of the resistance, first-noticed catch angle, clonus, and differences among joints and muscles that move at different velocities [52,53]. Nevertheless, MAS generally reflects muscle overactivity, including the elements of hypertonia and muscle stiffness, which are both the components of a positive sign of upper motor neuron syndrome, and they compose the resistance of passive stretch. These elements affecting the active or passive function of patients could be treated through pharmacologic treatment or other remedies. Therefore, it is reasonable to use the MAS as a scale for measuring muscle tone [54].

Finally, our results are limited to stroke survivors with mild–moderate upper-limb impairments. This dynamic splint can only be applied to stroke survivors who can extend their wrist and open their affected hand by passive movements. Therefore, the results cannot be generalized to other stroke populations, especially those with severe spasticity of the affected limb.

5. Conclusions

In conclusion, this new 3D-printed dynamic hand–wrist splint is a feasible and effective alternative modality for reducing muscle spasticity and improving hand motor function. The users gave very good satisfaction scores for muscle tone reduction, comfort, and ease of use. This splint can be a supplementary device for home exercises in addition to hospital-based rehabilitation for chronic stroke survivors with hemiparesis.

Author Contributions: Conceptualization, Y.-S.Y., C.-H.T. and S.-C.H.; methodology, Y.-S.Y. and S.-C.H.; validation, C.-H.T., W.-C.F. and I.-W.H.; investigation, W.-C.F. and I.-W.H.; data curation, Y.-S.Y. and C.-H.T.; writing—original draft preparation, Y.-S.Y.; writing—review and editing, S.-C.H.; project administration, Y.-S.Y.; funding acquisition, Y.-S.Y. All authors have read and agreed to the published version of the manuscript.

Funding: This research was funded by Ministry of Science and Technology, Taiwan, grant number MOST1092221E037002.

Institutional Review Board Statement: The study was conducted according to the guidelines of the Declaration of Helsinki, and approved by the Institutional Review Board of Kaohsiung Medical University Chung-Ho Memorial Hospital (protocol code KMUHIRB-F(I)-20200017, date of approval: 7 February 2020).

Informed Consent Statement: Informed consent was obtained from all subjects involved in the study.

Data Availability Statement: Data available on request due to privacy/ethical restrictions. The data presented in this study are available on request from the corresponding author.

Conflicts of Interest: The authors declare no conflict of interest.

References

1. Kong, K.H.; Chua, K.S.; Lee, J. Symptomatic upper limb spasticity in patients with chronic stroke attending a rehabilitation clinic: Frequency, clinical correlates and predictors. *J. Rehabil. Med.* **2010**, *42*, 453–457. [CrossRef]
2. Urban, P.P.; Wolf, T.; Uebele, M.; Marx, J.J.; Vogt, T.; Stoeter, P.; Bauermann, T.; Weibrich, C.; Vucurevic, G.D.; Schneider, A.; et al. Occurence and clinical predictors of spasticity after ischemic stroke. *Stroke* **2010**, *41*, 2016–2020. [CrossRef] [PubMed]
3. Pandyan, A.; Cameron, M.; Powell, J.; Stott, D.; Granat, M. Contractures in the post-stroke wrist: A pilot study of its time course of development and its association with upper limb recovery. *Clin. Rehabil.* **2003**, *17*, 88–95. [CrossRef] [PubMed]
4. Malhotra, S.; Pandyan, A.; Rosewilliam, S.; Roffe, C.; Hermens, H. Spasticity and contractures at the wrist after stroke: Time course of development and their association with functional recovery of the upper limb. *Clin. Rehabil.* **2011**, *25*, 184–191. [CrossRef]
5. Salazar, A.P.; Pinto, C.; Mossi, J.V.R.; Figueiro, B.; Lukrafka, J.L.; Pagnussat, A.S. Effectiveness of static stretching positioning on post-stroke upper-limb spasticity and mobility: Systematic review with meta-analysis. *Ann. Phys. Rehabil. Med.* **2019**, *62*, 274–282. [CrossRef] [PubMed]
6. O'dwyer, N.; Ada, L.; Neilson, P. Spasticity and muscle contracture following stroke. *Brain* **1996**, *119*, 1737–1749. [CrossRef] [PubMed]
7. Gracies, J.M. Pathophysiology of spastic paresis. I: Paresis and soft tissue changes. *Muscle Nerve* **2005**, *31*, 535–551. [CrossRef]
8. Franceschini, M.; La Porta, F.; Agosti, M.; Massucci, M. Is health-related-quality of life of stroke patients influenced by neurological impairments at one year after stroke? *Eur. J. Phys. Rehabil. Med.* **2010**, *46*, 389–399.
9. Schinwelski, M.; Sławek, J. Prevalence of spasticity following stroke and its impact on quality of life with emphasis on disability in activities of daily living. Systematic review. *Neurol. Neurochir. Pol.* **2010**, *44*, 404–411. [CrossRef]
10. Sonmez, I.; Karasel, S. Poor sleep quality i related to impaired functional status following stroke. *J. Stroke Cerebrovasc. Dis.* **2019**, *28*, 104349. [CrossRef]

11. Heijnen, I.; Franken, R.; Bevaart, B.; Meijer, J. Long-term outcome of superficialis-to-profundus tendon transfer in patients with clenched fist due to spastic hemiplegia. *Disabil. Rehabil.* **2008**, *30*, 675–678. [CrossRef] [PubMed]
12. Lieber, R.L.; Fridén, J. Spasticity causes a fundamental rearrangement of muscle–joint interaction. *Muscle Nerve* **2002**, *25*, 265–270. [CrossRef] [PubMed]
13. Boven'Eerdt, T.J.; Newman, M.; Barker, K.; Dawes, H.; Minelli, C.; Wade, D.T. The effects of stretching in spasticity: A systematic review. *Arch. Phys. Med. Rehabil.* **2008**, *89*, 1395–1406. [CrossRef] [PubMed]
14. Harvey, L.A.; Katalinic, O.M.; Herbert, R.D.; Moseley, A.M.; Lannin, N.A.; Schurr, K. Stretch for the treatment and prevention of contracture: An abridged republication of a cochrane systematic review. *J. Physiother.* **2017**, *63*, 67–75. [CrossRef]
15. Jung, Y.J.; Hong, J.H.; Kwon, H.G.; Song, J.C.; Kim, C.; Park, S.; Kim, Y.K.; Ahn, S.H.; Jang, S.H. The effect of a stretching device on hand spasticity in chronic hemiparetic stroke patients. *NeuroRehabilitation* **2011**, *29*, 53–59. [CrossRef]
16. Lannin, N.A.; Cusick, A.; Hills, C.; Kinnear, B.; Vogel, K.; Matthews, K.; Bowring, G. Upper limb motor training using a saebo™ orthosis is feasible for increasing task-specific practice in hospital after stroke. *Aust. Occup. Ther. J.* **2016**, *63*, 364–372. [CrossRef]
17. Andringa, A.S.; Van de Port, I.G.; Meijer, J.W. Tolerance and effectiveness of a new dynamic hand-wrist orthosis in chronic stroke patients. *NeuroRehabilitation* **2013**, *33*, 225–231. [CrossRef]
18. Kim, E.H.; Chang, M.C.; Seo, J.P.; Jang, S.H.; Song, J.C.; Jo, H.M. The effect of a hand-stretching device during the management of spasticity in chronic hemiparetic stroke patients. *Ann. Rehabil. Med.* **2013**, *37*, 235–240. [CrossRef]
19. Greg Pitts, D.; Peganoff O'Brien, S. Splinting the hand to enhance motor control and brain plasticity. *Top. Stroke. Rehabil.* **2008**, *15*, 456–467. [CrossRef]
20. Lannin, N.A.; Horsley, S.A.; Herbert, R.; McCluskey, A.; Cusick, A. Splinting the hand in the functional position after brain impairment: A randomized, controlled trial. *Arch. Phys. Med. Rehabil.* **2003**, *84*, 297–302. [CrossRef]
21. Lannin, N.A.; Cusick, A.; McCluskey, A.; Herbert, R.D. Effects of splinting on wrist contracture after stroke: A randomized controlled trial. *Stroke* **2007**, *38*, 111–116. [CrossRef] [PubMed]
22. Lannin, N.A.; Herbert, R.D. Is hand splinting effective for adults following stroke? A systematic review and methodologic critique of published research. *Clin. Rehabil.* **2003**, *17*, 807–816. [CrossRef] [PubMed]
23. Bianca, C.; Machuki, J.; Chen, W. A dynamic splint for the treatment of spasticity of the hand after stroke-recognition of its design, functionality and limitations: A narrative review article. *J. Neurol. Neurorehabil. Res.* **2018**, *3*, 17–19.
24. Andringa, A.; van de Port, I.; Meijer, J.-W. Long-term use of a static hand-wrist orthosis in chronic stroke patients: A pilot study. *Stroke. Res. Treat.* **2013**, *2013*, 546092. [CrossRef] [PubMed]
25. Lin, H.; Shi, L.; Wang, D. A rapid and intelligent designing technique for patient-specific and 3d-printed orthopedic cast. *3D Print. Med.* **2016**, *2*, 4. [CrossRef] [PubMed]
26. Lunsford, C.; Grindle, G.; Salatin, B.; Dicianno, B.E. Innovations with 3-dimensional printing in physical medicine and rehabilitation: A review of the literature. *PM&R* **2016**, *8*, 1201–1212.
27. Barry, J.G.; Ross, S.A.; Woehrle, J. Therapy incorporating a dynamic wrist-hand orthosis versus manual assistance in chronic stroke: A pilot study. *J. Neurol. Phys. Ther.* **2012**, *36*, 17–24. [CrossRef] [PubMed]
28. Huang, T.Y.; Pan, L.H.; Yang, W.W.; Huang, L.Y.; Sun, P.C.; Chen, C.S. Biomechanical evaluation of three-dimensional printed dynamic hand device for patients with chronic stroke. *IEEE Trans. Neural. Syst. Rehabil. Eng.* **2019**, *27*, 1246–1252. [CrossRef]
29. Dudley, D.R.; Knarr, B.A.; Siu, K.C.; Peck, J.; Ricks, B.; Zuniga, J.M. Testing of a 3d printed hand exoskeleton for an individual with stroke: A case study. *Disabil. Rehabil. Assist. Technol.* **2021**, *16*, 209–213. [CrossRef]
30. Sarlegna, F.R.; Sainburg, R.L. The roles of vision and proprioception in the planning of reaching movements. *Adv. Exp. Med. Biol.* **2009**, *629*, 317–335.
31. Scheidt, R.A.; Conditt, M.A.; Secco, E.L.; Mussa-Ivaldi, F.A. Interaction of visual and proprioceptive feedback during adaptation of human reaching movements. *J. Neurophysiol.* **2005**, *93*, 3200–3213. [CrossRef] [PubMed]
32. Yang, Y.S.; Emzain, Z.F.; Huang, S.C. Biomechanical evaluation of dynamic splint based on pulley rotation design for management of hand spasticity. *IEEE Trans. Neural. Syst. Rehabil. Eng.* **2021**, *29*, 683–689. [CrossRef] [PubMed]
33. Sands, D.; Pérez Gracia, A.; McCormack, J.; Wolbrecht, E.T. Design method for a reconfigurable mechanism for finger rehabilitation. In Proceedings of the 15th IASTED International Conference on Robotics and Applications, Cambridge, MA, USA, 1–3 November 2010; pp. 1–8.
34. Charalambous, C.P. Interrater reliability of a modified ashworth scale of muscle spasticity. In *Classic Papers in Orthopaedics*; Springer: New York, NY, USA, 2014; pp. 415–417.
35. Craven, B.; Morris, A. Modified ashworth scale reliability for measurement of lower extremity spasticity among patients with SCI. *SpinalCord* **2010**, *48*, 207–213. [CrossRef] [PubMed]
36. Meseguer-Henarejos, A.-B.; Sanchez-Meca, J.; Lopez-Pina, J.-A.; Carles-Hernandez, R. Inter-and intra-rater reliability of the modified ashworth scale: A systematic review and meta-analysis. *Eur. J. Phys. Rehabil. Med.* **2017**, *54*, 576–590. [PubMed]
37. Baker, K.; Cano, S.J.; Playford, E.D. Outcome measurement in stroke: A scale selection strategy. *Stroke* **2011**, *42*, 1787–1794. [CrossRef]
38. Kwakkel, G.; Lannin, N.A.; Borschmann, K.; English, C.; Ali, M.; Churilov, L.; Saposnik, G.; Winstein, C.; Van Wegen, E.E.; Wolf, S.L. Standardized measurement of sensorimotor recovery in stroke trials: Consensus-based core recommendations from the stroke recovery and rehabilitation roundtable. *Neurorehabil. Neural. Repair* **2017**, *31*, 784–792. [CrossRef]

39. Page, S.J.; Levine, P.; Hade, E. Psychometric properties and administration of the wrist/hand subscales of the fugl-meyer assessment in minimally impaired upper extremity hemiparesis in stroke. *Arch. Phys. Med. Rehabil.* **2012**, *93*, 2373–2376. [CrossRef]
40. Lundquist, C.B.; Maribo, T. The fugl–meyer assessment of the upper extremity: Reliability, responsiveness and validity of the danish version. *Disabil. Rehabil.* **2017**, *39*, 934–939. [CrossRef]
41. Hernandez, E.D.; Galeano, C.P.; Barbosa, N.E.; Forero, S.M.; Nordin, Å.; Sunnerhagen, K.S.; Alt Murphy, M. Intra-and inter-rater reliability of fugl-meyer assessment of upper extremity in stroke. *J. Rehabil. Med.* **2019**, *51*, 652–659. [CrossRef]
42. Chang, W.D.; Lai, P.T. New design of home-based dynamic hand splint for hemiplegic hands: A preliminary study. *J. Phys. Ther. Sci.* **2015**, *27*, 829–831. [CrossRef]
43. Page, S.J.; Fulk, G.D.; Boyne, P. Clinically important differences for the upper-extremity fugl-meyer scale in people with minimal to moderate impairment due to chronic stroke. *Phys. Ther.* **2012**, *92*, 791–798. [CrossRef] [PubMed]
44. Vaughan-Graham, J.; Cott, C.; Wright, F.V. The bobath (NDT) concept in adult neurological rehabilitation: What is the state of the knowledge? A scoping review. Part I: Conceptual perspectives. *Disabil. Rehabil.* **2015**, *37*, 1793–1807. [CrossRef] [PubMed]
45. Chae, J.; Yang, G.; Park, B.K.; Labatia, I. Muscle weakness and cocontraction in upper limb hemiparesis: Relationship to motor impairment and physical disability. *Neurorehabil. Neural. Repair* **2002**, *16*, 241–248. [CrossRef] [PubMed]
46. Gracies, J.M. Pathophysiology of spastic paresis. II: Emergence of muscle overactivity. *Muscle Nerve* **2005**, *31*, 552–571. [CrossRef]
47. Hu, X.L.; Tong, K.Y.; Song, R.; Zheng, X.J.; Leung, W.W. A comparison between electromyography-driven robot and passive motion device on wrist rehabilitation for chronic stroke. *Neurorehabil. Neural. Repair* **2009**, *23*, 837–846. [CrossRef] [PubMed]
48. Hung, C.S.; Hsieh, Y.W.; Wu, C.Y.; Lin, K.C.; Lin, J.C.; Yeh, L.M.; Yin, H.P. Comparative assessment of two robot-assisted therapies for the upper extremity in people with chronic stroke. *Am. J. Occup. Ther.* **2019**, *73*, 7301205010p1–7301205010p9. [CrossRef]
49. Lee, K.W.; Kim, S.B.; Lee, J.H.; Lee, S.J.; Yoo, S.W. Effect of upper extremity robot-assisted exercise on spasticity in stroke patients. *Ann. Rehabil. Med.* **2016**, *40*, 961. [CrossRef]
50. Ansari, N.N.; Naghdi, S.; Moammeri, H.; Jalaie, S. Ashworth scales are unreliable for the assessment of muscle spasticity. *Physiother. Theory Pract.* **2006**, *22*, 119–125. [CrossRef]
51. Pandyan, A.D.; Johnson, G.R.; Price, C.I.; Curless, R.H.; Barnes, M.P.; Rodgers, H. A review of the properties and limitations of the ashworth and modified ashworth scales as measures of spasticity. *Clin. Rehabil.* **1999**, *13*, 373–383. [CrossRef]
52. Patrick, E.; Ada, L. The tardieu scale differentiates contracture from spasticity whereas the ashworth scale is confounded by it. *Clin. Rehabil.* **2006**, *20*, 173–182. [CrossRef]
53. Haugh, A.B.; Pandyan, A.D.; Johnson, G.R. A systematic review of the tardieu scale for the measurement of spasticity. *Disabil. Rehabil.* **2006**, *28*, 899–907. [CrossRef] [PubMed]
54. Li, F.; Wu, Y.; Li, X. Test-retest reliability and inter-rater reliability of the modified tardieu scale and the modified ashworth scale in hemiplegic patients with stroke. *Eur. J. Phys. Rehabil. Med.* **2014**, *50*, 9–15. [PubMed]

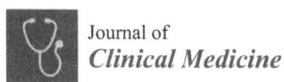

Article

Sensory Nerve Conduction Velocity Predicts Improvement of Hand Function with Nerve Gliding Exercise Following Carpal Tunnel Release Surgery

Yoshiki Tamaru [1], Akiyoshi Yanagawa [2] and Akiyoshi Matsugi [1,*]

[1] Faculty of Rehabilitation, Shijonawate-Gakuen University, Hojo 5-11-10, Daitou, Osaka 574-0011, Japan; eubrj601@ican.zaq.ne.jp
[2] Department of Rehabilitation, Tesseikai Neurosurgical Hospital, Nakano Honmachi 28-1, Shijonawate, Osaka 575-8511, Japan; akipara@yahoo.co.jp
* Correspondence: aki.pt0422@gmail.com; Tel.: +81-72-863-5043

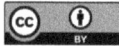

Citation: Tamaru, Y.; Yanagawa, A.; Matsugi, A. Sensory Nerve Conduction Velocity Predicts Improvement of Hand Function with Nerve Gliding Exercise Following Carpal Tunnel Release Surgery. J. Clin. Med. 2021, 10, 4121. https://doi.org/10.3390/jcm10184121

Academic Editor: Michael Sauerbier

Received: 31 July 2021
Accepted: 10 September 2021
Published: 13 September 2021

Publisher's Note: MDPI stays neutral with regard to jurisdictional claims in published maps and institutional affiliations.

Copyright: © 2021 by the authors. Licensee MDPI, Basel, Switzerland. This article is an open access article distributed under the terms and conditions of the Creative Commons Attribution (CC BY) license (https://creativecommons.org/licenses/by/4.0/).

Abstract: This study aims to investigate the effects of nerve gliding exercise following carpal tunnel release surgery (NGE-CTRS) and the probing factors affecting the effect of NGE-CTRS on hand function. A total of 86 patients after CTRS participated. Grip strength (grip-s), pinch strength (pinch-s), Semmes-Weinstein monofilament test (SWMT), two-point discrimination (2PD), numbness, pain, and Phalen test (Phalen) were measured and compared between pre- and post-NGE-CTRS. The results showed that the combination of surgery and NGE significantly improved the postoperative grip-s, pinch-s, SWMT, 2PD, numbness, and Phalen; however, no improvement was observed in pain. Background factors that influenced the improved grip-s and pinch-s included gender and preoperative sensory nerve conduction velocity (SCV). Additionally, numbness and Phalen were not affected by age, gender, fault side, bilateral, trigger finger, dialysis, thenar eminence atrophy, motor nerve conduction velocity, SCV, the start of treatment, and occupational therapy intervention. In conclusion, the combination of surgical procedures and NGE showed a high improvement. SCV and time-to-start treatment of intervention for carpal tunnel syndrome may be useful in predicting the function after the intervention.

Keywords: carpal tunnel syndrome; nerve gliding exercise; sensory nerve conduction velocity

1. Introduction

Carpal tunnel syndrome (CTS) caused by median nerve compression at the wrist is considered the most common entrapment neuropathy [1] with a prevalence of 2–4% in the general population [2,3]. CTS symptoms include pain, paresthesia, numbness, or tingling involving the fingers innervated by the median nerve. Symptoms are worst at night and upon waking up [4]. Patients with severe CTS present with thenar atrophy and loss of sensation [5], which results in gradual weakness and loss of hand function [6,7]. Treatment for CTS with severe symptoms involves surgical procedures to open the carpal tunnel and relieve pressure [8]. Moreover, non-surgical interventions, such as wrist splint [9–14], ultrasound [4,15–17], steroid injections [18–20], and nerve gliding exercise (NGE) [10–12,21], were administered for mild to moderate symptoms.

Recently, several systematic reviews have advocated nerve and tendon gliding exercises as a biologically plausible alternative for traditionally advocated treatment modalities in the conservative management for CTS [10–12,22,23].

Previous studies on NGE effects have reported improved pinch strength (pinch-s) [24], grip-strength (grip-s) [24,25], and pain [26]. Reports of the effect of no treatment, include pain [26,27], low functional performance [26–28], and sensation [15,24,25,27,29]. Thus, the effect of NGE on strength can be expected; however, it does not affect pain, functional performance, or sensation. Since conservative care is ineffective, surgical treatment should be considered. Although surgical treatment can improve symptoms, postoperative care is also important. Degnan et al. (1997) [30] described the importance of controlling edema early postoperatively for CTS. Furthermore, Cook et al. (1995) [31] reported that hand and wrist exercises should be started early in the postoperative period because splinting of the wrist after CTS surgery may cause bowstringing. Steyers et al. (2002) [32] reported that postoperative care should include early mobilization to encourage tendon and nerve gliding. The beneficial effects of these exercises may include direct mobilization of the nerve, facilitation of venous return, edema dispersal, decreased pressure inside the perineurium, and decreased carpal tunnel pressure [10,33]. Thus, it is recommended to surgically decompress the carpal tunnel in patients with severe CTS; however, NGE should be performed as part of the postoperative care.

Therefore, our research hypothesis is that the combination of surgery and NGE for CTS will improve symptoms and that background factors may contribute to the symptom improvement. Thus, this study aims to determine whether the combination of surgery and NGE improves CTS symptoms and what background factors affect the symptom improvement.

2. Materials and Methods

2.1. Participants

A total of 86 outpatients (31 men and 55 women; mean age 66.8 ± 14.1 years) participated in this study. Table 1 shows the patient characteristics. The inclusion category comprised of those who were prescribed occupational therapy after carpal tunnel release surgery. Exclusion criteria included those who were diagnosed with complex regional pain syndrome, difficulty with NGE due to severe pain, and difficulty understanding instructions.

Table 1. Attributes.

	n
Subjects	67
Hands (Rt/Lt)	86 (48/38)
Age (mean ± SD)	66.8 ± 14.1
Gender	M: 24; F: 43
Dialysis	4
Trigger finger	20
TEA [1] (Rt/Lt)	43 (26/17)

[1] TEA: thenar eminence atrophy; M: Male, F: Female.

All participants were informed of the aim of the study and were requested to provide signed informed consent before participation. This study was approved by the Shijonawate-Gakuen University of Faculty of Rehabilitation research ethics review committee (approval no. 21-2) and conducted in accordance with the Declaration of Helsinki.

2.2. NGE

This study used the NGE method by Nazarieh et al. [34]. Procedures for conducting an NGE (position 1: wrist in neutral and fingers and thumb in flexion; position 2: wrist in neutral and fingers and thumb extended; position 3: thumb in neutral and wrist and fingers extended; position 4: wrist, fingers, and thumb extended: position 5, the same as position 4 with the forearm in supination (palm up); and position 6: same as position 5 with the other hand gently stretching the thumb) were observed (Figure 1).

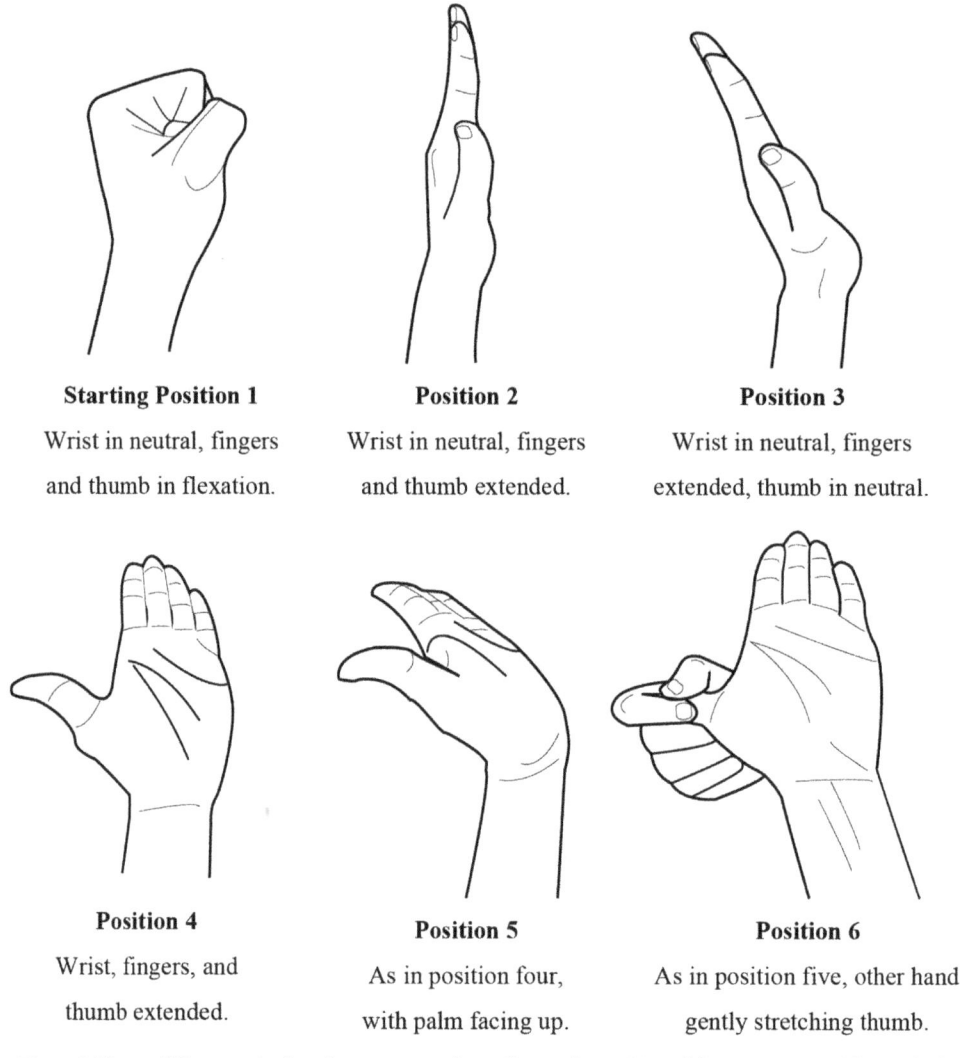

Figure 1. Nerve gliding exercise has six movements depending on the position of the wrist joint and fingers [34].

The NGE was started 4 days postop and performed three times a day during outpatient treatment and self-exercise at home. The NGE is performed in six positions, holding each position for 7 s. These were performed for five sets [35].

2.3. Outcome Measures

Basic information was collected on age, gender, fault side, with/without surgery on both sides (bilateral), with/without trigger finger (trigger finger) [11,15], with/without dialysis (dialysis), with/without thenar eminence atrophy (TEA) [11,15,36], preoperative motor nerve conduction velocity (MCS), and preoperative sensory nerve conduction velocity (SCV), time-to-start treatment (start-treat), and occupational therapy intervention period (OT-inter). Additionally, grip-strength (grip-s), pinch strength (pinch-s), Semmes-Weinstein Monofilament test (SWMT), two-point discrimination (2PD), numerical rating scale score for numbness, numerical rating scale score for pain (pain), and positive angle on Phalen test (Phalen). Each test was measured at a frequency of 1 week postoperatively.

2.3.1. Grip-s and Pinch-s

CTS reduces grip-s and pinch-s [37], which were evaluated with the use of dynamometry [5,15,24].

2.3.2. Semmes-Weinstein Monofilament Test (SWMT)

The SWMT is a noninvasive sensory testing method. Monofilaments of different thicknesses are applied to the test area for 1 s. Scoring is determined according to the thickness of the monofilament perceived to be touched [12,38,39].

2.3.3. Two-Point Discrimination (2PD)

A measure of sensory acuity and light touch—2PD—is tested by measuring the smallest distance in a patient to perceive two pinpricks as separate units. This is a commonly used method for assessing the sensory function of the median nerve [15,24,36].

2.3.4. Numerical Rating Scale (NRS) for Numbness and Pain

The NRS has a numerical range from 0 to 10, with 0 indicating nothing at all and 10 indicating the worst. In this study, we assessed the degree of pain and numbness according to the NRS [40].

2.4. Statistical Analysis

Paired Student's t-test was used to compare whether the combination of CTS surgery and NGE improves grip-s (kgf), pinch-s (kgf), SWMT, 2PD (mm), numbness (NRS), pain (NRS), and Phalen test (angle) at pre- and post-intervention. This test can reveal the effect of CTS surgery and NGE on these parameters that reflect hand function. Multiple regression analysis was performed with endpoints of the effect of combined surgery and NGE as dependent variables and fault side, gender, age, trigger finger, dialysis, bilateral, TEA, MCS, SCV, Start-treat, and OT-inter as independent variables to determine which of the basic characteristics (age, gender, fault side, bilateral, trigger finger, dialysis, TEA, MCV, SCV, start-treat, and OT-inter) affect the parameters associated with hand function at the end of the treatment. The alpha level was set at 0.05.

3. Results

3.1. Comparison between Preintervention and Final Assessments

Comparison between the two groups of preoperative and final evaluations showed significant improvement in grip-s ($p = 0.04$), pinch-s ($p = 0.007$), SWMT ($p = 0.001$), 2PD ($p = 0.005$), numb ($p = 0.001$), and Phalen ($p = 0.001$); Pain was not significantly different ($p = 0.143$) (Table 2).

Table 2. Comparison between preoperative and final assessments.

	Difference between Pre vs. Post		95% CL		p-Value	
	Average	Standard Error	Lower	Upper		
Grip-s (kgf)	1.13	4.45	0.05	2.21	0.04	**
Pinch-s (kgf)	0.45	1.33	0.13	0.77	0.007	**
SWMT	0.96	1.26	0.66	1.26	0.001	**
2PD (mm)	1.71	4.99	0.52	2.91	0.005	**
Numb (score)	4.18	2.38	3.60	4.75	0.001	**
Pain (score)	0.56	3.19	−0.20	1.33	0.14	
Phalen (angle)	16.01	19.49	11.37	20.66	0.001	**

** $p < 0.01$.

3.2. Multiple Regression Analysis

Background factors of each assessment that were significantly different in Result 1 were analyzed using multiple regression analysis. These results of multiple regression analysis showed significant differences in grip-s (F = 1.120, $p < 0.366$, R = 0.437, and $R^2 = 0.192$), and pinch-s (F = 1.513, $p = 0.155$, R = 0.492, and $R^2 = 0.242$) for gender and SCV. SWMT (F = 2.18, $p < 0.03$) in the start-treat and OT-inter. 2PD (F = 1.14, $p < 0.35$) in Start-treat. Pain (F = 1.77, $p = 0.08$), numb (F = 1.77, $p = 0.08$), and Phalen (F = 1.32, $p = 0.24$) were not affected by independent variables set in this study (Tables 3–9).

Table 3. Independent variable for grip-s.

	B	Standard Error	β	B (95% CI) Lower	B (95% CI) Upper	F	t	p-Value		VIF
Age	0.03	0.09	0.05	−0.14	0.20	0.12	0.35	0.727		1.43
Gender	−6.03	2.53	−0.33	−11.10	−0.96	5.70	−2.39	0.021	*	1.20
Fault side	2.42	2.36	0.14	−2.33	7.16	1.05	1.02	0.311		1.21
Bilateral	0.55	2.57	0.03	−4.61	5.70	0.05	0.21	0.832		1.28
Trigger finger	−2.19	1.98	−0.14	−6.17	1.78	1.22	−1.11	0.274		1.09
Dialysis	−4.64	5.54	−0.12	−15.76	6.47	0.70	−0.84	0.406		1.23
TEA	−0.34	2.43	−0.02	−5.23	4.54	0.02	−0.14	0.888		1.33
MCV	−0.08	0.14	−0.08	−0.36	0.20	0.34	−0.58	0.562		1.24
SCV	0.24	0.12	0.30	0.00	0.48	4.11	2.03	0.048	*	1.38
Start-treat	0.04	0.03	0.18	−0.02	0.09	1.83	1.35	0.182		1.15
OT-inter	−0.01	0.10	−0.02	−0.21	0.19	0.01	−0.11	0.914		1.23
Constant	−0.05	13.03		−26.20	26.10	0.00	0.00	0.997		

B: partial regression coefficient; β: standardized partial regression coefficient. 95% CI: 95% confidence interval; VIF: Variance inflation factor; * $p < 0.05$.

Table 4. Independent variable for pinch-s.

	B	Standard Error	β	B (95% CI) Lower	B (95% CI) Upper	F	t	p-Value		VIF
Age	0.00	0.02	−0.03	−0.04	0.03	0.05	−0.23	0.822		1.43
Gender	−1.40	0.48	−0.39	−2.36	−0.44	8.54	−2.92	0.005	**	1.20
Fault side	0.25	0.45	0.07	−0.65	1.14	0.30	0.55	0.587		1.21
Bilateral	0.24	0.49	0.07	−0.74	1.21	0.24	0.49	0.629		1.28
Trigger finger	−0.20	0.38	−0.07	−0.96	0.55	0.29	−0.54	0.594		1.09
Dialysis	−0.77	1.05	−0.10	−2.87	1.34	0.53	−0.73	0.468		1.23
TEA	−0.44	0.46	−0.13	−1.37	0.48	0.92	−0.96	0.343		1.33
MCV	−0.02	0.03	−0.11	−0.07	0.03	0.64	−0.80	0.428		1.24
SCV	0.05	0.02	0.29	0.00	0.09	4.18	2.04	0.046	*	1.38
Start-treat	0.01	0.01	0.21	0.00	0.02	2.65	1.63	0.109		1.15
OT-inter	−0.02	0.02	−0.15	−0.06	0.02	1.22	−1.10	0.275		1.23
Constant	2.18	2.47		−2.78	7.13	0.78	0.88	0.383		

B: partial regression coefficient; β: standardized partial regression coefficient. 95% CI: 95% confidence interval; VIF: Variance inflation factor; * $p < 0.05$, ** $p < 0.01$.

Table 5. Independent variable for SWMT.

	B	Standard Error	β	B (95% CI) Lower	B (95% CI) Upper	F	t	p-Value		VIF
Age	−0.01	0.02	−0.06	−0.04	0.02	0.22	−0.47	0.640		1.43
Gender	−0.62	0.44	−0.18	−1.50	0.26	1.99	−1.41	0.164		1.20
Fault side	0.45	0.41	0.14	−0.38	1.27	1.18	1.08	0.283		1.21
Bilateral	−0.25	0.45	−0.07	−1.15	0.64	0.32	−0.56	0.576		1.28
Trigger finger	0.07	0.34	0.03	−0.62	0.76	0.05	0.21	0.831		1.09
Dialysis	−0.19	0.96	−0.03	−2.12	1.73	0.04	−0.20	0.840		1.23
TEA	0.20	0.42	0.06	−0.65	1.05	0.22	0.47	0.639		1.33
MCV	0.03	0.02	0.14	−0.02	0.08	1.28	1.13	0.263		1.24
SCV	0.03	0.02	0.19	−0.01	0.07	2.03	1.42	0.161		1.38
Start-treat	0.01	0.00	0.30	0.00	0.02	5.81	2.41	0.019	*	1.15
OT-inter	−0.05	0.02	−0.33	−0.08	−0.01	6.82	−2.61	0.012	*	1.23
Constant	−1.46	2.26		−6.00	3.09	0.41	−0.64	0.523		

B: partial regression coefficient; β: standardized partial regression coefficient. 95% CI: 95% confidence interval; VIF: Variance inflation factor; * $p < 0.05$.

Table 6. Independent variable for 2PD.

	B	Standard Error	β	B (95% CI) Lower	B (95% CI) Upper	F	t	p-Value		VIF
Age	0.02	0.05	0.08	−0.07	0.12	0.26	0.51	0.611		1.43
Gender	−0.92	1.38	−0.09	−3.69	1.86	0.44	−0.66	0.509		1.20
Fault side	1.55	1.29	0.16	−1.04	4.15	1.44	1.20	0.236		1.21
Bilateral	1.82	1.41	0.18	−1.00	4.65	1.68	1.30	0.201		1.28
Trigger finger	0.55	1.09	0.07	−1.63	2.73	0.26	0.51	0.616		1.09
Dialysis	−1.54	3.03	−0.07	−7.62	4.55	0.26	−0.51	0.614		1.23
TEA	−0.75	1.33	−0.08	−3.43	1.92	0.32	−0.57	0.574		1.33
MCV	0.10	0.08	0.18	−0.05	0.25	1.68	1.30	0.201		1.24
SCV	0.08	0.06	0.18	−0.05	0.21	1.52	1.23	0.224		1.38
Start-treat	0.03	0.01	0.27	0.00	0.06	4.23	2.06	0.045	*	1.15
OT-intere	0.03	0.05	0.07	−0.08	0.14	0.25	0.50	0.618		1.23
Constant	−16.28	7.14		−30.60	−1.96	5.20	−2.28	0.027	*	

B: partial regression coefficient; β: standardized partial regression coefficient. 95% CI: 95% confidence interval; VIF: Variance inflation factor; * $p < 0.05$.

Table 7. Independent variable for pain.

	B	Standard Error	β	B (95% CI) Lower	B (95% CI) Upper	F	t	p-Value	VIF
Age	0.01	0.03	0.05	−0.05	0.07	0.21	0.35	0.73	1.43
Gender	−1.80	0.89	−0.26	−3.59	−0.01	4.07	−2.02	0.07	1.20
Fault side	1.31	0.84	0.20	−0.36	2.99	2.47	1.57	0.12	1.21
Bilateral	−0.24	0.91	−0.04	−2.07	1.58	0.07	−0.27	0.79	1.28
Trigger finger	−0.02	0.70	0.00	−1.43	1.39	0.00	−0.03	0.98	1.09
Dialysis	−0.81	1.96	−0.05	−4.74	3.12	0.17	−0.42	0.68	1.23
TEA	1.62	0.86	0.26	−0.11	3.35	3.55	1.88	0.07	1.33
MCV	−0.02	0.05	−0.05	−0.12	0.08	0.16	−0.40	0.69	1.24
SCV	0.07	0.04	0.24	−0.01	0.16	3.14	1.77	0.08	1.38
Start-treat	0.02	0.01	0.22	0.00	0.04	3.07	1.75	0.09	1.15
OT-intere	−0.06	0.04	−0.21	−0.13	0.01	2.51	−1.58	0.12	1.23
Constant	−1.76	4.61		−11.01	7.49	0.15	−0.38	0.70	

B: partial regression coefficient; β: standardized partial regression coefficient. 95% CI: 95% confidence interval; VIF: Variance inflation factor.

Table 8. Independent variable for numb.

	B	Standard Error	β	B (95% CI) Lower	B (95% CI) Upper	F	t	p-Value	VIF
Age	−0.03	0.03	−0.12	−0.09	0.04	0.71	−0.84	0.404	1.43
Gender	0.21	0.90	0.03	−1.59	2.02	0.06	0.24	0.812	1.20
Fault side	0.77	0.84	0.12	−0.92	2.46	0.84	0.92	0.363	1.21
Bilateral	−0.87	0.91	−0.13	−2.71	0.96	0.91	−0.96	0.343	1.28
Trigger finger	0.85	0.70	0.15	−0.56	2.27	1.47	1.21	0.232	1.09
Dialysis	−0.07	1.97	0.00	−4.02	3.88	0.00	−0.03	0.973	1.23
TEA	−0.08	0.87	−0.01	−1.82	1.65	0.01	−0.09	0.926	1.33
MCV	0.08	0.05	0.21	−0.02	0.18	2.47	1.57	0.122	1.24
SCV	0.08	0.04	0.27	0.00	0.17	3.83	1.96	0.056	1.38
Start-treat	0.01	0.01	0.18	−0.01	0.03	2.12	1.45	0.152	1.15
OT-intere	−0.03	0.04	−0.11	−0.10	0.04	0.72	−0.85	0.399	1.23
Constant	−9.51	4.63		−18.81	−0.22	4.22	−2.05	0.045 *	

B: partial regression coefficient; β: standardized partial regression coefficient. 95% CI: 95% confidence interval; VIF: Variance inflation factor; * $p < 0.05$.

Table 9. Independent variable for Phalen.

	B	Standard Error	β	B (95% CI) Lower	B (95% CI) Upper	F	t	p-Value	VIF
Age	0.39	0.24	0.24	−0.09	0.88	2.64	1.63	0.110	1.43
Gender	−3.52	7.07	−0.07	−17.71	10.66	0.25	−0.50	0.620	1.20
Fault side	5.10	6.62	0.10	−8.18	18.38	0.59	0.77	0.444	1.21
Bilateral	7.56	7.19	0.15	−6.87	21.99	1.11	1.05	0.298	1.28
Trigger finger	−7.77	5.55	−0.18	−18.90	3.37	1.96	−1.40	0.168	1.09
Dialysis	2.62	15.50	0.02	−28.49	33.72	0.03	0.17	0.867	1.23
TEA	−7.04	6.81	−0.15	−20.72	6.63	1.07	−1.03	0.306	1.33
MCV	0.11	0.39	0.04	−0.68	0.90	0.08	0.28	0.781	1.24
SCV	0.42	0.33	0.18	−0.24	1.09	1.63	1.28	0.207	1.38
Start-treat	0.13	0.08	0.22	−0.03	0.28	2.76	1.66	0.102	1.15
OT-intere	−0.33	0.28	−0.16	−0.88	0.23	1.37	−1.17	0.247	1.23
Constant	−36.69	36.48		−109.88	36.51	1.01	−1.01	0.319	

B: partial regression coefficient; β: standardized partial regression coefficient. 95% CI: 95% confidence interval; VIF: Variance inflation factor.

4. Discussion

4.1. Effectiveness of Surgical Treatment Combined with NGE

In this study, a significant treatment effect was observed for grip-s, pinch-s, SWMT, 2PD, numb, and Phalen, but no effect for pain. The pathophysiology of CTS is a combination of mechanical and ischemic injury of the median nerve in the carpal tunnel [39]. This type of strangulation neuropathy, CTS, can be greatly improved by surgically releasing the pressure on the carpal tunnel. However, the effectiveness of symptom improvement greatly varies depending on the postoperative care method [30–32]. Degnan et al. (1997) reported that early control of edema is important after surgery for CTS [30]. Cook et al. (1995) reported that splint immobilization of the wrist joint postoperatively causes deformity, therefore, early exercise of the fingers and wrist joint is important [31]. Steyers et al. (2002) reported that mobilization should be performed early postoperatively to promote gliding of tendons and nerves [32]. Effects of early mobilization are expected to include nerve stimulation, promotion of venous return, edema resolution and prevention, and reduction of carpal tunnel pressure [10,33,38]. The study results showed that CTS treatment with surgery and NGE can improve hand function, and this finding is in agreement with those of previous studies. Additionally, the positive angle of the Phalen test may have been affected.

Conversely, the pain was not affected by the combination of surgery and NGE as a background factor. This result may be because we did not specify the type or cause of pain evaluated in this study.

4.2. Functions and Factors Improved by Surgery and NGE

Surgical treatment combined with NGE significantly improved grip-s, Pinch-s, SWMT, 2PD, Numb, and Phalen. Regression analysis revealed the possible factors associated with the improvement of these parameters. Grip-s and pinch-s were affected by gender and SCV, SWMT by start-treat and OT-inter, and 2PD by start-treat and OT-inter. Pain, numbness and Phalen are the factors without effect on these. Results of this study showed that SCV and gender affected grip-s and pinch-s. SWMT and 2PD were influenced by start-treat. In contrast, numb and Phalen were not affected by factors as independent variables. Furthermore, SCV and organic factors such as gender were involved in the background of intervention effects in grip-sand pinch-s. Werner et al. (2011) reported that in mild CTS, SCV was delayed but MCV was normal; when CTS was moderate, MCV was delayed in addition to SCV [41]. In other words, SCV was impaired earlier than MCV, and myelin lesion was impaired earlier than the axon lesion. Lew et al. reported that SCV is a sensitive test for CTS [42]. The results of this study also suggest that the involvement of SCV in muscle strength, such as grip-s and pinch-s, sensitively reflects the degree of disability before the MCV effect is achieved.

In both SWMT and 2PD results, start-treat was involved. Gelberman et al. (1981) reported that delayed surgery for CTS could damage the median nerve [43]. Additionally, Choi et al. and Townshend et al. reported that prolonged and severe compression of the median nerve can cause axonal degeneration, rendering SCV immeasurable [44,45]. In other words, we thought that the duration of compression and damage to the median nerve would be a background factor behind the improved SWMT and 2PD.

Of note, pain could not be explained by any factor. Neuropathic pain is a very important target of treatment, but pain improvement is difficult because of the wide variety of causes, not just in CTS [46]. Therefore, to address pain caused by CTS, we should perform a further study, such as a study to explore the cause of pain in patients with CTS.

4.3. Limitation

In this study, the combination of surgery and NGE improved the treatment for muscle strength and sensation, and background factors were identified. However, background factors of numb and Phalen were not identified, which had an improved effect in variables considered as factors, and pain. The present study is limited in its pain examination due to the various possible causes for the pain mechanism.

There was another concern about the interpretation of our data. We did not collect affectable parameters that affect the results, including smoking [47] or alcohol habits [48], physical sporting performance [49], and kinesiophobia [50]. In interpreting the results of this study, it should be noted that the influence of these factors has not been considered. A further study including these parameters is needed.

4.4. Clinical Implications

The results of our current study indicate the positive effect of combination of surgery for CTS and NGE on motor and sensory function in the affected hand, as in previous studies [10–12,22,23]. Therefore, occupational or physical therapy can be recommended as after-therapy to improve motor and sensory function. However, for pain, our result indicates that this combination therapy cannot be enough. If pain remains a crucial problem, other treatments need to be considered.

5. Conclusions

Treatment with NGE after CTS surgery increased the treatment effect on grip-s, pinch-s, SWMT, 2PD, numbness, and Phalen-positive angle. Furthermore, SCV was a background factor for muscle strength, and time-to-treatment initiation was a background factor for sensation.

Author Contributions: Conceptualization, Y.T., A.Y. and A.M.; Data curation, A.Y.; Formal analysis, Y.T. and A.M.; Funding acquisition, Y.T.; Investigation, A.Y.; Methodology, Y.T., A.Y. and A.M.; Project administration, A.Y.; Resources, Y.T. and A.Y.; Software application, Y.T.; Supervision, A.M.; Validation, Y.T. and A.M.; Visualization, Y.T.; Writing—original draft, Y.T.; Writing—review and editing, Y.T., A.Y. and A.M. All authors have read and agreed to the published version of the manuscript.

Funding: This research was funded by JSPS KAKENHI (grant number 21K17418). The APC was funded by JSPS KAKENHI (grant number 21K17418).

Institutional Review Board Statement: The study was conducted according to the guidelines of the Declaration of Helsinki, and approved by the research ethics review committee of the Shijonawate-Gakuen University of Faculty of Rehabilitation (Approval No. 21-2).

Informed Consent Statement: Informed consent was obtained from all subjects involved in the study. Written informed consent has been obtained from the patient(s) to publish this paper.

Data Availability Statement: The data presented in this study are openly available in Mendeley Data at doi:10.17632/dpyg8dw49n.2, reference number [51].

Conflicts of Interest: The authors declare no conflict of interest.

References

1. Gerritsen, A.A.; de Krom, M.C.; Struijs, M.A.; Scholten, R.J.; de Vet, H.C.; Bouter, L.M. Conservative treatment options for carpal tunnel syndrome: A systematic review of randomised controlled trials. *J. Neurol.* **2002**, *249*, 272–280. [CrossRef]
2. Atroshi, I.; Gummesson, C.; Johnsson, R.; Ornstein, E.; Ranstam, J.; Rosén, I. Prevalence of carpal tunnel syndrome in a general population. *JAMA* **1999**, *282*, 153–158. [CrossRef]
3. Papanicolaou, G.D.; McCabe, S.J.; Firrell, J. The prevalence and characteristics of nerve compression symptoms in the general population. *J. Hand Surg.* **2001**, *26*, 460–466. [CrossRef]
4. Bakhtiary, A.H.; Rashidy-Pour, A. Ultrasound and laser therapy in the treatment of carpal tunnel syndrome. *Aust. J. Physiother.* **2004**, *50*, 147–151. [CrossRef]
5. Vogt, T.; Scholz, J. Clinical outcome and predictive value of electrodiagnostics in endoscopic carpal tunnel surgery. *Neurosurg. Rev.* **2002**, *25*, 218–221. [CrossRef] [PubMed]
6. Fernández-de-Las-Peñas, C.; Pérez-de-Heredia-Torres, M.; Martínez-Piédrola, R.; de la Llave-Rincón, A.I.; Cleland, J.A. Bilateral deficits in fine motor control and pinch grip force in patients with unilateral carpal tunnel syndrome. *Exp. Brain Res.* **2009**, *194*, 29–37. [CrossRef]
7. Li, K.; Evans, P.J.; Seitz, W.H., Jr.; Li, Z.M. Carpal tunnel syndrome impairs sustained precision pinch performance. *Clin. Neurophysiol.* **2015**, *126*, 194–201. [CrossRef]
8. Huisstede, B.M.; Randsdorp, M.S.; Coert, J.H.; Glerum, S.; van Middelkoop, M.; Koes, B.W. Carpal tunnel syndrome. Part II: Effectiveness of surgical treatments—A systematic review. *Arch. Phys. Med. Rehabil.* **2010**, *91*, 1005–1024. [CrossRef] [PubMed]
9. Burke, D.T.; Burke, M.M.; Stewart, G.W.; Cambré, A. Splinting for carpal tunnel syndrome: In search of the optimal angle. *Arch. Phys. Med. Rehabil.* **1994**, *75*, 1241–1244. [CrossRef]
10. Burke, F.D.; Ellis, J.; McKenna, H.; Bradley, M.J. Primary care management of carpal tunnel syndrome. *Postgrad. Med. J.* **2003**, *79*, 433–437. [CrossRef]
11. Michlovitz, S.L. Conservative interventions for carpal tunnel syndrome. *J. Orthop. Sports Phys. Ther.* **2004**, *34*, 589–600. [CrossRef] [PubMed]
12. Osterman, A.L.; Whitman, M.; Porta, L.D. Nonoperative carpal tunnel syndrome treatment. *Hand Clin.* **2002**, *18*, 279–289. [CrossRef]
13. Ucan, H.; Yagci, I.; Yilmaz, L.; Yagmurlu, F.; Keskin, D.; Bodur, H. Comparison of splinting, splinting plus local steroid injection and open carpal tunnel release outcomes in idiopathic carpal tunnel syndrome. *Rheumatol. Int.* **2006**, *27*, 45–51. [CrossRef] [PubMed]
14. Verdugo, R.J.; Salinas, R.A.; Castillo, J.L.; Cea, J.G. Surgical versus non-surgical treatment for carpal tunnel syndrome. *Cochrane Database Syst. Rev.* **2008**, *2008*, Cd001552. [CrossRef]
15. Baysal, O.; Altay, Z.; Ozcan, C.; Ertem, K.; Yologlu, S.; Kayhan, A. Comparison of three conservative treatment protocols in carpal tunnel syndrome. *Int. J. Clin. Pract.* **2006**, *60*, 820–828. [CrossRef] [PubMed]
16. Page, M.J.; O'Connor, D.; Pitt, V.; Massy-Westropp, N. Exercise and mobilisation interventions for carpal tunnel syndrome. *Cochrane Database Syst. Rev.* **2012**, *2012*, Cd009899. [CrossRef] [PubMed]
17. Page, M.J.; O'Connor, D.; Pitt, V.; Massy-Westropp, N. Therapeutic ultrasound for carpal tunnel syndrome. *Cochrane Database Syst. Rev.* **2013**, *2013*, Cd009601. [CrossRef] [PubMed]
18. Hui, A.C.; Wong, S.; Leung, C.H.; Tong, P.; Mok, V.; Poon, D.; Li-Tsang, C.W.; Wong, L.K.; Boet, R. A randomized controlled trial of surgery vs steroid injection for carpal tunnel syndrome. *Neurology* **2005**, *64*, 2074–2078. [CrossRef]

19. Ly-Pen, D.; Andréu, J.L.; de Blas, G.; Sánchez-Olaso, A.; Millán, I. Surgical decompression versus local steroid injection in carpal tunnel syndrome: A one-year, prospective, randomized, open, controlled clinical trial. *Arthritis Rheum.* **2005**, *52*, 612–619. [CrossRef]
20. Marshall, S.; Tardif, G.; Ashworth, N. Local corticosteroid injection for carpal tunnel syndrome. *Cochrane Database Syst. Rev.* **2007**, *2007*, Cd001554. [CrossRef]
21. McKeon, J.M.M.; Yancosek, K.E. Neural gliding techniques for the treatment of carpal tunnel syndrome: A systematic review. *J. Sport Rehabil.* **2008**, *17*, 324–341. [CrossRef] [PubMed]
22. Lim, Y.H.; Chee, D.Y.; Girdler, S.; Lee, H.C. Median nerve mobilization techniques in the treatment of carpal tunnel syndrome: A systematic review. *J. Hand Ther.* **2017**, *30*, 397–406. [CrossRef] [PubMed]
23. Muller, M.; Tsui, D.; Schnurr, R.; Biddulph-Deisroth, L.; Hard, J.; MacDermid, J.C. Effectiveness of hand therapy interventions in primary management of carpal tunnel syndrome: A systematic review. *J. Hand Ther.* **2004**, *17*, 210–228. [CrossRef]
24. Akalin, E.; El, O.; Peker, O.; Senocak, O.; Tamci, S.; Gülbahar, S.; Cakmur, R.; Oncel, S. Treatment of carpal tunnel syndrome with nerve and tendon gliding exercises. *Am. J. Phys. Med. Rehabil.* **2002**, *81*, 108–113. [CrossRef]
25. Pinar, L.; Enhos, A.; Ada, S.; Güngör, N. Can we use nerve gliding exercises in women with carpal tunnel syndrome? *Adv. Ther.* **2005**, *22*, 467–475. [CrossRef]
26. Heebner, M.L.; Roddey, T.S. The effects of neural mobilization in addition to standard care in persons with carpal tunnel syndrome from a community hospital. *J. Hand Ther.* **2008**, *21*, 229–241. [CrossRef] [PubMed]
27. Coppieters, M.W.; Alshami, A.M. Longitudinal excursion and strain in the median nerve during novel nerve gliding exercises for carpal tunnel syndrome. *J. Orthop. Res.* **2007**, *25*, 972–980. [CrossRef]
28. Tal-Akabi, A.; Rushton, A. An investigation to compare the effectiveness of carpal bone mobilisation and neurodynamic mobilisation as methods of treatment for carpal tunnel syndrome. *Man. Ther.* **2000**, *5*, 214–222. [CrossRef]
29. Horng, Y.S.; Hsieh, S.F.; Tu, Y.K.; Lin, M.C.; Horng, Y.S.; Wang, J.D. The comparative effectiveness of tendon and nerve gliding exercises in patients with carpal tunnel syndrome: A randomized trial. *Am. J. Phys. Med. Rehabil.* **2011**, *90*, 435–442. [CrossRef]
30. Degnan, G.G. Postoperative management following carpal tunnel release surgery: Principles of rehabilitation. *Neurosurg. Focus* **1997**, *3*, e8. [CrossRef]
31. Cook, A.C.; Szabo, R.M.; Birkholz, S.W.; King, E.F. Early mobilization following carpal tunnel release. A prospective randomized study. *J. Hand Surg.* **1995**, *20*, 228–230. [CrossRef]
32. Steyers, C.M. Recurrent carpal tunnel syndrome. *Hand Clin.* **2002**, *18*, 339–345. [CrossRef]
33. Seradge, H.; Jia, Y.C.; Owens, W. In Vivo measurement of carpal tunnel pressure in the functioning hand. *J. Hand Surg.* **1995**, *20*, 855–859. [CrossRef]
34. Nazarieh, M.; Hakakzadeh, A.; Ghannadi, S.; Maleklou, F.; Tavakol, Z.; Alizadeh, Z. Non-Surgical Management and Post-Surgical Rehabilitation of Carpal Tunnel Syndrome: An Algorithmic Approach and Practical Guideline. *Asian J. Sports Med.* **2020**, *11*, e102631. [CrossRef]
35. Rozmaryn, L.M.; Dovelle, S.; Rothman, E.R.; Gorman, K.; Olvey, K.M.; Bartko, J.J. Nerve and tendon gliding exercises and the conservative management of carpal tunnel syndrome. *J. Hand Ther.* **1998**, *11*, 171–179. [CrossRef]
36. Wolny, T.; Linek, P. Reliability of two-point discrimination test in carpal tunnel syndrome patients. *Physiother. Theory Pract.* **2019**, *35*, 348–354. [CrossRef] [PubMed]
37. Simovic, D.; Weinberg, D.H. Carpal tunnel syndrome. *Arch. Neurol.* **2000**, *57*, 754–755. [CrossRef] [PubMed]
38. Feng, Y.; Schlösser, F.J.; Sumpio, B.E. The Semmes Weinstein monofilament examination as a screening tool for diabetic peripheral neuropathy. *J. Vasc. Surg.* **2009**, *50*, 675–682.e671. [CrossRef] [PubMed]
39. Werner, R.A.; Andary, M. Carpal tunnel syndrome: Pathophysiology and clinical neurophysiology. *Clin. Neurophysiol.* **2002**, *113*, 1373–1381. [CrossRef]
40. Phan, N.Q.; Blome, C.; Fritz, F.; Gerss, J.; Reich, A.; Ebata, T.; Augustin, M.; Szepietowski, J.C.; Ständer, S. Assessment of pruritus intensity: Prospective study on validity and reliability of the visual analogue scale, numerical rating scale and verbal rating scale in 471 patients with chronic pruritus. *Acta Derm.-Venereol.* **2012**, *92*, 502–507. [CrossRef] [PubMed]
41. Werner, R.A.; Andary, M. Electrodiagnostic evaluation of carpal tunnel syndrome. *Muscle Nerve* **2011**, *44*, 597–607. [CrossRef]
42. Lew, H.L.; Date, E.S.; Pan, S.S.; Wu, P.; Ware, P.F.; Kingery, W.S. Sensitivity, specificity, and variability of nerve conduction velocity measurements in carpal tunnel syndrome. *Arch. Phys. Med. Rehabil.* **2005**, *86*, 12–16. [CrossRef]
43. Gelberman, R.H.; Hergenroeder, P.T.; Hargens, A.R.; Lundborg, G.N.; Akeson, W.H. The carpal tunnel syndrome. A study of carpal canal pressures. *J. Bone Jt. Surgery. Am. Vol.* **1981**, *63*, 380–383. [CrossRef]
44. Choi, S.J.; Ahn, D.S. Correlation of clinical history and electrodiagnostic abnormalities with outcome after surgery for carpal tunnel syndrome. *Plast. Reconstr. Surg.* **1998**, *102*, 2374–2380. [CrossRef] [PubMed]
45. Townshend, D.N.; Taylor, P.K.; Gwynne-Jones, D.P. The outcome of carpal tunnel decompression in elderly patients. *J. Hand Surg.* **2005**, *30*, 500–505. [CrossRef]
46. Serrano Afonso, A.; Carnaval, T.; Videla Ces, S. Combination Therapy for Neuropathic Pain: A Review of Recent Evidence. *J. Clin. Med.* **2021**, *10*, 3533. [CrossRef] [PubMed]
47. Hulkkonen, S.; Auvinen, J.; Miettunen, J.; Karppinen, J.; Ryhanen, J. Smoking as risk factor for carpal tunnel syndrome: A birth cohort study. *Muscle Nerve* **2019**, *60*, 299–304. [CrossRef]

48. Nathan, P.A.; Keniston, R.C.; Lockwood, R.S.; Meadows, K.D. Tobacco, caffeine, alcohol, and carpal tunnel syndrome in American industry. A cross-sectional study of 1464 workers. *J. Occup. Environ. Med.* **1996**, *38*, 290–298. [CrossRef]
49. Meirelles, L.M.; Fernandes, C.H.; Ejnisman, B.; Cohen, M.; dos Santos, J.B.G.; Albertoni, W.M. The prevalence of carpal tunnel syndrome in adapted Sports athletes based on clinical diagnostic. *Orthop. Traumatol. Surg. Res.* **2020**, *106*, 751–756. [CrossRef]
50. Bartlett, O.; Farnsworth, J.L. The Influence of Kinesiophobia on Perceived Disability in Patients With an Upper-Extremity Injury: A Critically Appraised Topic. *J. Sport Rehabil.* **2021**, *30*, 818–823. [CrossRef]
51. Tamaru, Y.; Yanagawa, A.; Matsugi, A. Dataset_CTS, Mendeley Data, Version 2. 2021. Available online: https://data.mendeley.com/research-data/?search=doi:10.17632/dpyg8dw49n.2 (accessed on 9 September 2021).

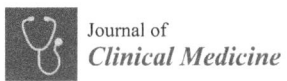

Article

Effect of Posterior Pelvic Tilt Taping on Pelvic Inclination, Muscle Strength, and Gait Ability in Stroke Patients: A Randomized Controlled Study

Tae-sung In [1,†], Jin-hwa Jung [2,†], May Kim [3], Kyoung-sim Jung [1,*] and Hwi-young Cho [4,*]

1. Department of Physical Therapy, Gimcheon University, Gimcheon 39528, Korea; 20160072@gimcheon.ac.kr
2. Department of Occupational Therapy, Semyung University, Jecheon 27136, Korea; otsalt@semyung.ac.kr
3. Department of Physical Education, College of Education, Korea University, Seoul 02841, Korea; kimmay@korea.ac.kr
4. Department of Physical Therapy, College of Health Science, Gachon University, Incheon 21936, Korea
* Correspondence: 20190022@gimcheon.ac.kr (K.-s.J.); hwiyoung@gachon.ac.kr (H.-y.C.)
† These two authors contributed equally to this study as co-first author.

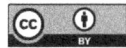

Citation: In, T.-s.; Jung, J.-h.; Kim, M.; Jung, K.-s.; Cho, H.-y. Effect of Posterior Pelvic Tilt Taping on Pelvic Inclination, Muscle Strength, and Gait Ability in Stroke Patients: A Randomized Controlled Study. J. Clin. Med. 2021, 10, 2381. https://doi.org/10.3390/jcm10112381

Academic Editors: Akiyoshi Matsugi, Naoki Yoshida, Hideki Nakano and Yohei Okada

Received: 30 April 2021
Accepted: 25 May 2021
Published: 28 May 2021

Publisher's Note: MDPI stays neutral with regard to jurisdictional claims in published maps and institutional affiliations.

Copyright: © 2021 by the authors. Licensee MDPI, Basel, Switzerland. This article is an open access article distributed under the terms and conditions of the Creative Commons Attribution (CC BY) license (https:// creativecommons.org/licenses/by/ 4.0/).

Abstract: Objective: Pelvic alignment asymmetry in stroke patients negatively affects postural control ability. This study aimed to investigate the effect of posterior pelvic tilt taping on pelvic inclination, muscle strength, and gait ability in stroke patients. Methods: Forty stroke patients were recruited and randomly divided into the following two groups: the posterior pelvic tilt taping (PPTT) group ($n = 20$) and the control group ($n = 20$). All participants underwent sitting-to-standing, indoor walking, and stair walking training (30 min per day, 5 days per week, for 6 weeks). The PPTT group applied posterior pelvic tilt taping during the training period, while the control group did not receive a tape intervention. Pelvic inclination was measured using a palpation meter (PALM). A hand-held dynamometer and the 10-meter walk test were used to measure muscle strength and gait ability. Results: Significantly greater improvements in the pelvic anterior tilt were observed in the PPTT group than in the control group ($p < 0.05$). Muscle strength in the PPTT group was significantly increased compared to the control group ($p < 0.05$). Significantly greater improvements in gait speed were observed in the PPTT group than the control group. Conclusions: According to our results, posterior pelvic tilt taping may be used to improve the anterior pelvic inclination, muscle strength, and gait ability in stroke patients.

Keywords: pelvic inclination; taping; gait; stroke

1. Introduction

The pelvis is an important structure that connects the torso and lower limbs to support and transmit weight to the lower limbs when performing various functional movements. In addition, the pelvis is a part of the lower trunk in the sitting position but becomes a functional element of the lower limb when standing or walking [1]. Therefore, changes in pelvic alignment in a standing position also affect balance, gait, and functional performance [2]. In addition, proper pelvic control is essential for the establishment of more economical movements and gait [3], and if this is not properly controlled during gait, the speed, stability, and efficiency decrease [4–6].

In order to properly perform functional movements, such as sitting-to-standing [7] or walking [8], the ability to move weight to the affected lower limb must be preceded. However, in stroke patients, body deficits such as loss of sensation, impaired motor function of the upper and lower extremities, spasticity, and muscle weakness are caused by damage to the blood vessels in the brain. This results in a secondary damage in body control and a change in pelvic alignment, resulting in decreased weight support on the paralyzed side [9]. In addition, stroke patients show a forward tilted posture alignment compared to a healthy person when maintaining a standing posture [10] or show a posture in which the pelvis is tilted anteriorly and to the affected side [9].

Kinesio taping was introduced by Kenzo Kase as a method of attaching an elastic adhesive tape with elasticity similar to that of the skin and is currently used in rehabilitation for various purposes [11]. Taping is applied in combination with other therapeutic techniques to strengthen weakened muscles, regulate joint instability, assist postural alignment, reduce pain, improve blood flow and lymphatic circulation, relieve spasticity, and strengthen muscle function [12–14]. Additionally, studies have reported that pelvic inclination decreases when taping is applied for posture correction [15–19]. Lee et al. reported that a significant difference occurred in the pelvic inclination angle when seated workers were divided into a group in which anterior pelvic tilt taping was applied and a group in which it was not, and a slumped sitting posture was maintained for 30 min [16]. Therefore, it was determined that taping can help prevent the musculoskeletal problems caused by an awkward sitting posture [16]. In a study in which posterior pelvic tilt taping was applied for a week to patients experiencing lower-back pain with hyperlordosis, it was found that lumbar lordosis, pain, disability, and abdominal thickness were improved compared to the control group [18]. They said that the skin irritation due to the tape would have improved the abdominal strength by allowing more units of exercise to be mobilized [18]. These studies were also conducted in stroke patients. Mehta et al. reported that when taping was attached to the thoracic and abdomen of stroke patients, the pelvic obliquity and anterior pelvic tilt in a sitting position were improved compared to the control group, which resulted in improved balance [20]. In addition, one study reported that posterior pelvic tilt taping significantly improved pelvic anterior tilt, gait speed, and step length in stroke patients, but further studies are needed as the long-term effects have not been confirmed [21].

Therefore, this study aimed to investigate the effect of posterior pelvic tilt taping on pelvic inclination, lower extremity muscle strength, and gait ability in stroke patients.

2. Experimental Section

2.1. Participants

We used G*power 3.1.9.2 software (Heinrich-Heine-University Düsseldorf, version 3.1.9.4, Düsseldorf, Germany) to calculate the sample size. In the present study, the mean power was set to 0.8 and the alpha error was set to 0.05. In addition, the effect size was set to 0.8148 based on a pilot study (10 subjects). The analysis of G*power software showed that at least 18 participants would make an acceptable group sample size for each group; thus, 42 participants were recruited in consideration of dropout.

Participants were recruited from the H rehabilitation centers in Gyeonggi-do. The inclusion criteria were as follows: (1) first episode of unilateral stroke with hemiparalysis caused by hemicerebrum damage; (2) an anterior pelvic inclination greater than $15°$ (normal range, $11 \pm 4°$) [22–24]; (3) the ability to understand and follow verbal commands; (4) the ability to independently walk for at least 15 m without assistance; and (5) Brunnstrom stage 3 or higher motor recovery of the lower extremity. The exclusion criteria included the following: (1) hemianopia, dizziness, or other symptoms indicating vestibular impairment; (2) neglect and sensory loss; and (3) an orthopedic disease influencing gait.

This trial was approved by the Gachon University Institutional Review Board (1044396-202006-HR-112-01) and was registered (WHO International Clinical Trials Registry Platform, KCT0005215). Prior to enrollment in the study, the content of the study was explained to all of the participants and written consent was obtained. Table 1 shows the characteristics of the subjects in the posterior pelvic tilt taping (PPTT) and control groups. The subjects were randomly assigned to the PPTT group ($n = 21$) or control group ($n = 21$) using a selection envelope. Before the post-evaluation, one person from each group dropped out due to skin redness and a change of address. A total of 40 subjects were evaluated for pelvic inclination, muscle strength, and gait ability after 6 weeks of training (Figure 1).

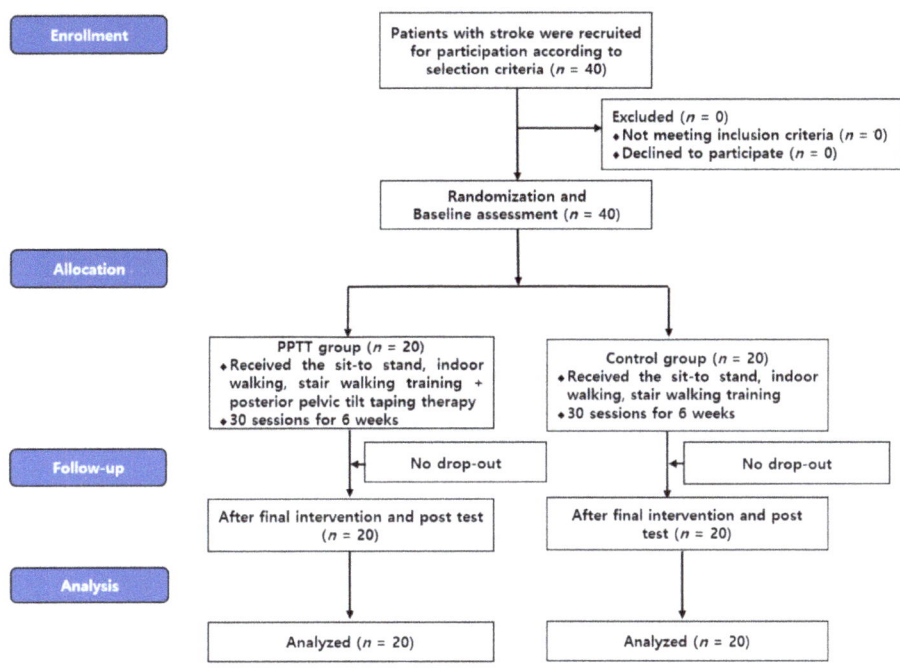

Figure 1. CONSORT flow diagram.

Table 1. Common and clinical characteristics of the subjects (N = 40).

Variables	PPTT Group (n = 20)	Control Group (n = 20)	p
Sex (male/female)	14/6	15/5	0.723 [b]
Affected side (right/left)	12/8	11/9	0.749 [b]
Age (years)	55.8 ± 8.5 [a]	54.4 ± 9.9	0.361 [c]
Height (cm)	165.9 ± 9.1	166.5 ± 9.9	0.856 [c]
Weight (kg)	62.4 ± 8.7	63.9 ± 8.4	0.758 [c]
Stroke duration (months)	8.0 ± 1.9	7.1 ± 2.6	0.315 [c]
Disease (diabetes/hypercholesterolemia/hypertension/ ≥ 2)	1/1/12/6	1/2/10/7	
Work (engineer/white-collar jobs/etc.)	5/10/5	6/8/6	
Sport activities (none/running/golf/tennis)	14/3/3/2	12/4/3/1	

PPTT, Posterior pelvic tilt taping. [a] mean ± standard deviation, [b] chi–square test, [c] independent t-test.

2.2. Intervention

In both the PPTT group and the control group, sit-to-stand, indoor walking, and stair walking training were performed for 30 min per day, 5 times per week, for 6 weeks. In sit-to-stand training, to increase the weight support for the affected side, the big toe of the affected foot was placed in the middle of the healthy foot, and the subjects were then instructed to stand up without supporting their arm. Indoor walking training included straight walking and S-shaped walking; for stair walking, the subjects were instructed to go up and down stairs that had a height of 10 cm each. All of the training sessions were supervised by a physiotherapist with more than 5 years of rehabilitation experience. In addition, the PPTT group applied posterior pelvic tilt taping. For mechanical correction, a 5-centimeter-wide tape was extended to 50–75% of its original length and attached to both rectus abdominis (RA) and external oblique (EO) muscles [18]. First, the pelvis was tilted posteriorly in the side-lying position and then attached to the EO muscle from the inguinal region to the spinous process of T12. For mechanical correction of the posterior pelvic tilt, the pelvis from the anterior superior iliac spine (ASIS) to the posterior superior iliac spine (PSIS) was attached while tilting in the posterior direction. Finally, the RA muscle was attached from the pubic symphysis to the xiphoid process in the knee bent and supine positions (Figure 2). The tape was changed once every 3 days.

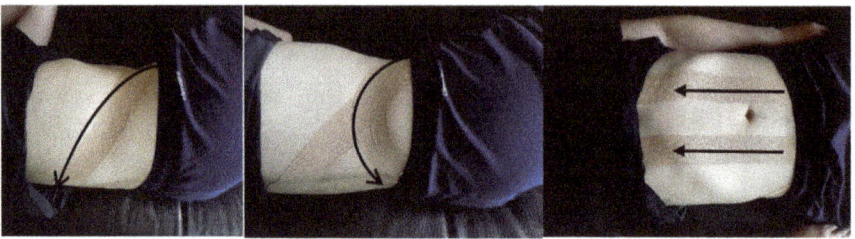

Figure 2. Application of the posterior pelvic tilt taping.

2.3. Outcome Measurements

Pelvic inclination was measured using an inclinometer and a palpation meter (PALM; Performance Attainment Associations, St. Paul, MN, USA) consisting of two caliper arms. This measurement tool was reported to be highly reliable for measuring height differences between landmarks [25]. In this study, before measurement, the subjects stood upright with the front of their thigh in contact with a fixed table, then the caliper tip of the PALM was positioned on the ASIS and PSIS on the paralytic side, respectively, to measure the anterior tilt angle.

The isometric strength of the hip extensor was measured using a handheld dynamometer (Model 01163; Lafayette Inc., IN, USA). The subjects were instructed to stretch their hip joint, flex their knee joints by 90°, and to extend their legs backwards against the hand-held dynamometer for 5 seconds in a side-lying position. The average value of three measurements was used. The handheld dynamometer is known to have high intra-rater and inter-rater reliability in patients with nervous system damage [26].

Gait ability was measured using the 10-meter walk test (10MWT). This measurement tool measures the time it takes to walk 10 meters, and the intra-rater and inter-rater reliabilities have been reported to be high [27].

2.4. Data Analysis

Statistical analysis was performed using SPSS 21.0 (IBM, Armonk, NY, USA). The Shapiro–Wilk test was used to evaluate the normality of the variables. Independent t-tests and chi–square tests were used to compare the baseline characteristics of the two groups of continuous and categorical variables. A paired t-test was performed to examine the changes in pelvic inclination, strength, and gait speed within a group. An independent t-test was used to determine any significant differences between the two groups in the amount of change in pelvic inclination, strength, and gait speed before and after 6 weeks of training. The significance level was set at $p < 0.05$.

3. Results

3.1. General Characteristics of Participants

No significant difference was found in the general characteristics between the PPTT and control groups before treatment (Table 1). In this study, there was one person who complained of redness due to the tape, but no other person complained of any special side effects.

3.2. Changes in Pelvic Inclination

The PPTT group (mean change, each 18.2 ± 3.6 vs. 14.2 ± 2.8, $p < 0.05$) showed a greater degree of improvement in pelvic inclination than the control group (mean change, each 16.9 ± 2.8 vs. 15.5 ± 2.8, $p < 0.05$) (Table 2).

Table 2. Changes in pelvic inclination of the study participants (N = 40).

	PPTT Group			Control Group			
	Pre-Test	Post-Test	Difference	Pre-Test	Post-Test	Difference	p-Value
Pelvic inclination (°)	18.2 ± 3.6	14.2 ± 2.8 *	−4.0 ± 2.8	16.9 ± 2.8	15.5 ± 2.8 *	−1.4 ± 1.2	<0.001

PPTT, Posterior pelvic tilt taping. * Significant difference between pre-test and post-test ($p < 0.05$).

3.3. Changes in Muscle Strength

Significantly greater improvements in hip extensor muscle strength were observed in the PPTT group (mean change, each 9.9 ± 2.4, 14.6 ± 3.0, $p < 0.05$) than in the control group (mean change, each 10.7 ± 1.7, 12.6 ± 1.6, $p < 0.05$) (Table 3).

Table 3. Changes in the muscle strength of the study participants (N = 40).

	PPTT Group			Control Group			
	Pre-Test	Post-Test	Difference	Pre-Test	Post-Test	Difference	p-Value
Muscle strength (kg)	9.9 ± 2.4	14.6 ± 3.0 *	4.7 ± 2.3	10.7 ± 1.7	12.6 ± 1.6 *	1.8 ± 1.7	<0.001

PPTT, Posterior pelvic tilt taping. * Significant difference between pre-test and post-test ($p < 0.05$).

3.4. Changes in Gait Speed

After training, the PPTT group (26.0 ± 5.1 vs. 21.1 ± 4.1, $p < 0.05$) showed a more significant improvement in gait speed than the control group (24.6 ± 4.6 vs. 22.3 ± 4.0, $p < 0.05$) (Table 4).

Table 4. Changes in the gait speed of the study participants (N = 40).

	PPTT Group			Control Group			
	Pre-Test	Post-Test	Difference	Pre-Test	Post-Test	Difference	p-Value
10MWT (sec)	26.0 ± 5.1	21.1 ± 4.1 *	−4.9 ± 1.6	24.6 ± 4.6	22.3 ± 4.0 *	−2.3 ± 2.8	0.003

PPTT, Posterior pelvic tilt taping; 10MWT, 10 m walk test. * Significant difference between pre-test and post-test ($p < 0.05$).

4. Discussion

In this study, we investigated whether the application of posterior pelvic tilt taping in stroke patients with an anterior pelvic inclination affected pelvic inclination. As a result, the anterior pelvic tilt angle in the PPTT group was significantly decreased compared to the control group. Unlike traditional methods, taping applied to the pelvis has elasticity that exceeds the original length [11], and this elasticity increases overall joint movement, skin deformation [28], and stimulation of cutaneous mechanoreceptors [29]. In a study that investigated the effect of taping in lower-back pain patients with increased lordosis, the anterior pelvic tilt was reduced by applying tape to the RA and EO. They reported that as stimulation to mechanoreceptors activates nerve impulses, the strength of the abdominal muscles increases, and consequently, the anterior pelvic tilt decreases [17]. In addition, Bozorgmehr et al. argued that the length–tension relationship of the muscle could be optimized as the application of taping can continuously pull the fascia concentrically and shorten the distance between the muscle origin and insertion, and this could have a positive effect on the joint alignment [18]. The reason the anterior pelvic tilt decreased in this study is thought to be because, as in the previous study, the attachment method, which increases the elasticity of the tape, stimulates the skin's mechanoreceptors to activate the muscles involved in the posterior tilt of the pelvis, such as the RA and EO. Trunk muscle attaches to the pelvis and provides core stability, which is an important factor in the normal postural alignment of the pelvis [30,31]. Since the trunk is bilaterally innervated and connected by the linea alba with fascia, damage to one side of the brain affects all of the abdominal muscles, which in turn affects the position of the anterior superior iliac spines [9]. The normal anterior pelvic tilt angle was reported as $11 \pm 4°$ [22–24]. In this study, a stroke patient with a pelvic anterior tilt angle of $15°$ or more was targeted. After training, the anterior pelvic tilt angle of the PPTT group was $14.2°$, which was within the normal range, indicating clinically significant results.

In addition, in this study, as a result of examining the effect on the muscle strength of the hip extensor involved in the posterior tilt of the pelvis after training, it was confirmed that the PPTT group had a significant improvement compared to the control group. In stroke patients, altered pelvic alignment makes trunk–pelvic dissociation difficult or decreases control of the hip muscles around the pelvis, resulting in asymmetrical weight distribution on the affected side during gait [32], which in turn leads to a weakening of the affected limb due to non-use. In a study on the pelvic alignment of stroke patients, pelvic asymmetry was reported to have a significant correlation with weight-bearing asymmetry [9]. In addition, Verheyden et al. reported that the posture of stroke patients is forward leaning compared to healthy adults, and that posture control ability decreased significantly as the bent increased [10]. In this study, in the case of the PPTT group, posterior pelvic tilt taping was applied during sitting-to-standing, indoor walking, and stair walking training. Although the change in the center of mass was not measured in this study, it is thought that as the alignment of the pelvis was improved, the center of mass was moved backward, thereby promoting the muscle activity of the hip extensor. Dubey et al. reported that the hip extensor's muscle strength and gait speed were improved after pelvic stability training, which is related to the recruitment of more motor units and the reorganization of the muscle fiber structure as an adaptive response to postural alignment [1].

Previous studies reported that stroke patients exhibit low temporal synchronization between the pelvis and lower extremities when walking or performing functional postures and showed anterior pelvic tilt with impaired motor function [5,6]. Moreover, Kim et al. confirmed that the anterior pelvic tilt in stroke patients had significant negative correlations with gait velocity, cadence, and step length [22]. In addition, in stroke patients, weakening of the hip extensor, which is most involved in the terminal stance of the gait, affects the movement control of the hip and knee flexion during the ipsilateral swing phase, resulting in a decrease in walking speed [33,34]. In this study, the gait speed of the PPTT group significantly increased after training compared to the control group, which is thought to be due to the improvement of the anterior pelvic tilt and the resulting increase in the muscle strength of the hip extensor, resulting in an improved posture in the stance phase.

In this study, we confirmed that posterior pelvic tilt taping has a significant effect on pelvic inclination, muscle strength, and gait ability in stroke patients. Pelvic asymmetry causes a negative effect on postural control in stroke patients, but there is no exercise specifically designed for this, and it is more difficult to correct the patient. If the taping attachment method used in this study is used during weight support training, which is widely used for the rehabilitation of stroke patients, it will help to correct the pelvic alignment easily at home by activating the muscles that posteriorly tilt the pelvis. However, it is difficult to generalize due to the small number of subjects, and it was not confirmed whether activation of the trunk muscle was increased, or the center of gravity was changed. Therefore, in a future study, it will be necessary to examine the effects on various gait variables such as cadence, step length, and gait symmetry, as well as the angle of the trunk and lower limb joints whilst walking using a 3D motion analyzer, along with the activation of the trunk muscles.

5. Conclusions

The results of this study demonstrated that posterior pelvic tilt taping can improve pelvic tilt, leg muscle strength, and gait in stroke patients with excessive anterior pelvic tilt.

Author Contributions: T.-s.I., conceptualization; K.-s.J., writing—original draft preparation; H.-y.C., methodology; J.-h.J. and M.K., investigation and measurement visualization; T.-s.I. and H.-y.C., writing–review and editing. All authors have read and agreed to the published version of the manuscript.

Funding: This work was supported by the Ministry of Education of the Republic of Korea and the National Research Foundation of Korea (NRF-2020S1A5A2A03042018).

Institutional Review Board Statement: This trial was approved by the Gachon University Institutional Review Board (1044396-202006-HR-112-01) and was registered (WHO International Clinical Trials Registry Platform, KCT0005215).

Informed Consent Statement: Prior to enrollment in the study, the content of the study was explained to all of the participants and written consent was obtained.

Data Availability Statement: The data presented in this study are available on request from the corresponding author.

Conflicts of Interest: All authors declare no potential conflicts of interest.

References

1. Dubey, L.; Karthikbabu, S.; Mohan, D. Effects of Pelvic Stability Training on Movement Control, Hip Muscles Strength, Walking Speed and Daily Activities after Stroke: A Randomized Controlled Trial. *Ann. Neurosci.* **2018**, *25*, 80–89. [CrossRef]
2. Verheyden, G.; Vereeck, L.; Truijen, S.; Troch, M.; Herregodts, I.; Lafosse, C.; Nieuwboer, A.; De Weerdt, W. Trunk performance after stroke and the relationship with balance, gait and functional ability. *Clin. Rehabil.* **2006**, *20*, 451–458. [CrossRef]
3. Staszkiewicz, R.; Chwala, W.; Forczek, W.; Laska, J. Three-dimensional analysis of the pelvic and hip mobility during gait on a treadmill and on the ground. *Acta. Bioeng. Biomech.* **2012**, *14*, 83–89.
4. Chen, C.L.; Chen, H.C.; Tang, S.F.T.; Wu, C.Y.; Cheng, P.T.; Hong, W.H. Gait performance with compensatory adaptations in stroke patients with different degrees of motor recovery. *Am. J. Phys. Med. Rehabil.* **2003**, *82*, 925–935. [CrossRef]
5. Dickstein, R.; Abulaffio, N. Postural sway of the affected and nonaffected pelvis and leg in stance of hemiparetic patients. *Arch. Phys. Med. Rehabil.* **2000**, *81*, 364–367. [CrossRef]
6. Titianova, E.B.; Tarkka, I.M. Asymmetry in walking performance and postural sway in patients with chronic unilateral cerebral infarction. *J. Rehabil. Res. Dev.* **1995**, *32*, 236–244.
7. Lomaglio, M.J.; Eng, J.J. Muscle strength and weight-bearing symmetry relate to sit-to-stand performance in individuals with stroke. *Gait. Posture* **2005**, *22*, 126–131. [CrossRef]
8. Tyson, S.F. Trunk kinematics in hemiplegic gait and the effect of walking aids. *Clin. Rehabil.* **1999**, *13*, 295–300. [CrossRef]
9. Karthikbabu, S.; Chakrapani, M.; Ganesan, S.; Ellajosyula, R. Relationship between Pelvic Alignment and Weight-bearing Asymmetry in Community-dwelling Chronic Stroke Survivors. *J. Neurosci. Rural Pract.* **2016**, *7*, S37–S40. [CrossRef]
10. Verheyden, G.; Ruesen, C.; Gorissen, M.; Brumby, V.; Moran, R.; Burnett, M.; Ashburn, A. Postural alignment is altered in people with chronic stroke and related to motor and functional performance. *J. Neurol. Phys. Ther.* **2014**, *38*, 239–245. [CrossRef]
11. Briem, K.; Eythörsdöttir, H.; Magnúsdóttir, R.G.; Pálmarsson, R.; Rúnarsdóttir, T.; Sveinsson, T. Effects of kinesio tape compared with nonelastic sports tape and the untapped ankle during a sudden inversion perturbation in male athletes. *J. Orthop. Sports Phys. Ther.* **2011**, *41*, 328–335. [CrossRef]
12. Kase, K.; Wallis, J.; Kase, T. *Clinical Therapeutic Applications of the Kinesio Taping Method*, 2nd ed.; Kinesio Taping Association: Tokyo, Japan, 2003; pp. 19–39.
13. Lee, H.; Lim, H. Effects of Double-Taped Kinesio Taping on Pain and Functional Performance due to Muscle Fatigue in Young Males: A Randomized Controlled Trial. *Int. J. Environ. Res. Public. Health* **2020**, *17*, 2364. [CrossRef] [PubMed]
14. Paoloni, M.; Bernetti, A.; Fratocchi, G.; Mangone, M.; Parrinello, L.; Cooper, M.D.P.; Sesto, L.; Di Sante, L.; Santilli, V. Kinesio taping applied to lumbar muscles influences clinical and electromyographic characteristics in chronic low back pain patients. *Eur. J. Phys. Rehabil. Med.* **2011**, *47*, 237–244. [PubMed]
15. Lee, J.H.; Yoo, W.G.; Gak, H.B. The immediate effect of anterior pelvic tilt taping on pelvic inclination. *J. Phys. Ther. Sci.* **2011**, *23*, 201–203. [CrossRef]
16. Lee, J.H.; Yoo, W.G. The mechanical effect of anterior pelvic tilt taping on slump sitting by seated workers. *Ind. Health* **2011**, *49*, 403–409. [CrossRef]
17. Lee, J.H.; Yoo, W.G. Application of posterior pelvic tilt taping for the treatment of chronic low back pain with sacroiliac joint dysfunction and increased sacral horizontal angle. *Phys. Ther. Sport* **2012**, *13*, 279–285. [CrossRef]

18. Bozorgmehr, A.; Takamjani, E.I.; Akbari, M.; Salehi, R.; Mohsenifar, H.; Rasouli, O. Effect of Posterior Pelvic Tilt Taping on Abdominal Muscle Thickness and Lumbar Lordosis in Individuals With Chronic Low Back Pain and Hyperlordosis: A Single-Group, Repeated-Measures Trial. *J. Chiropr. Med.* **2020**, *19*, 213–221. [CrossRef]
19. Lee, J.H.; Yoo, W.G.; Kim, M.H.; Oh, J.S.; Lee, K.S.; Han, J.T. Effect of posterior pelvic tilt taping in women with sacroiliac joint pain during active straight leg raising who habitually wore high-heeled shoes: A preliminary study. *J. Manip. Physiol. Ther.* **2014**, *37*, 260–268. [CrossRef]
20. Mehta, M.; Joshua, A.M.; Karthikbabu, S.; Misri, Z.; Unnikrishnan, B.; Mithra, P.; Nayak, A. Effect of Taping of Thoracic and Abdominal Muscles on Pelvic Alignment and Forward Reach Distance Among Stroke Subjects: A Randomized Controlled Trial. *Ann. Neurosci.* **2019**, *26*, 10–16. [CrossRef]
21. Ting, W.Y. The Immediate Effect of Posterior Pelvic Tilt Taping on Gait Function and Balance in Chronic Stroke Patients. Master's Thesis, Daegu University, Daegu, Korea, 2017.
22. Kim, M.K.; Kim, S.G.; Shin, Y.J.; Choi, E.H.; Choe, Y.W. The relationship between anterior pelvic tilt and gait, balance in patient with chronic stroke. *J. Phys. Ther. Sci.* **2018**, *30*, 27–30. [CrossRef]
23. Hagins, M.; Brown, M.; Cook, C.; Gstalder, K.; Kam, M.; Kominer, G.; Strimbeck, K. Intratester and intertester reliability of the palpation meter (PALM) in measuring pelvic position. *J. Manual. Manip. Ther.* **1998**, *6*, 130–136. [CrossRef]
24. Levine, D.; Whittle, M.W. The effects of pelvic movement on lumbar lordosis in the standing position. *J. Orthop. Sports Phys. Ther.* **1996**, *24*, 130–135. [CrossRef]
25. Gnat, R.; Saulicz, E.; Bialy, M.; K1aptocz, P. Does pelvic asymmetry always mean pathology? Analysis of mechanical factors leading to the asymmetry. *J. Hum. Kinet.* **2009**, *21*, 23–35. [CrossRef]
26. Bohannon, R.W. Test-retest reliability of hand-held dynamometry during a single session of strength assessment. *Phys. Ther.* **1986**, *66*, 206–209. [CrossRef]
27. Steffen, T.M.; Hacker, T.A.; Mollinger, L. Age- and gender-related test performance in community-dwelling elderly people: Six-Minute Walk Test, Berg Balance Scale, Timed up & Go Test, and gait speeds. *Phys. Ther.* **2002**, *82*, 128–137.
28. Shim, J.Y.; Lee, H.R.; Lee, D.C. The use of elastic adhesive tape to promote lymphatic flow in the rabbit hind leg. *Yonsei Med. J.* **2003**, *44*, 1045–1052. [CrossRef]
29. Chang, H.Y.; Chou, K.Y.; Lin, J.J.; Lin, C.F.; Wang, C.H. Immediate effect of forearm Kinesio taping on maximal grip strength and force sense in healthy collegiate athletes. *Phys. Ther. Sport* **2010**, *11*, 122–127. [CrossRef]
30. Lee, D. *The Pelvic Girdle: An Integration of Clinical Expertise and Research*, 3rd ed.; Churchill Livingstone: London, UK, 2004.
31. Yu, S.H.; Park, S.D. The effects of core stability strength exercise on muscle activity and trunk impairment scale in stroke patients. *J. Exerc. Rehabil.* **2013**, *9*, 362–367. [CrossRef]
32. Patterson, K.K.; Parafianowicz, I.; Danells, C.J.; Closson, V.; Verrier, M.C.; Staines, W.R.; Black, S.E.; McIlroy, W.E. Gait asymmetry in community-ambulating stroke survivors. *Arch. Phys. Med. Rehabil.* **2008**, *89*, 304–310. [CrossRef]
33. Moore, S.; Schurr, K.; Wales, A.; Moseley, A.; Herbert, R. Observation and analysis of hemiplegic gait: Swing phase. *Aust. J. Physiother.* **1993**, *39*, 271–278. [CrossRef]
34. Cruz, T.H.; Lewek, M.D.; Dhaher, Y.Y. Biomechanical impairments and gait adaptations post-stroke: Multi-factorial associations. *J. Biomech.* **2009**, *42*, 1673–1677. [CrossRef]

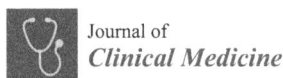

Review

Neurorehabilitation in Multiple Sclerosis—A Review of Present Approaches and Future Considerations

Carmen Adella Sîrbu [1], Dana-Claudia Thompson [2,3], Florentina Cristina Plesa [1,4,*], Titus Mihai Vasile [1,5,*], Dragoș Cătălin Jianu [6], Marian Mitrica [4], Daniela Anghel [7,†] and Constantin Stefani [8,9,†]

1. Department of Neurology, 'Dr. Carol Davila' Central Military Emergency University Hospital, 010242 Bucharest, Romania
2. Department of Rehabilitation Medicine, Elias Emergency University Hospital, 011461 Bucharest, Romania
3. Alessandrescu-Rusescu National Institute for Mother and Child Health, Fetal Medicine Excellence Research Center, 020395 Bucharest, Romania
4. Department of Preclinical Disciplines, Titu Maiorescu University, 031593 Bucharest, Romania
5. Clinical Neurosciences Department, University of Medicine and Pharmacy "Carol Davila", 050474 Bucharest, Romania
6. Centre for Cognitive Research in Neuropsychiatric Pathology (Neuropsy-Cog), Department of Neurology, Faculty of Medicine, "Victor Babeș" University of Medicine and Pharmacy, 300041 Timișoara, Romania
7. Department of Medico-Surgical and Prophylactic Disciplines, Titu Maiorescu University, 031593 Bucharest, Romania
8. Department of Family Medicine and Clinical Base, 'Dr. Carol Davila' Central Military Emergency University Hospital, 010242 Bucharest, Romania
9. Department No. 5, University of Medicine and Pharmacy "Carol Davila", 050474 Bucharest, Romania
* Correspondence: plesacristina@yahoo.com (F.C.P.); mtvasile@yahoo.com (T.M.V.)
† These authors contributed equally to this work as co-last authors.

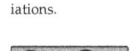

Abstract: Multiple sclerosis is an increasingly prevalent disease, representing the leading cause of non-traumatic neurological disease in Europe and North America. The most common symptoms include gait deficits, balance and coordination impairments, fatigue, spasticity, dysphagia and an overactive bladder. Neurorehabilitation therapeutic approaches aim to alleviate symptoms and improve the quality of life through promoting positive immunological transformations and neuroplasticity. The purpose of this study is to evaluate the current treatments for the most debilitating symptoms in multiple sclerosis, identify areas for future improvement, and provide a reference guide for practitioners in the field. It analyzes the most cited procedures currently in use for the management of a number of symptoms affecting the majority of patients with multiple sclerosis, from different training routines to cognitive rehabilitation and therapies using physical agents, such as electrostimulation, hydrotherapy, cryotherapy and electromagnetic fields. Furthermore, it investigates the quality of evidence for the aforementioned therapies and the different tests applied in practice to assess their utility. Lastly, the study looks at potential future candidates for the treatment and evaluation of patients with multiple sclerosis and the supposed benefits they could bring in clinical settings.

Keywords: multiple sclerosis; rehabilitation; gait; balance; fatigue; spasticity; dysphagia; overactive bladder; neurorehabilitation

1. Introduction

Multiple sclerosis (MS) is an immunologically driven pathology affecting the central nervous system, characterized by chronic inflammation and progressive demyelinating lesions, with an unidentified etiology [1]. MS is currently affecting 2.8 million people worldwide, while in North America and Europe it is the leading cause of chronic non-traumatic neurological disease in young adults [2]. The prevalence is higher in women (69%) than in men (31%), and the number of children below the age of 18 reported to suffer from MS is continuously increasing [2].

The symptoms caused by multiple sclerosis cover a wide spectrum of neurological impairments, due to the nature of the lesions, which can be located in various areas of the central nervous system. However, the most common of them include diplopia (double vision), loss of sight in one or more areas of the visual field, nystagmus, dysphagia (difficulty swallowing solids, liquids or both), dysphonia, cognitive function impairments, alterations in all types of sensitive perception, fatigue, gait and balance disorders, ataxia, spasticity, and bowel and bladder disorders [3,4]. In addition to the above-mentioned impairments, walking is also gradually affected, specifically the speed and distance covered without the occurrence of fatigue, leading to an increased dependence in the activities of daily living (ADL) and a decreased quality of life (QoL) [5,6]. To assess the level of disability and therapeutic approaches in clinical settings for patients suffering from multiple sclerosis, Dr. John Kurtzke developed in the 1950s the Kurtzke Disability Status Scale (DSS), which has since been modified several times and led to the currently used 10-point Expanded Disability Status Scale (EDSS) [7]. The EDSS measures gait and eight additional functional systems (FS): pyramidal (motor function), cerebellar, brainstem, sensory, bowel and bladder, visual, cerebral or mental and other. The scores start at 0, which translates into a normal neurological exam; 1–3 corresponds to a mild disability, without signs of affected ambulation; 3.5–5.5 represents a moderate disability, with patients starting to display ambulation restrictions; a score of 6–6.5 requires walking aids; 7–8 refers to the need to use a wheelchair; in the 8.5 to 9.5 range, the patient is generally restricted to bed and a score of 10 corresponds to death due to MS [8].

One of the treatments used for multiple sclerosis consists of drug therapies that have the capacity to positively influence the rate of relapses, the progression of lesions on MRI (magnetic resonance imaging) scans, as well as the overall evolution of the disease [9]. However, while the majority of these medicines are able to improve certain parameters, such as ambulation capability, fatigue, and spasticity to various degrees, studies show they have little effect on pre-existing neurological deficits [10,11].

Neurorehabilitation has only recently been considered a treatment option in the context of multiple sclerosis, and is generally being used either as a supportive therapy for the control of symptoms or as a preventive approach for the consequences related to a sedentary lifestyle [12–14]. Studies show that MS patients that are included in rehabilitation programs improved their quality of life and are more independent in their activities of daily living [15,16]. Furthermore, several symptoms associated with MS are beneficially impacted through exercise, such as cardiovascular capacity [17], neuromuscular function [18], ambulation [19], depression [20], and cognitive performance [21]. Recently, neuroimaging techniques have also revealed the positive effects of neurorehabilitation on the anatomy and physiology of the brain, together with markers of inflammation [22–25].

Neurorehabilitation is a therapeutic option for all multiple sclerosis patients that is constantly adapting and improving together with the advancement of technology, making it an increasingly affordable and easy-to-self-administer approach [26]. With the advent of the COVID-19 pandemic, professionals have made more use of novel techniques to allow patients to participate remotely in programs through telerehabilitation [27]. Moreover, various types of passive exercise technologies, which can target specific brain areas involved in MS, are being implemented in everyday practice, such as noninvasive brain stimulation (NIBS) and robot-assisted therapy devices [28]. More specifically, repetitive transcranial magnetic stimulation (rTMS) as a form of NIBS has proven its utility in the treatment of cognitive deficits, spasticity and fatigue in the context of multiple sclerosis [29,30].

2. The Effect of Neurorehabilitation on the Neurobiological Particularities of Multiple Sclerosis Patients

The central nervous system (CNS) possesses a characteristic called neuroplasticity, which can be defined by its ability to adapt and remodel as a result of environmental pressure, exerted upon itself by disease or injury [31]. This adaptive response triggers alterations in the neuroglia (changes of number and size), the grey matter (the building of new synapses, dendritic branching modifications and axonal sprouting) and the white matter (myelin production, fiber density alterations) [31]. Neuroplasticity can be noticed subsequent to neurological lesions such as stroke, and has also been documented in patients with MS, potentially compensating for the damage caused by the demyelination processes [11]. Research involving functional magnetic resonance imaging (fMRI) highlights the ability of MS patients' brains to continuously reorganize, but in an apparently limited manner in severe cases of MS, possibly due to the extension of the underlying lesions [31]. A study conducted by Bonzano et al. demonstrated that the neuroplasticity in MS could be preserved through neurorehabilitation programs designed to extend over predetermined periods of time [32]. Moreover, other research involving fMRI scans showed that in comparison to the control groups, non-disabled MS patients used more energy when asked to perform simple tasks and presented more activated areas in the brain [33]. Neuroplasticity influences a variety of functions, such as memory, cognition, and motor function [34–37].

The literature regarding the fMRI changes in the brains of MS patients also analyzed the impacts of cognitive rehabilitation [38]. Following cognitive rehabilitation programs, resting-state MRI neuroimaging revealed an improvement in the patterns of brain synchronization and cognitive performance, involving areas in the right frontal middle orbital gyrus and the visual medial resting state network (RSN), from the cerebellum crus 1 region, which corresponded to the clinically observed improved performances [38]. Furthermore, other studies achieved similar results when using the classic block-design fMRI technique [39–42], thus underlining the importance of the cerebellum in performing executive tasks and in the process of cognition.

Nevertheless, changes occurring in the architecture of the brain through neuroplasticity can also be detrimental to the individual, by sustaining or contributing to the preexisting disability [43,44]. To exemplify this, a number of studies have suggested that brain plasticity is preserved regardless of the severity of the cerebral pathology, as long as rehabilitation focuses on repeating a task for a sufficient amount of time [43–45], while others report a decreased or potentially absent adaptive capacity in patients suffering from a primary progressive form of MS, as opposed to those with relapsing–remitting MS [46]. Furthermore, research shows that the newly formed network connections in the brains of MS patients have a higher complexity level than the previous architecture of the healthy brain, unlike other conditions, such as stroke, where brain tissue restoration follows its original network patterns [47–52]. In addition, the neuroplasticity of patients with MS could decline after two years of an initial increase, thus leading to a progression of the disease and disability [53,54].

Besides the changes in neuroplasticity determined by neurorehabilitation programs, the exercises involved can also induce peripheral immunomodulatory responses [55,56]. Research focusing on experimental autoimmune encephalomyelitis (EAE) in mice found that endurance and resistance training protocols could enhance the immunosuppressive functions by elevating the markers of regulatory T lymphocytes (Treg), therefore leading to an improvement in neurological disability [57], and this was further confirmed through passive immunization [58,59]. Consequential benefits were also observed regarding cytokine levels, infiltrating immune cells, astrogliosis, and microgliosis [55,56]. Recently, a novel regulatory connection between the peripheral immune system and the hypothalamus was discovered in EAE mice through environmental enrichment. The research highlights the immunomodulatory activity determined by the effect of the brain-derived neurotrophic factor (BDNF), produced in the hypothalamus, upon the glucocorticoid receptor in thymocytes [60]. Likewise, demyelinating models in mice, using cuprizone (CPZ) and lysolecithin (LCT), showed the potential of voluntary exercise to determine myelination and direct anti-inflammatory effects, through reduced microgliosis, astrogliosis and the loss of myelin, and enhanced myelin production capacity and the proliferation of oligodendrocyte precursor cells (OPCs), respectively [61,62].

Lastly, neurorehabilitation programs may have beneficial effects on the gut microbiota of patients with a long history of MS, which could improve the level of inflammation related to the disease [63]. Past studies observed various levels of dysbiosis in patients suffering from multiple sclerosis when compared to healthy individuals, with a severe depletion in short-chain fatty acids (SCFAs)-producing bacteria from the Lachnospiraceae family [64–66]. One of the SCFAs that is of particular importance in the context of multiple sclerosis is butyrate, a bacterial metabolite that is involved in preserving the integrity of the intestinal barrier, and also in the process of Treg differentiation [67–71]. Furthermore, higher levels of bacteria involved in pro-inflammatory responses were detected in the case of MS patients, with gut microbiota enriched in species such as Prevotella and Collinsella [63,72,73]. The reassessment of the individuals involved in the study following a complex rehabilitation routine revealed an improved clinical status, namely, improved fatigue and gait, in tight correlation with reduced inflammatory markers, particularly the pro-inflammatory cytokine IL-17 and a more balanced gut microbiota [63].

3. Present Therapeutic Approaches

Multiple sclerosis causes a wide range of symptoms determined by various lesional patterns in the central nervous system that lead to a degree of handicap. While the relapsing–remitting form most commonly displays visual and sensory deficiencies (46% and 41% respectively), primary–progressive MS typically displays gait impairments (88%) and various degrees of paresis (38%) [74]. Symptoms may have a variable influence on the quality of life of each patient, with fatigue being the most commonly reported disturbance of everyday life activities [75]. The median survival time is around 40 years from the moment it was diagnosed; therefore, many MS patients report a variable degree of disability throughout the course of the disease. About 29% of patients require a wheelchair and 50% are using walking aids 15 years following the diagnosis [76]. Furthermore, the median time of retirement is 11.1 years from diagnosis, which is significantly lower than in the average population [77]. Treatments that aim to improve the symptoms of multiple sclerosis are therefore essential, and must take a multidisciplinary approach between a number of medical specialties, requiring medication, neurorehabilitation, and psychological therapy.

3.1. Disease-Modifying Therapies and Symptomatic Medication in Multiple Sclerosis

Patients diagnosed with multiple sclerosis are required to follow a strict drug therapy course for the rest of their lives. The gold standard treatment for acute relapses is represented by intravenous steroids administered in high doses to diminish the inflammatory damage and accelerate the recovery process [78]. Pro-inflammatory metabolite clearance through plasmapheresis could also be considered in cases that do not show an improvement after steroids [79]. Chronic medical treatment includes various classes of drugs, amongst which immunomodulatory medicines represent the first-line agents [80]. Beta interferons (IFNβ) were the first disease-modifying therapies to be approved in 1993, offering clinicians a valuable tool to reduce the number of relapses and to postpone the onset of disability in relapsing–remitting MS patients [81]. Other drugs utilized for the treatment of relapsing–remitting MS include injectable therapies such as glatiramer acetate and oral therapies such as fingolimod, dimethyl fumarate, diroximel fumarate, teriflunomide, Siponimod, and cladribine [82]. The only available treatment for primary–progressive MS is ocrelizumab [82]. Other lines of treatment aim at improving the debilitating symptoms associated with the progression of the disease. Therefore, drug therapies with gabapentin, tizanidine or baclofen have been proven effective in reducing spasticity [83,84]; botulinum toxin injections or oral oxybutynin could improve overactive bladder symptoms [85,86]; fatigue management could be achieved using modafinil or amantadine [87], while lamotrigine, gabapentin and carbamazepine could alleviate sudden pain attacks [88,89]. However, while effective in managing the disease, the above-mentioned treatments do not stop the progression of multiple sclerosis.

3.2. Physical Rehabilitation Strategies

The focus of rehabilitation is to help patients with multiple sclerosis acquire the best possible recovery, allowing them to reduce their physical and mental impairments and offering them the possibility to remain completely or partially integrated in society. For instance, the current guidelines of the National Health Service (NHS) in the UK offer patients suffering from MS a two-week rehabilitation program, consisting of a personalized number of daily sessions of the following therapies: physiotherapy, occupational therapy, speech and language therapy, diet and nutrition advice and neuropsychology [90]. Further, this paper will discuss the current approaches to neurorehabilitation for the most common symptoms of multiple sclerosis. It is worth mentioning that patients with multiple sclerosis might present a variety of the following symptoms in different degrees of severity. Various techniques can be used for treating multiple symptoms. The goal of rehabilitation is to improve the quality of life of MS patients, by targeting the most debilitating symptoms for each individual, without overexerting them. Thus, when putting together a neurorehabilitation routine for a specific MS patient, the practitioner should consider using techniques that are both efficient and target more than one symptom that particular patient is presenting. The symptoms and overlapping techniques used for their treatment are presented in Figure 1.

Treatment Type	Gait Management	Balance & Coordination	Fatigue Management	Spasticity Management	Dysphagia Management	Bladder Management	Cognitive Rehabilitation
Physical Training							
Hydrotherapy							
Proprioceptive Neuromuscular Facilitation							
Therapeutic Standing on An Oswestry Standing Frame							
Hippotherapy							
Transcranial Direct Current Stimulation							
Botulinum Toxin Injections							
Virtual Reality							
Robotic Exoskeletons							
Robotic-Assisted Gait Training							
Ankle-Foot Orthoses							
Cryotherapy							
Pulsed Electromagnetic Field Therapy							
Functional Electrical Stimulation							
Occupational Therapy							
Speed-Intensive Gait Training							
Frenkel Exercises							
Stabilometric Platform							
The Bobath Concept							
Breathing Exercises							
Vibration Therapy							
Transcutaneous Electrical Nerve Stimulation							
Neuromuscular Electrical Stimulation							
Speech-Language Therapy							
Pelvic Floor Muscle Training							
Bladder Training							
Cognitive-Behavioral Therapy							
Neurocognitive Rehabilitation							
Computer-Assisted Cognitive Rehabilitation							

Figure 1. Multiple sclerosis symptoms and rehabilitation treatments. Caption: Rehabilitation treatments ordered by number of symptoms addressed in multiple sclerosis patients.

3.2.1. Gait Management

Walking impairment is one of the most frequent and debilitating symptoms experienced by people diagnosed with multiple sclerosis, with up to 93% of them experiencing a variable degree of gait limitation 10 years after diagnosis [91,92]. Objectively, walking disabilities can be measured in a clinical setting using well-established tests, such as the 2-Minute Walk Test (2MWT), the 6-Minute Walk Test (6MWT) [93], the Timed 25-Foot Walk test (T25FW) [94] and the 12-Item Multiple Sclerosis Walking Scale (MSWS-12) [95]. These tests are useful tools for assessing the activity of the disease, and offer the possibility of evaluating treatment efficacy.

The majority of patients with multiple sclerosis present muscle weakness, more frequently in the trunk and lower limbs. This is considered one of the most important contributing factors that determine gait impairment [96–98]. Strength training is therefore crucial, and should be performed at least twice every week in the process of rehabilitation for people with MS [99]. Moreover, studies have shown that this type of physical activity is beneficial for maintaining neuroplasticity through the activation of motor units and firing rate synchronization [100]. Strength training exercises can be performed using a variety of techniques, machines and weight levels, and can target different muscle groups, with all of these different approaches offering similar outcomes [101]. When it comes to weights, some clinicians prefer using solely the body weight of the patient performing the exercises [102,103], while others choose weight machines, resistance bands [104] or cuff weights [105]. The weight machines most commonly utilized are the traditional ones [106–108], or may include isokinetic dynamometers [109]. Finally, the typically targeted muscle groups include the ones involved in knee extension [105–108], knee flexion [106,110,111], hip extension, flexion [104,106,108] and abduction [103,104], and ankle flexion [109] and extension [110], with most programs consisting of a combination of the abovementioned.

A complementary type of exercise for people with gait deficiencies is endurance training—for example, walking and cycling, which aim to improve aerobic capacity and allow MS patients to walk increasingly longer distances [112]. However, due to the increased risk of falling, body weight-supported treadmill training (BWSTT) is preferred—an exercise that can be useful in the early initiation phase [113]. A novel and more efficient way of performing BWSTT is through robotic-assisted gait training (RAGT), which is more stable, provides a reduced workload for the physiotherapist and is more physiological and reproducible [114]. While most studies focus on progressive resistance training, there is also an alternative approach to gait training. One particular exercise that can be replicated on body weight-supported devices is speed-intensive gait training, involving alternating short intervals of walking at faster speeds with longer periods of walking at a normal pace [115]. This can enhance endurance, speed and other measurable parameters, both in the healthy population [116,117] and in patients suffering from neurological impairments [118,119].

Ankle–foot orthoses (AFOs) represent a frequently recommended solution for gait, balance and strength improvement [120]. Previous studies suggest that their utility is more pronounced in people with higher levels of disability [121]. Recently, clinicians have also started recommending textured insoles for similar purposes, which have shown promising results after repeated plantar stimulation for more than two weeks [122,123].

3.2.2. Balance and Coordination Management

Balance and coordination impairments are some of the most common issues reported by patients suffering from multiple sclerosis. Exercises that focus on balance improvement should aim at preventing falls, and enhancing walking stability and posture control, while those targeted at improving coordination should reduce energy requirements and increase the continuity of movement. Frenkel exercises are commonly used for this purpose. They consist of slow repetitions of each stage of movement that gradually increase in complexity and require high levels of concentration. For instance, the action of sitting up is split into three phases—withdrawing the feet, bending the trunk forward, straightening the legs while getting up [124]. In order to improve the accuracy of exercises for each individual case, patients that are capable of standing without support can be required to perform the exercises on a stabilometric platform [125]. Balance and coordination training can be complemented by proprioception exercises, which further decrease the risk of injury in patients affected by balance impairments [126]. An alternative to the abovementioned is hippotherapy, which uses the natural movement of a horse to improve balance and gait in people suffering from various neurological conditions [127].

A certain degree of variation is required during the rehabilitation process of people with MS, due to the lengthy periods of time involved, which could determine a lower level of motivation and compliance to treatment. Therefore, the Bobath concept could be used as an option to improve the outcomes of these patients [128]. The Bobath concept, also known as neurodevelopmental treatment, is a problem-solving approach, which assumes dysfunctional postural reflexes needed for movement coordination and equilibrium are the essential cause of motor deficits in people with central nervous system lesions [124]. It focuses on inhibiting pathological tonic reflexes in order to achieve appropriate active motion and muscle tension. The approach is also more convenient for people with higher EDSS scores, thanks to the fact that it can be applied in a multitude of positions, including supine and prone positions.

Proprioceptive neuromuscular facilitation (PNF) is a rehabilitation technique that can also be used to improve balance and coordination, together with mobility and spasticity [129,130]. It enhances the muscle function through stimulation of the proprioceptive organs present in tendons and muscles, thus improving postural reflexes and increasing balance, strength and flexibility [131,132]. The method has been extensively studied and proven efficient in patients with post-stroke impairments, and requires further assessment in patients with MS, as it could provide a valuable addition to their treatment.

3.2.3. Fatigue Management

Another frequent symptom reported by MS patients is fatigue, which is encountered in 75–95% of cases [133–135] and is considered a key factor affecting the quality of life in these people [136,137]. Fatigue is defined as a perceived reduction in physical and mental energy that hinders everyday activities [135]. Physical exercise, especially aerobic training, can improve both primary and secondary fatigue in MS patients, through direct changes in the central nervous system and inflammation reduction, but also by improving depression symptoms and quality of sleep [138]. Physical exercises for fatigue management should be adapted to each individual, taking into consideration the patient's degree of disability [139]. These include strength exercises, aerobic training (walking, running, swimming, cycling), neuromotor exercises (dancing, tai chi, yoga, pilates) and breathing exercises [138].

In addition to physical training, physiotherapy procedures should be used to enhance the effects of exercise. Approaches using high temperatures should be avoided, considering the negative impact of heat on nerve conductivity and fatigue [140]. Cryotherapy has proven its potential benefits on fatigue management in several instances, either through whole-body cryotherapy, which involves short sessions of whole-body exposure to ultra-low temperatures ($-110\ °C$) [141], or by using a cooling garment [142]. However, patients with certain conditions, such as hypertension, cardiovascular diseases, a history of blood clotting or thyroid sufferance, should not be exposed to cryotherapy [141].

Another procedure for MS patients with fatigue is pulsed electromagnetic field therapy (PEMF). One of the advantages of this technique is that it offers the option of using it at home, through a small, portable device [143]. One of the routines studied involved 8 min sessions, two times a day for 12 weeks, which resulted in significant improvements in the level of perceived fatigue [144].

Training programs can also be enhanced by functional electrical stimulation (FES) in patients with MS [145,146]. One study analyzed the effects of muscular electrical stimulation through FES during cycling. The researchers observed an amelioration of pain, fatigue and cognitive impairment after 24 weeks of training [145]. In another paper, FES was applied on the quadricep muscles during training, showing beneficial effects on fatigue levels after 8 weeks [146].

3.2.4. Spasticity Management

A symptom that is particularly debilitating in MS is spasticity. This can involve all four limbs, with an increased predilection towards the lower extremities, and it is measured by the Modified Ashworth Scale (MAS) that ranges from 0 (no increase in tone) to 4 (flexion and extension are limited in the examined part). In moderation, spasticity can exert beneficial effects on blood circulation and can counter muscle atrophy. However, beyond a certain level, it leads to joint malformations, contractures and pressure ulcers. Spasticity is present in 40–60% of MS patients [124].

The management of spasticity requires a spectrum of therapies including medication (baclofen administered through intrathecal or oral route), transcranial magnetic stimulation, botulinum toxin injections and physiotherapy [147–149]. Of the abovementioned, physiotherapy is the most utilized treatment applied to patients living with spasticity [150]. The approaches taken by rehabilitation programs to treat this impairment range from physical training to vibration therapy (focal muscle vibration or whole-body vibration), hydrotherapy, electrical stimulation, radial shock wave therapy, electromagnetic fields, cryotherapy, and therapeutic standing on an Oswestry standing frame [149]. Their aim is to maintain neuroplasticity, prevent contracture and preserve the length of muscles [151].

Rehabilitation plans should not employ intense physical efforts, which can aggravate spasticity, and instead should prioritize the use of physical agents ahead of exercise training, for enhancing the efficiency of the latter [124]. Cryotherapy is one of the procedures that can be used prior to exercise initiation, and is utilized either systemically through whole-body cryotherapy and ice baths, or locally through cryo cuffs, cooling garments and ice massage [152,153]. Its purpose is to induce local anesthesia and reduce the reaction to active stretching.

Physical training to alleviate spasticity should be introduced gradually, starting with lighter exercises and avoiding intense stretching, and should concentrate on improving the range of motion of the ankle dorsiflexion, decreasing the muscle tone in the calf, and enhancing the strength of the antigravity muscles [154,155]. Literature reviews have found significant improvements in spasticity and MAS in patients engaged in BWSTT and RAGT [156,157], and in those performing outpatient exercises, such as walking, endurance, aquatic, active and passive stretching exercises [149].

Electrotherapy is another physiotherapeutic method for alleviating spasticity. It can be applied in the form of transcutaneous electrical nerve stimulation (TENS), functional electrical stimulation (FES), neuromuscular electrical stimulation (NMES), and Hufschmidt electrical stimulation. TENS is typically used for the treatment of pain; however, it can provide an alternative treatment for spasticity, if used prior to physical training [158,159]. The method uses electrodes placed on dermatomes or along the nerves, delivering frequencies that range between 1 and 100 Hz. The frequency can be adapted to every individual level of feeling, yet most studies involving spastic paresis used frequencies of 99–100 Hz [159]. The intensity ranged between 15 and 50 mA and the impulse duration between 0.06 and 0.2 ms [159]. In contrast, FES uses rectangular pulse currents with lower frequencies of 20–50 Hz and pulse widths of 0.1–0.2 ms, applied on paretic muscles [124]. NMES is a more efficient procedure that is not influenced by motor neuron damage. It uses electrical impulses that are stronger and wider than the ones used in TENS. The functional parameters are usually established through electromyography (EMG) investigations [160].

Electromagnetic fields represent a further type of therapeutic intervention that improves spasticity in MS patients. According to the literature, they can be delivered through either transcranial magnetic stimulation [161,162], pulsed electromagnetic field therapy (PEMF) [143,163] or repetitive peripheral magnetic nerve stimulation (RPMS) [164,165]. The advantages of using peripheral electromagnetic fields in the treatment of spasticity reside in the fact that they induce significantly less pain than other types of electrotherapy, such as

NMES [166], they are permeable through human tissues, and they do not produce heat [124]. The frequencies cited by various studies are placed within the 1–150 Hz range [167], with impulses having trapezoidal, sinusoidal, rectangular, or triangular shapes [124].

Water can provide a good environment, and presents a multitude of benefits, for MS patients. Hydrotherapy decreases the activity of gamma neurons, and limits the afferent impulses, leading to a relaxing and analgesic effect, and finally to a reduction in spasticity. The preferred temperature is between 34 and 36 °C, and hot baths are not permitted in order to avoid the occurrence of the Uhthoff effect [168]. Water also acts as a supportive medium for physical exercises, without presenting the risk of falling, therefore increasing mobility in patients with multiple sclerosis. In addition, hydrotherapy improves fatigue and depression symptoms [169].

3.2.5. Dysphagia Management

Dysphagia is a symptom that occurs in around 43% of MS patients [170], and is the result of a number of factors such as cognitive impairment, cranial nerves paresis and accumulated lesions in the brainstem, cerebellum and the corticobulbar tracts [171]. If left untreated, it can seriously impact the quality of life and lead to life-threatening consequences such as malnutrition, dehydration and aspiration pneumonia [172]. Since it can be associated with speech disorders, the utilized therapies often focus on treating the two symptoms assosciatively, through physiotherapy, occupational therapy and speech–language therapy (SLT) [173].

SLT is an essential tool in the rehabilitation of MS patients suffering from dysphagia, which aims at re-teaching swallowing in order to prevent food aspiration. The therapy includes exercises that strengthen the muscle structures involved in swallowing, the stimulation of the deglutition and cough reflexes (for defense purposes), posture training for the head and trunk, and the establishment of compensatory actions for more natural swallowing [174]. For example, in a case study described by Farazi et al., which rendered positive results, SLT procedures were provided two to three times every day, for two weeks. One of the techniques involved was compensatory swallow therapy through progressively increasing the quantity and consistency of the intake. Further, oral motor exercises including passive and active movements, as well as massage, were included. Chin-down posture training and the Mandelson method were also part of the program [173].

Physiotherapy can provide useful tools for managing dysphagia through physical exercises, botulinum toxin injections and electrotherapy [174]. Weight management and appetite stimulation are some of the beneficial effects of increased physical activity. Botulinum toxin treatment is administered in the cryopharingeus muscle under general or local anesthesia for upper esophageal sphincter dysfunctions [175]. It can be injected either through esophagoscopy [176] or percutaneously through electromyographic guidance [177]. Lastly, transcranial direct current stimulation is another viable therapeutic approach for MS patients with swallowing difficulties. Recent studies have demonstrated a mild and transient improvement in deglutition scores when the current was applied over the right swallowing motor cortex for five consecutive days [178].

3.2.6. Overactive Bladder Management

Between 63% and 68% of patients with multiple sclerosis develop neurogenic bladder dysfunction during the course of the disease [179]. Therapeutic strategies that target it include pelvic floor muscle training (PFMT), also known as Kegel exercises, bladder training, drug therapies, electrostimulation therapy and botulinum toxin injections [74].

Pelvic floor muscle training is aimed at increasing the resting tension of the pelvic diaphragm, through a series of repetitions of tensing and relaxing the groups of muscles in the region [180]. Strengthening these muscles allows them to contract for prolonged periods, therefore enhancing the control over the mechanism of urination. Other muscle groups, such as the adductor, the gluteal and the transversus abdominis muscles, should be strengthened together with PFMT, as they present a reduced activation in patients with urinary incontinence [181]. Bladder training programs that aim to increase the capacity of the bladder through behavioral changes [182] can also be associated, and if necessary, weight loss should be considered in order to reduce physical stress over the bladder [183].

Electrostimulation therapy is another alternative for the management of an overactive bladder. Electrostimulation can be vaginal or anal, and it is directed at stimulating the pudendal nerves while inhibiting hyperreflexia [74]. Moreover, botulinum toxin injected in the detrusor muscle via cystoscopy also has the ability to suppress hyperreflexia. Studies have shown that doses of 100–150 units were effective for 3–6 months [180].

3.3. Cognitive Rehabilitation

Besides the physical disabilities caused by the brain lesions in multiple sclerosis, cognitive impairments are also associated in 34–65% of cases, depending on the duration of the disease and the age at onset [184]. These include memory deficits, diminished speed of processing and attention, and other symptoms linked with a decreased cognitive reserve. The brain structures that show a particularly affected connectivity are the cortical prefrontal lobe and the amygdala in the limbic system, responsible for emotional control [185]. Together with cognitive deficits, this leads to the further development of depression and other emotional disorders [186].

In treating these afflictions, neurocognitive rehabilitation needs to be associated with psychotherapy for the optimal therapeutic outcome. Disease severity or duration seem to be less related to the development of emotional disorders than inadequate acceptance and coping mechanisms, therefore downgrading medication to a second-line treatment option [187]. Cognitive reappraisal, coping improvement and stress management are all effective strategies for treating depression and improving the quality of life of these patients [188,189]. Cognitive behavioral therapy (CBT) is an example of psychotherapy that enables cortical prefrontal structures to mitigate negative emotional responses by adjusting the patients' perception and stress levels in situations outside their control [190]. Neurocognitive rehabilitation is a useful tool in ameliorating cognitive impairments in MS patients [191]. It is targeted at the brain's neuroplasticity through retraining certain functions, such as memory, attention, learning and executive functions [186]. Thanks to the development of knowledge regarding neuroplasticity, new and improved methods are now available for the treatment and diagnosis of cognitive deficits, including aerobic exercises and transcranial direct current stimulation (tDCS) [192].

4. Subjective and Objective Measures of Improvement after Neurorehabilitation

The internet medical databases contain numerous studies on a variety of rehabilitation procedures applied to MS patients, with the aim of alleviating their diverse symptoms. However, while some of them provide moderate- to high-quality evidence for their benefits, others do not offer such reliability. This may be due to the difficulty in designing double-blinded studies in the area of rehabilitation, or to the subjective nature of some of the tests used for assessment. Further, this paper will analyze some of the evidence provided for the neurorehabilitation procedures involved in treating MS, together with the reliability of the tests and scales that are applied.

Quality of life (QoL) is a complex assessment test that encompasses a wide spectrum of domains covering the elaborate definition of health provided by the World Health Organization [193]. In multiple sclerosis, QoL is impacted by a multitude of factors, such as impairments affecting everyday activities, level of dependency on caregivers, employment status, social support, or mental health [194–198]. In this context, QoL assessment provides useful information concerning the progression of the disease or the impact of therapy [199,200]. Various rehabilitation interventions have been evaluated using QoL, mostly in the areas of cognitive rehabilitation, psychotherapy, and the treatment of fatigue [201–204], all of which have shown success in improving QoL scores. Furthermore, other studies that focused on improving social support also enhanced the QoL [205,206].

The activities of daily living (ADL) scale is another useful measure for multiple sclerosis patients, which focuses more on the physical impairment aspect, but it can also provide insights related to cognition [207,208]. Rehabilitation programs aimed at improving mobility, fatigue and cognitive deficits have been assessed using the ADL scale. In 2019, a comprehensive Cochrane meta-analysis was published, with the purpose of evaluating the quality of evidence (according to the GRADE framework) provided by previous review papers that analyzed the impacts of various rehabilitation techniques on ADL [16]. Three randomized control studies from one review, comprising a total of 217 participants, provided a moderate quality of evidence that multidisciplinary inpatient rehabilitation is beneficial for improving mobility, functional independence (ADL) and locomotion (for patients using a wheelchair) [209–211]. However, the authors note that these studies provided strong evidence for ADL (and the similar Barthel index) improvement due to rehabilitation, but the quality of evidence was downgraded because different outcome measures were used. A moderate quality of evidence was also provided regarding the efficacy of inpatient or outpatient rehabilitation on improving bladder impairment, and the ability of exercise training to enhance mobility, muscle strength and effort tolerance [16]. Evidence for balance improvement using whole-body vibration techniques and for the short-term benefits of telerehabilitation on functional activities was graded as low quality, due to the increased risk of bias and the use of different outcome measures in the analyzed studies [16].

Gait rehabilitation is among the main goals in the treatment of multiple sclerosis. The deficits are caused by a range of factors including sensory disturbances, cerebellar impairments, spasticity, and muscle weakness that lead to a markedly decreased quality of life [212]. In clinical settings, gait assessment is commonly performed using timed walking tests (2MWT, 6MWT, T25FW) or standardized scales (EDSS). However, these measures do not offer great reliability, due to the limits of timed walking tests used for evaluating gait quality [213–215] or to the low sensitivity of EDSS to short-term changes [216]. A more accurate method to assess the effect of neurorehabilitation on gait deficits is represented by novel technologies in the form of wearable sensors [217]. These devices are able to track the subtle changes in gait kinematics while performing a surface electromyography (sEMG) that detects spasticity through muscle activation patterns [218,219]. In a study performed by Huang et al., a 4-week multidisciplinary gait rehabilitation program was assessed using wearable technology. They reported significant progress in gait speed, kinematics, spasticity and balance, in alignment with improved results in the standard clinical tests [220]. Moreover, wearable accelerometers could also be a useful tool in monitoring gait kinematics in MS patients, even in non-clinical settings. Researchers suggest that the future benefits of accelerometers reside in their potential to become a biomarker for disease severity and progression [221].

Various neurorehabilitation strategies have been evaluated for balance and coordination improvement in MS patients. Currently, there are a number of tests that are used to track different static and dynamic parameters that influence these two functions. The trunk impairment scale (TIS), Berg balance scale (BBS), international cooperative ataxia rating scale (ICARS) and nine-hole peg test (NHPT) are among the tests performed in clinical settings. TIS is a reliable test applied to patients with multiple sclerosis that uses a selection of movements to evaluate three parameters: coordination, static sitting balance and dynamic sitting balance [222]. The Berg balance scale represents another widely utilized test comprising 14 items that provide information on the patient's balance abilities and the changes induced in them by rehabilitation programs [223]. Ataxia is an MS symptom that can be assessed using ICARS, a valid and reliable scale containing four subscales targeting posture and gait disorders, limb ataxia, dysarthria and oculomotor impairments [224]. Lastly, NHPT is a test that evaluates manual dexterity, affecting up to 75% of MS patients [225], and it is currently considered the gold standard in its field [226]. Previous studies demonstrated significant improvements in all the above-mentioned tests after both exercises based on the Bobath method and traditional rehabilitation routines [227]. In order to improve the objectiveness of measurement, some authors have developed innovative solutions, such as video processing of the Berg balance scale parameters [228,229]. In these studies, the assessments of 360-degree turning and the one-leg stance (both part of BBS) are performed using a video camera, without any additional garments. As the authors state, besides increased accuracy, the method could also provide a solution for self-monitoring to patients. Furthermore, another study that used a mobile app based on the Romberg test found it to have 80% sensitivity and 87% specificity in detecting balance disorders [230].

Although wearable devices performing sEMG are a sensitive and accurate way of measuring changes in spasticity determined by neurorehabilitation, they are not a widely available technology. Therefore, in most clinical settings, spasticity is evaluated using standardized tests, such as the Ashworth scale (AS) or the modified Ashworth scale (MAS). Most studies show an improvement in spasticity for patients with stable MS, measured on these scales, especially after electrostimulation, RAGT and BWSTT [149]. However, using H-reflex as a comparison, some authors have suggested MAS and AS are not able to differentiate reflex from non-reflex forms of spasticity [231]. More research is required to address the impact of rehabilitation on spasticity, and novel tests need to be designed for this challenge.

Treatment for dysphagia can be assessed using either the Mann assessment of swallowing ability (MASA) scale [232] or the penetration–aspiration scale (PAS) [233]. The MASA scale comprises 24 items and has 73% sensitivity and 89% specificity for predicting dysphagia [232]. PAS is used to evaluate the functional improvement of deglutition through the fiber optic endoscopic evaluation of swallowing (FEES). Tarameshlu et al. found significant and sustained improvements in both scores for MS patients following a program of oral motor exercises and swallowing compensation techniques in comparison to those who engaged solely in posture reeducation and diet prescription [232]. Other tests recommended by different authors, which could provide useful insights, are the eating assessment tool (EAT-10) and the more specific Dysphagia in multiple sclerosis (DYMUS) questionnaire [174,234].

The findings regarding the therapeutic goals, approaches and assessment scales for the most common symptoms in multiple sclerosis are summarized in Table 1.

Table 1. Neurorehabilitation for the most common symptoms in multiple sclerosis.

Symptom	Rehabilitation Goals	Method	Assessment Test
Gait management (up to 93% of patients after 10 years of diagnosis [91,92])	Increasing lower limb and trunk strength Enhancing gait speed and endurance Improving gait kinematics Maintaining neuroplasticity	Strength training [5] Endurance Training [6] Robotic-assisted gait training [7] Speed-intensive gait training [115] Ankle–foot orthoses [8] Proprioceptive neuromuscular facilitation [130,131] Virtual Reality [235] Robotic Exoskeletons [236]	*Subjective methods:* 2-Minute Walk Test (2MWT) [9] 6-Minute Walk Test (6MWT) [9] Timed 25-Foot Walk test (T25FW) [10] 12-Item Multiple Sclerosis Walking Scale (MSWS-12) [11] Expanded Disability Status Scale (EDSS) *Objective methods:* Wearable sensors combined with surface electromyography (sEMG) [217] Accelerometers [221]
Balance and coordination management (80% of cases [237,238])	Preventing falls Enhancing walking stability Posture control Reduce energy requirements Increase continuity of movement	Frenkel exercises [14] Stabilometric platform [15] Hippotherapy [127] The Bobath concept [128] Proprioceptive neuromuscular facilitation [130,131] Virtual Reality [239] Robotic Exoskeletons [236]	*Subjective methods:* Trunk impairment scale (TIS) [222] Berg balance scale (BBS) [223] International cooperative ataxia rating scale (ICARS) [224] *Objective methods:* Video processed BBS [228,229] Mobile apps [230] Nine-hole peg test (NHPT) [226]

Table 1. Cont.

Symptom	Rehabilitation Goals	Method	Assessment Test
Fatigue management (75–95% of cases [133–135])	Improve mental and physical energy Inflammation reduction Improving depressive symptoms Quality of sleep improvement	Aerobic training [138] Strength exercises [138] Neuromotor exercises (dancing, tai chi, yoga, pilates) [138] Breathing exercises [138] Cryotherapy [141] Pulsed electromagnetic field therapy [143] Functional electrical stimulation [145,146] Hydrotherapy [169]	*Subjective methods:* Quality of Life (QoL) [202,204]
Spasticity Management (40–60% of patients [124])	Maintain neuroplasticity Prevent contracture Prevent joint malformation Preserve muscle length Improve ROM of ankle dorsiflexion Decrease hypertonia in the calf muscles Enhance strength of the antigravity muscles	Physical training Vibration therapy Hydrotherapy [168,169] Electrotherapy [158,159] Electromagnetic fields [161,162] Cryotherapy [152,153] Therapeutic standing on an Oswestry standing frame [149] Proprioceptive neuromuscular facilitation [130,131]	*Subjective methods:* Ashworth scale (AS) [149,231] Modified Ashworth Scale (MAS) [149,231] *Objective methods:* Wearable sensors combined with surface electromyography (sEMG) [217]
Dysphagia management (around 43% of patients [170])	Speech improvement Avoid malnutrition, dehydration and aspiration pneumonia Maintain healthy weight	Speech–language therapy [173,174] Physical exercises [174] Botulinum toxin injections [174,176,177] Electrotherapy [174] Occupational therapy [174] Transcranial direct current stimulation [178]	*Subjective methods:* Mann assessment of swallowing ability (MASA) [232] Eating assessment tool (EAT-10) [174,234] Dysphagia in multiple sclerosis (DYMUS) [174,234] *Objective methods:* Penetration-aspiration scale (PAS) [233]
Overactive bladder management (between 63% and 68% of cases [179])	Increasing resting tension of the pelvic diaphragm Enhanced control over urination mechanism Increase bladder capacity	Pelvic floor muscle training [178,180] Bladder training [182] Weight loss [183] Electrostimulation therapy [74] Botulinum toxin injections [174,180]	*Subjective methods:* Activities of Daily Living (ADL) [16]
Cognitive Rehabilitation (34–65% of cases [184])	Reduce emotional disorders Improve emotional control Improve memory, attention and learning Enhance stress management	Cognitive behavioral therapy Neurocognitive rehabilitation [186] Aerobic exercises Transcranial direct current stimulation [192] Computer-assisted cognitive rehabilitation [240]	*Subjective methods:* Quality of Life (QoL) [201,203] Activities of Daily Living (ADL) [208] *Objective methods:* Montreal Cognitive Assessment Test (MoCA)

Neurorehabilitation goals, approaches and assessment tests for the management of the most common symptoms in multiple sclerosis.

5. Emerging Techniques and Future Considerations

Technological development opens up new possibilities in the area of neurorehabilitation, for treatment, diagnosis and progress tracking. The mass production of virtual reality devices started in the 1990s and ever since, the technology has gained attention in various fields of work, including healthcare [241]. In medical rehabilitation, virtual reality has brought novel solutions for a variety of afflictions. VR headsets (HMD or head-mounted displays) have been trialed for patients suffering from Parkinson's disease, in order to improve their gait pattern [242], and for children with cerebral palsy with the purpose of operating motorized wheelchairs [243] and enhancing their spatial awareness [244]. In multiple sclerosis, VR could provide an alternative to traditional rehabilitation programs, through increasing adherence and motivation in patients [235]. Previous studies revealed the ability of VR-based training to enhance gait [245], balance [239] and upper limb mobility and control [246]. Furthermore, MS patients that are dependent on a wheelchair could benefit from this type of technology [247]. In an inpatient setting, VR exercises can also be combined with other neurorehabilitation procedures, such as FES and robot-assisted training [246]. This technology could be especially beneficial for people that are restricted by their location or financial means, or who are reliant on different types of caregivers [248]. Another important aspect that supports the adoption of VR in neurorehabilitation is that the system is able to receive feedback in real time and automatically adapt the intensity to every individual case [249,250]. The clinician can also access the feedback, and is therefore able to track the progress of every patient and change the settings accordingly [236].

Another novel approach to the treatment of multiple sclerosis is represented by robotic exoskeletons [251]. This represents an alternative to BWSTT and RAGT that brings additional benefits, such as offering severely disabled MS patients the option to engage in over-ground walking, therefore enhancing their chances of functional adaptation through neuroplasticity [252–254]. Recent literature provides increasing evidence for the efficacy of robotic exoskeletons, with more pronounced results for gait, balance and mobility improvement in MS patients suffering from more advanced forms of the disease [240,255,256].

Cognitive rehabilitation could also benefit from the introduction of new technologies. Computer-assisted cognitive rehabilitation aims to re-train the residual neurological capacity by creating individualized strategies through cognitive models [257]. It targets the improvement of processing speed, language, attention and memory by making use of specific software and multimedia libraries [40,258,259]. The advantages of computer-assisted cognitive rehabilitation reside in its ability to perform cognitive recovery while providing visual and auditory feedback in real time. Furthermore, it increases adherence and motivation through a diversity of immersive scenarios, and it offers the option for patients to engage in it from home [257].

6. Conclusions

Multiple sclerosis is a disease with a wide range of symptoms that has seen an increasing prevalence in recent years and requires a multidisciplinary approach. While neurorehabilitation plays a significant part in the management of symptoms and employs a vast number of approaches for achieving this target, there is a continuous need for updates in the most efficacious therapeutic approaches. More research is required to establish better study designs in order to avoid the current biases related to subjectivity and the impossibility of double blinding. There is also a further need to evaluate the validity and reliability of the tests used to assess the status of the disease and the efficacy of the treatment. Moreover, international collaboration could be useful for establishing protocols comprising rigorously tested and approved exercise programs and physiotherapeutic approaches. In this regard, technological innovation could benefit the area of rehabilitation by introducing the more accurate tracking of treatment responses and novel therapeutic solutions.

Author Contributions: Conceptualization, C.A.S., F.C.P., D.-C.T. and D.C.J.; methodology, D.A., F.C.P., C.A.S., C.S. and M.M.; software, D.-C.T. and T.M.V.; validation, M.M., D.C.J., F.C.P., T.M.V. and C.A.S.; formal analysis, M.M., T.M.V., D.A. and C.S.; resources, M.M., D.A., C.S. and D.-C.T.; data curation, C.A.S., D.C.J. and T.M.V.; writing—original draft preparation, D.-C.T. and D.C.J.; writing—review and editing, C.A.S., F.C.P., T.M.V., D.A. and C.S. All authors have read and agreed to the published version of the manuscript.

Funding: This research received no external funding.

Institutional Review Board Statement: Not applicable.

Informed Consent Statement: Not applicable.

Data Availability Statement: Not applicable.

Conflicts of Interest: The authors declare no conflict of interest.

Abbreviations

2MWT	2-min walk test
6MWT	6-min walk test
ADL	Activities of daily living
AFOs	Ankle-foot orthoses
AS	Ashworth scale
BBS	Berg balance scale
BDNF	Brain-derived neurotrophic factor
BWSTT	Body-weight supported treadmill training
CBT	Cognitive-behavioral therapy
CNS	Central nervous system
CPZ	Cuprizone
DSS	Disability status scale
DYMUS	Dysphagia in multiple sclerosis
EAE	Experimental autoimmune encephalomyelitis
EAT-10	Eating assessment tool
EDSS	Expanded disability status scale
EMG	Electromyography
FEES	Fiber optic endoscopic evaluation of swallowing
FES	Functional electrical stimulation
fMRI	Functional magnetic resonance imaging
FS	Functional systems
HMD	Head-mounted displays
ICARS	International cooperative ataxia rating scale
LCT	Lysolecithin
MAS	Modified Ashworth scale
MASA	Mann assessment of swallowing ability
MoCA	Montreal cognitive assessment test
MRI	Magnetic resonance imaging
MS	Multiple sclerosis
MSWS-12	12-item multiple sclerosis walking scale
NHPT	Nine-hole peg test
NHS	National health service
NIBS	Noninvasive brain stimulation
NMES	Neuromuscular electrical stimulation
OPC	Oligodendrocyte precursor cells
PAS	Penetration-aspiration scale
PEMF	Pulsed electromagnetic field therapy
PFMT	Pelvic floor muscle training
PNF	Proprioceptive neuromuscular facilitation
QoL	Quality of life
RAGT	Robotic-assisted gait training
ROM	Range of motion
RPMS	Repetitive peripheral magnetic nerve stimulation
RSN	Resting state network
SCFAs	Short chain fatty acids
sEMG	Surface electromyography
SLT	Speech–language therapy

T25FW	Timed 25-foot walk test
tDCS	Transcranial direct current stimulation
TENS	Transcutaneous electrical nerve stimulation
TIS	Trunk impairment scale
Treg	Regulatory T lymphocytes
VR	Virtual reality

References

1. Miller, E. Multiple sclerosis. *Adv. Exp. Med. Biol.* **2012**, *724*, 222–238. [CrossRef]
2. Federation, M.I. Atlas of MS 3rd Edition. Available online: https://www.msif.org/wp-content/uploads/2020/10/Atlas-3rd-Edition-Epidemiology-report-EN-updated-30-9-20.pdf (accessed on 10 October 2022).
3. Di Cara, M.; Lo Buono, V.; Corallo, F.; Cannistraci, C.; Rifici, C.; Sessa, E.; D'Aleo, G.; Bramanti, P.; Marino, S. Body image in multiple sclerosis patients: A descriptive review. *Neurol. Sci.* **2019**, *40*, 923–928. [CrossRef]
4. Macias Islas, M.A.; Ciampi, E. Assessment and Impact of Cognitive Impairment in Multiple Sclerosis: An Overview. *Biomedicines* **2019**, *7*, 22. [CrossRef]
5. Matsuda, P.N.; Hoffman, J.M. Patient perspectives on falls in persons with multiple sclerosis. *PM R* **2021**. [CrossRef]
6. Zasadzka, E.; Trzmiel, T.; Pieczynska, A.; Hojan, K. Modern Technologies in the Rehabilitation of Patients with Multiple Sclerosis and Their Potential Application in Times of COVID-19. *Medicina* **2021**, *57*, 549. [CrossRef]
7. Kurtzke, J.F. On the origin of EDSS. *Mult. Scler. Relat. Disord.* **2015**, *4*, 95–103. [CrossRef]
8. Pirko, I.; Noseworthy, J.H. Chapter 48—Demyelinating Disorders of the Central Nervous System. In *Textbook of Clinical Neurology*, 3rd ed.; Goetz, C.G., Ed.; W.B. Saunders: Philadelphia, PA, USA, 2007; pp. 1103–1133. [CrossRef]
9. Kamm, C.P.; Uitdehaag, B.M.; Polman, C.H. Multiple sclerosis: Current knowledge and future outlook. *Eur. Neurol.* **2014**, *72*, 132–141. [CrossRef]
10. de Sa, J.C.; Airas, L.; Bartholome, E.; Grigoriadis, N.; Mattle, H.; Oreja-Guevara, C.; O'Riordan, J.; Sellebjerg, F.; Stankoff, B.; Vass, K.; et al. Symptomatic therapy in multiple sclerosis: A review for a multimodal approach in clinical practice. *Ther. Adv. Neurol. Disord.* **2011**, *4*, 139–168. [CrossRef]
11. Vanbellingen, T.; Kamm, C.P. Neurorehabilitation Topics in Patients with Multiple Sclerosis: From Outcome Measurements to Rehabilitation Interventions. *Semin. Neurol.* **2016**, *36*, 196–202. [CrossRef]
12. Baird, J.F.; Sandroff, B.M.; Motl, R.W. Therapies for mobility disability in persons with multiple sclerosis. *Expert Rev. Neurother.* **2018**, *18*, 493–502. [CrossRef]
13. Riemenschneider, M.; Hvid, L.G.; Stenager, E.; Dalgas, U. Is there an overlooked "window of opportunity" in MS exercise therapy? Perspectives for early MS rehabilitation. *Mult. Scler.* **2018**, *24*, 886–894. [CrossRef]
14. Dalgas, U.; Langeskov-Christensen, M.; Stenager, E.; Riemenschneider, M.; Hvid, L.G. Exercise as Medicine in Multiple Sclerosis-Time for a Paradigm Shift: Preventive, Symptomatic, and Disease-Modifying Aspects and Perspectives. *Curr. Neurol. Neurosci. Rep.* **2019**, *19*, 88. [CrossRef]
15. Tollár, J.; Nagy, F.; Tóth, B.E.; Török, K.; Szita, K.; Csutorás, B.; Moizs, M.; Hortobágyi, T. Exercise Effects on Multiple Sclerosis Quality of Life and Clinical-Motor Symptoms. *Med. Sci. Sports Exerc.* **2020**, *52*, 1007–1014. [CrossRef]
16. Amatya, B.; Khan, F.; Galea, M. Rehabilitation for people with multiple sclerosis: An overview of Cochrane Reviews. *Cochrane Database Syst. Rev.* **2019**, *1*, Cd012732. [CrossRef]
17. Barclay, A.; Paul, L.; MacFarlane, N.; McFadyen, A.K. The effect of cycling using active-passive trainers on spasticity, cardiovascular fitness, function and quality of life in people with moderate to severe Multiple Sclerosis (MS); a feasibility study. *Mult. Scler. Relat. Disord.* **2019**, *34*, 128–134. [CrossRef]
18. Rooney, S.; Riemenschneider, M.; Dalgas, U.; Jørgensen, M.K.; Michelsen, A.S.; Brønd, J.C.; Hvid, L.G. Physical activity is associated with neuromuscular and physical function in patients with multiple sclerosis independent of disease severity. *Disabil. Rehabil.* **2021**, *43*, 632–639. [CrossRef] [PubMed]
19. Yazgan, Y.Z.; Tarakci, E.; Tarakci, D.; Ozdincler, A.R.; Kurtuncu, M. Comparison of the effects of two different exergaming systems on balance, functionality, fatigue, and quality of life in people with multiple sclerosis: A randomized controlled trial. *Mult. Scler. Relat. Disord.* **2019**, *39*, 101902. [CrossRef]
20. Bahmani, D.S.; Kesselring, J.; Papadimitriou, M.; Bansi, J.; Pühse, U.; Gerber, M.; Shaygannejad, V.; Holsboer-Trachsler, E.; Brand, S. In Patients With Multiple Sclerosis, Both Objective and Subjective Sleep, Depression, Fatigue, and Paresthesia Improved after 3 Weeks of Regular Exercise. *Front. Psychiatry* **2019**, *10*, 265. [CrossRef] [PubMed]
21. Zimmer, P.; Bloch, W.; Schenk, A.; Oberste, M.; Riedel, S.; Kool, J.; Langdon, D.; Dalgas, U.; Kesselring, J.; Bansi, J. High-intensity interval exercise improves cognitive performance and reduces matrix metalloproteinases-2 serum levels in persons with multiple sclerosis: A randomized controlled trial. *Mult. Scler.* **2018**, *24*, 1635–1644. [CrossRef]
22. Tavazzi, E.; Bergsland, N.; Cattaneo, D.; Gervasoni, E.; Laganà, M.M.; Dipasquale, O.; Grosso, C.; Saibene, F.L.; Baglio, F.; Rovaris, M. Effects of motor rehabilitation on mobility and brain plasticity in multiple sclerosis: A structural and functional MRI study. *J. Neurol.* **2018**, *265*, 1393–1401. [CrossRef] [PubMed]

23. Kjølhede, T.; Siemonsen, S.; Wenzel, D.; Stellmann, J.P.; Ringgaard, S.; Pedersen, B.G.; Stenager, E.; Petersen, T.; Vissing, K.; Heesen, C.; et al. Can resistance training impact MRI outcomes in relapsing-remitting multiple sclerosis? *Mult. Scler. J.* **2018**, *24*, 1356–1365. [CrossRef]
24. Sandroff, B.M.; Wylie, G.R.; Sutton, B.P.; Johnson, C.L.; DeLuca, J.; Motl, R.W. Treadmill walking exercise training and brain function in multiple sclerosis: Preliminary evidence setting the stage for a network-based approach to rehabilitation. *Mult. Scler. J. Exp. Transl. Clin.* **2018**, *4*, 2055217318760641. [CrossRef] [PubMed]
25. Joisten, N.; Rademacher, A.; Bloch, W.; Schenk, A.; Oberste, M.; Dalgas, U.; Langdon, D.; Caminada, D.; Purde, M.T.; Gonzenbach, R.; et al. Influence of different rehabilitative aerobic exercise programs on (anti-) inflammatory immune signalling, cognitive and functional capacity in persons with MS—Study protocol of a randomized controlled trial. *BMC Neurol.* **2019**, *19*, 37. [CrossRef] [PubMed]
26. Centonze, D.; Leocani, L.; Feys, P. Advances in physical rehabilitation of multiple sclerosis. *Curr. Opin. Neurol.* **2020**, *33*, 255–261. [CrossRef] [PubMed]
27. Galea, M.D. Telemedicine in Rehabilitation. *Phys. Med. Rehabil. Clin. N. Am.* **2019**, *30*, 473–483. [CrossRef] [PubMed]
28. Leocani, L.; Chieffo, R.; Gentile, A.; Centonze, D. Beyond rehabilitation in MS: Insights from non-invasive brain stimulation. *Mult. Scler.* **2019**, *25*, 1363–1371. [CrossRef]
29. Nasios, G.; Messinis, L.; Dardiotis, E.; Papathanasopoulos, P. Repetitive Transcranial Magnetic Stimulation, Cognition, and Multiple Sclerosis: An Overview. *Behav. Neurol.* **2018**, *2018*, 8584653. [CrossRef]
30. Şan, A.U.; Yılmaz, B.; Kesikburun, S. The Effect of Repetitive Transcranial Magnetic Stimulation on Spasticity in Patients with Multiple Sclerosis. *J. Clin. Neurol.* **2019**, *15*, 461–467. [CrossRef]
31. Zeller, D.; Classen, J. Plasticity of the motor system in multiple sclerosis. *Neuroscience* **2014**, *283*, 222–230. [CrossRef]
32. Bonzano, L.; Tacchino, A.; Brichetto, G.; Roccatagliata, L.; Dessypris, A.; Feraco, P.; De Carvalho, M.L.L.; Battaglia, M.A.; Mancardi, G.L.; Bove, M. Upper limb motor rehabilitation impacts white matter microstructure in multiple sclerosis. *Neuroimage* **2014**, *90*, 107–116. [CrossRef]
33. Filippi, M.; Rocca, M.A. Cortical reorganisation in patients with MS. *J. Neurol. Neurosurg. Psychiatry* **2004**, *75*, 1087–1089. [CrossRef] [PubMed]
34. Hillary, F.G.; Chiaravalloti, N.D.; Ricker, J.H.; Steffener, J.; Bly, B.M.; Lange, G.; Liu, W.C.; Kalnin, A.J.; DeLuca, J. An investigation of working memory rehearsal in multiple sclerosis using fMRI. *J. Clin. Exp. Neuropsychol.* **2003**, *25*, 965–978. [CrossRef] [PubMed]
35. Filippi, M.; Rocca, M.A. Present and future of fMRI in multiple sclerosis. *Expert. Rev. Neurother.* **2013**, *13*, 27–31. [CrossRef] [PubMed]
36. Valsasina, P.; Rocca, M.A.; Absinta, M.; Sormani, M.P.; Mancini, L.; De Stefano, N.; Rovira, A.; Gass, A.; Enzinger, C.; Barkhof, F.; et al. A multicentre study of motor functional connectivity changes in patients with multiple sclerosis. *Eur. J. Neurosci.* **2011**, *33*, 1256–1263. [CrossRef]
37. Rocca, M.A.; Valsasina, P.; Hulst, H.E.; Abdel-Aziz, K.; Enzinger, C.; Gallo, A.; Pareto, D.; Riccitelli, G.; Muhlert, N.; Ciccarelli, O.; et al. Functional correlates of cognitive dysfunction in multiple sclerosis: A multicenter fMRI Study. *Hum. Brain. Mapp.* **2014**, *35*, 5799–5814. [CrossRef]
38. Pareto, D.; Sastre-Garriga, J.; Alonso, J.; Galán, I.; Arévalo, M.J.; Renom, M.; Montalban, X.; Rovira, À. Classic Block Design "Pseudo"-Resting-State fMRI Changes After a Neurorehabilitation Program in Patients with Multiple Sclerosis. *J. Neuroimaging* **2018**, *28*, 313–319. [CrossRef]
39. Sastre-Garriga, J.; Alonso, J.; Renom, M.; Arévalo, M.J.; González, I.; Galán, I.; Montalban, X.; Rovira, A. A functional magnetic resonance proof of concept pilot trial of cognitive rehabilitation in multiple sclerosis. *Mult. Scler.* **2011**, *17*, 457–467. [CrossRef]
40. Cerasa, A.; Gioia, M.C.; Valentino, P.; Nisticò, R.; Chiriaco, C.; Pirritano, D.; Tomaiuolo, F.; Mangone, G.; Trotta, M.; Talarico, T.; et al. Computer-assisted cognitive rehabilitation of attention deficits for multiple sclerosis: A randomized trial with fMRI correlates. *Neurorehabil. Neural Repair* **2013**, *27*, 284–295. [CrossRef]
41. Enzinger, C.; Pinter, D.; Rocca, M.A.; De Luca, J.; Sastre-Garriga, J.; Audoin, B.; Filippi, M. Longitudinal fMRI studies: Exploring brain plasticity and repair in MS. *Mult. Scler.* **2016**, *22*, 269–278. [CrossRef]
42. Chiaravalloti, N.D.; Genova, H.M.; DeLuca, J. Cognitive rehabilitation in multiple sclerosis: The role of plasticity. *Front. Neurol.* **2015**, *6*, 67. [CrossRef]
43. Tomassini, V.; Matthews, P.M.; Thompson, A.J.; Fuglø, D.; Geurts, J.J.; Johansen-Berg, H.; Jones, D.K.; Rocca, M.A.; Wise, R.G.; Barkhof, F.; et al. Neuroplasticity and functional recovery in multiple sclerosis. *Nat. Rev. Neurol.* **2012**, *8*, 635–646. [CrossRef] [PubMed]
44. Tomassini, V.; Johansen-Berg, H.; Jbabdi, S.; Wise, R.G.; Pozzilli, C.; Palace, J.; Matthews, P.M. Relating brain damage to brain plasticity in patients with multiple sclerosis. *Neurorehabil. Neural Repair* **2012**, *26*, 581–593. [CrossRef] [PubMed]
45. Tomassini, V.; Johansen-Berg, H.; Leonardi, L.; Paixão, L.; Jbabdi, S.; Palace, J.; Pozzilli, C.; Matthews, P.M. Preservation of motor skill learning in patients with multiple sclerosis. *Mult. Scler.* **2011**, *17*, 103–115. [CrossRef]
46. Mori, F.; Rossi, S.; Piccinin, S.; Motta, C.; Mango, D.; Kusayanagi, H.; Bergami, A.; Studer, V.; Nicoletti, C.G.; Buttari, F.; et al. Synaptic plasticity and PDGF signaling defects underlie clinical progression in multiple sclerosis. *J. Neurosci.* **2013**, *33*, 19112–19119. [CrossRef] [PubMed]

47. Dobryakova, E.; Rocca, M.A.; Valsasina, P.; Ghezzi, A.; Colombo, B.; Martinelli, V.; Comi, G.; DeLuca, J.; Filippi, M. Abnormalities of the executive control network in multiple sclerosis phenotypes: An fMRI effective connectivity study. *Hum. Brain Mapp.* **2016**, *37*, 2293–2304. [CrossRef]
48. Calautti, C.; Baron, J.C. Functional neuroimaging studies of motor recovery after stroke in adults: A review. *Stroke* **2003**, *34*, 1553–1566. [CrossRef]
49. Rocca, M.A.; Pagani, E.; Ghezzi, A.; Falini, A.; Zaffaroni, M.; Colombo, B.; Scotti, G.; Comi, G.; Filippi, M. Functional cortical changes in patients with multiple sclerosis and nonspecific findings on conventional magnetic resonance imaging scans of the brain. *Neuroimage* **2003**, *19*, 826–836. [CrossRef]
50. Rocca, M.A.; Matthews, P.M.; Caputo, D.; Ghezzi, A.; Falini, A.; Scotti, G.; Comi, G.; Filippi, M. Evidence for widespread movement-associated functional MRI changes in patients with PPMS. *Neurology* **2002**, *58*, 866–872. [CrossRef]
51. Reddy, H.; Narayanan, S.; Arnoutelis, R.; Jenkinson, M.; Antel, J.; Matthews, P.M.; Arnold, D.L. Evidence for adaptive functional changes in the cerebral cortex with axonal injury from multiple sclerosis. *Brain* **2000**, *123*, 2314–2320. [CrossRef]
52. Rocca, M.A.; Valsasina, P.; Martinelli, V.; Misci, P.; Falini, A.; Comi, G.; Filippi, M. Large-scale neuronal network dysfunction in relapsing-remitting multiple sclerosis. *Neurology* **2012**, *79*, 1449–1457. [CrossRef]
53. Faivre, A.; Robinet, E.; Guye, M.; Rousseau, C.; Maarouf, A.; Le Troter, A.; Zaaraoui, W.; Rico, A.; Crespy, L.; Soulier, E.; et al. Depletion of brain functional connectivity enhancement leads to disability progression in multiple sclerosis: A longitudinal resting-state fMRI study. *Mult. Scler.* **2016**, *22*, 1695–1708. [CrossRef] [PubMed]
54. Kesselring, J. Neurorehabilitation in Multiple Sclerosis—Resilience in Practice. *Eur. Neurol. Rev.* **2017**, *12*, 31. [CrossRef]
55. Gentile, A.; Musella, A.; De Vito, F.; Rizzo, F.R.; Fresegna, D.; Bullitta, S.; Vanni, V.; Guadalupi, L.; Stampanoni Bassi, M.; Buttari, F.; et al. Immunomodulatory Effects of Exercise in Experimental Multiple Sclerosis. *Front. Immunol.* **2019**, *10*, 2197. [CrossRef] [PubMed]
56. Guo, L.Y.; Lozinski, B.; Yong, V.W. Exercise in multiple sclerosis and its models: Focus on the central nervous system outcomes. *J. Neurosci. Res.* **2020**, *98*, 509–523. [CrossRef]
57. Souza, P.S.; Gonçalves, E.D.; Pedroso, G.S.; Farias, H.R.; Junqueira, S.C.; Marcon, R.; Tuon, T.; Cola, M.; Silveira, P.C.L.; Santos, A.R.; et al. Physical Exercise Attenuates Experimental Autoimmune Encephalomyelitis by Inhibiting Peripheral Immune Response and Blood-Brain Barrier Disruption. *Mol. Neurobiol.* **2017**, *54*, 4723–4737. [CrossRef]
58. Fainstein, N.; Tyk, R.; Touloumi, O.; Lagoudaki, R.; Goldberg, Y.; Agranyoni, O.; Navon-Venezia, S.; Katz, A.; Grigoriadis, N.; Ben-Hur, T.; et al. Exercise intensity-dependent immunomodulatory effects on encephalomyelitis. *Ann. Clin. Transl. Neurol.* **2019**, *6*, 1647–1658. [CrossRef]
59. Einstein, O.; Fainstein, N.; Touloumi, O.; Lagoudaki, R.; Hanya, E.; Grigoriadis, N.; Katz, A.; Ben-Hur, T. Exercise training attenuates experimental autoimmune encephalomyelitis by peripheral immunomodulation rather than direct neuroprotection. *Exp. Neurol.* **2018**, *299*, 56–64. [CrossRef]
60. Xiao, R.; Bergin, S.M.; Huang, W.; Mansour, A.G.; Liu, X.; Judd, R.T.; Widstrom, K.J.; Queen, N.J.; Wilkins, R.K.; Siu, J.J.; et al. Enriched environment regulates thymocyte development and alleviates experimental autoimmune encephalomyelitis in mice. *Brain Behav. Immun.* **2019**, *75*, 137–148. [CrossRef] [PubMed]
61. Mandolesi, G.; Bullitta, S.; Fresegna, D.; De Vito, F.; Rizzo, F.R.; Musella, A.; Guadalupi, L.; Vanni, V.; Stampanoni Bassi, M.; Buttari, F.; et al. Voluntary running wheel attenuates motor deterioration and brain damage in cuprizone-induced demyelination. *Neurobiol. Dis.* **2019**, *129*, 102–117. [CrossRef] [PubMed]
62. Jensen, S.K.; Michaels, N.J.; Ilyntskyy, S.; Keough, M.B.; Kovalchuk, O.; Yong, V.W. Multimodal Enhancement of Remyelination by Exercise with a Pivotal Role for Oligodendroglial PGC1α. *Cell Rep.* **2018**, *24*, 3167–3179. [CrossRef]
63. Barone, M.; Mendozzi, L.; D'Amico, F.; Saresella, M.; Rampelli, S.; Piancone, F.; La Rosa, F.; Marventano, I.; Clerici, M.; d'Arma, A.; et al. Influence of a High-Impact Multidimensional Rehabilitation Program on the Gut Microbiota of Patients with Multiple Sclerosis. *Int. J. Mol. Sci.* **2021**, *22*, 7173. [CrossRef]
64. Cryan, J.F.; O'Riordan, K.J.; Sandhu, K.; Peterson, V.; Dinan, T.G. The gut microbiome in neurological disorders. *Lancet Neurol.* **2020**, *19*, 179–194. [CrossRef]
65. Tremlett, H.; Fadrosh, D.W.; Faruqi, A.A.; Zhu, F.; Hart, J.; Roalstad, S.; Graves, J.; Lynch, S.; Waubant, E. Gut microbiota in early pediatric multiple sclerosis: A case-control study. *Eur. J. Neurol.* **2016**, *23*, 1308–1321. [CrossRef] [PubMed]
66. Saresella, M.; Marventano, I.; Barone, M.; La Rosa, F.; Piancone, F.; Mendozzi, L.; d'Arma, A.; Rossi, V.; Pugnetti, L.; Roda, G.; et al. Alterations in Circulating Fatty Acid Are Associated With Gut Microbiota Dysbiosis and Inflammation in Multiple Sclerosis. *Front. Immunol.* **2020**, *11*, 1390. [CrossRef] [PubMed]
67. Peng, L.; He, Z.; Chen, W.; Holzman, I.R.; Lin, J. Effects of butyrate on intestinal barrier function in a Caco-2 cell monolayer model of intestinal barrier. *Pediatr. Res.* **2007**, *61*, 37–41. [CrossRef] [PubMed]
68. Mizuno, M.; Noto, D.; Kaga, N.; Chiba, A.; Miyake, S. The dual role of short fatty acid chains in the pathogenesis of autoimmune disease models. *PLoS ONE* **2017**, *12*, e0173032. [CrossRef] [PubMed]
69. Buscarinu, M.C.; Cerasoli, B.; Annibali, V.; Policano, C.; Lionetto, L.; Capi, M.; Mechelli, R.; Romano, S.; Fornasiero, A.; Mattei, G.; et al. Altered intestinal permeability in patients with relapsing-remitting multiple sclerosis: A pilot study. *Mult. Scler.* **2017**, *23*, 442–446. [CrossRef]
70. Atarashi, K.; Tanoue, T.; Oshima, K.; Suda, W.; Nagano, Y.; Nishikawa, H.; Fukuda, S.; Saito, T.; Narushima, S.; Hase, K.; et al. Treg induction by a rationally selected mixture of Clostridia strains from the human microbiota. *Nature* **2013**, *500*, 232–236. [CrossRef]

71. Furusawa, Y.; Obata, Y.; Fukuda, S.; Endo, T.A.; Nakato, G.; Takahashi, D.; Nakanishi, Y.; Uetake, C.; Kato, K.; Kato, T.; et al. Commensal microbe-derived butyrate induces the differentiation of colonic regulatory T cells. *Nature* **2013**, *504*, 446–450. [CrossRef]
72. Huang, Y.; Tang, J.; Cai, Z.; Zhou, K.; Chang, L.; Bai, Y.; Ma, Y. Prevotella Induces the Production of Th17 Cells in the Colon of Mice. *J. Immunol. Res.* **2020**, *2020*, 9607328. [CrossRef]
73. Cekanaviciute, E.; Yoo, B.B.; Runia, T.F.; Debelius, J.W.; Singh, S.; Nelson, C.A.; Kanner, R.; Bencosme, Y.; Lee, Y.K.; Hauser, S.L.; et al. Gut bacteria from multiple sclerosis patients modulate human T cells and exacerbate symptoms in mouse models. *Proc. Natl. Acad. Sci. USA* **2017**, *114*, 10713–10718. [CrossRef] [PubMed]
74. Kesselring, J.; Beer, S. Symptomatic therapy and neurorehabilitation in multiple sclerosis. *Lancet Neurol.* **2005**, *4*, 643–652. [CrossRef] [PubMed]
75. Amtmann, D.; Bamer, A.M.; Kim, J.; Chung, H.; Salem, R. People with multiple sclerosis report significantly worse symptoms and health related quality of life than the US general population as measured by PROMIS and NeuroQoL outcome measures. *Disabil. Health J.* **2018**, *11*, 99–107. [CrossRef]
76. Kantarci, O.H.; Weinshenker, B.G. Natural history of multiple sclerosis. *Neurol. Clin.* **2005**, *23*, 17–38. [CrossRef]
77. Landfeldt, E.; Castelo-Branco, A.; Svedbom, A.; Löfroth, E.; Kavaliunas, A.; Hillert, J. The long-term impact of early treatment of multiple sclerosis on the risk of disability pension. *J. Neurol.* **2018**, *265*, 701–707. [CrossRef] [PubMed]
78. Sinha, A.; Bagga, A. Pulse steroid therapy. *Indian J. Pediatr.* **2008**, *75*, 1057–1066. [CrossRef]
79. Geng, T.; Mark, V. Clinical neurorestorative progress in multiple sclerosis. *J. Neurorestoratology* **2015**, *3*, 83. [CrossRef]
80. Minagar, A. Current and future therapies for multiple sclerosis. *Scientifica* **2013**, *2013*, 249101. [CrossRef]
81. Sirbu, C.A.; Furdu-Lungut, E.; Plesa, C.F.; Nicolae, A.C.; Dragoi, C.M. Pharmacological Treatment of Relapsing Remitting Multiple Sclerosis—Where Are We? *Farmacia* **2016**, *64*, 651–655.
82. Tobin, O. Multiple Sclerosis. Available online: https://www.mayoclinic.org/diseases-conditions/multiple-sclerosis/diagnosis-treatment/drc-20350274 (accessed on 7 October 2022).
83. Bass, B.; Weinshenker, B.; Rice, G.P.A.; Noseworthy, J.H.; Cameron, M.G.P.; Hader, W.; Bouchard, S.; Ebers, G.C. Tizanidine Versus Baclofen in the Treatment of Spasticity in Patients with Multiple Sclerosis. *Can. J. Neurol. Sci. J. Can. Des. Sci. Neurol.* **1988**, *15*, 15–19. [CrossRef]
84. Tullman, M.J. A review of current and emerging therapeutic strategies in multiple sclerosis. *Am. J. Manag. Care* **2013**, *19*, S21–S27.
85. Cameron, M.H.; Bethoux, F.; Davis, N.; Frederick, M. Botulinum toxin for symptomatic therapy in multiple sclerosis. *Curr. Neurol. Neurosci. Rep.* **2014**, *14*, 463. [CrossRef]
86. Nicholas, R.S.; Friede, T.; Hollis, S.; Young, C.A. Anticholinergics for urinary symptoms in multiple sclerosis. *Cochrane Database Syst. Rev.* **2009**, *1*. [CrossRef]
87. Ledinek, A.H.; Sajko, M.C.; Rot, U. Evaluating the effects of amantadin, modafinil and acetyl-L-carnitine on fatigue in multiple sclerosis—Result of a pilot randomized, blind study. *Clin. Neurol. Neurosurg.* **2013**, *115* (Suppl. S1), S86–S89. [CrossRef]
88. Solaro, C.; Uccelli, M.M.; Uccelli, A.; Leandri, M.; Mancardi, G.L. Low-dose gabapentin combined with either lamotrigine or carbamazepine can be useful therapies for trigeminal neuralgia in multiple sclerosis. *Eur. Neurol.* **2000**, *44*, 45–48. [CrossRef]
89. Leandri, M. Therapy of trigeminal neuralgia secondary to multiple sclerosis. *Expert Rev. Neurother.* **2003**, *3*, 661–671. [CrossRef]
90. East Kent Hospital University NHS Foundation Trust. Inpatient Neuro-Rehabilitation for People with Multiple Sclerosis (MS). Available online: https://www.ekhuft.nhs.uk/EasySiteWeb/GatewayLink.aspx?alId=214554 (accessed on 10 October 2022).
91. Minden, S.L.; Frankel, D.; Hadden, L.; Perloffp, J.; Srinath, K.P.; Hoaglin, D.C. The Sonya Slifka Longitudinal Multiple Sclerosis Study: Methods and sample characteristics. *Mult. Scler.* **2006**, *12*, 24–38. [CrossRef]
92. Asch, P. Impact of mobility impairment in multiple sclerosis 2—Patient perspectives. *Eur. Neurol. Rev.* **2011**, *6*, 115–120. [CrossRef]
93. Goldman, M.D.; Marrie, R.A.; Cohen, J.A. Evaluation of the six-minute walk in multiple sclerosis subjects and healthy controls. *Mult. Scler.* **2008**, *14*, 383–390. [CrossRef]
94. Bethoux, F.A.; Palfy, D.M.; Plow, M.A. Correlates of the timed 25 foot walk in a multiple sclerosis outpatient rehabilitation clinic. *Int. J. Rehabil. Res.* **2016**, *39*, 134–139. [CrossRef]
95. Hobart, J.C.; Riazi, A.; Lamping, D.L.; Fitzpatrick, R.; Thompson, A.J. Measuring the impact of MS on walking ability: The 12-Item MS Walking Scale (MSWS-12). *Neurology* **2003**, *60*, 31–36. [CrossRef]
96. Jørgensen, M.; Dalgas, U.; Wens, I.; Hvid, L.G. Muscle strength and power in persons with multiple sclerosis—A systematic review and meta-analysis. *J. Neurol. Sci.* **2017**, *376*, 225–241. [CrossRef] [PubMed]
97. Hoang, P.; Gandevia, S.; Herbert, R. Prevalence of joint contractures and muscle weakness in people with multiple sclerosis. *Disabil. Rehabil.* **2013**, *36*, 1588–1593. [CrossRef] [PubMed]
98. Mañago, M.M.; Hebert, J.R.; Schenkman, M. Psychometric Properties of a Clinical Strength Assessment Protocol in People with Multiple Sclerosis. *Int. J. MS Care* **2017**, *19*, 253–262. [CrossRef] [PubMed]
99. Latimer-Cheung, A.E.; Ginis, K.A.M.; Hicks, A.L.; Motl, R.W.; Pilutti, L.A.; Duggan, M.; Wheeler, G.; Persad, R.; Smith, K.M. Development of evidence-informed physical activity guidelines for adults with multiple sclerosis. *Arch. Phys. Med. Rehabil.* **2013**, *94*, 1829–1836.E7. [CrossRef] [PubMed]
100. Frontera, W.R.; Hughes, V.A.; Krivickas, L.S.; Kim, S.K.; Foldvari, M.; Roubenoff, R. Strength training in older women: Early and late changes in whole muscle and single cells. *Muscle Nerve* **2003**, *28*, 601–608. [CrossRef]

101. Mañago, M.M.; Glick, S.; Hebert, J.R.; Coote, S.; Schenkman, M. Strength Training to Improve Gait in People with Multiple Sclerosis: A Critical Review of Exercise Parameters and Intervention Approaches. *Int. J. MS Care* **2019**, *21*, 47–56. [CrossRef]
102. Eftekhari, E.; Mostahfezian, M.; Etemadifar, M.; Zafari, A. Resistance training and vibration improve muscle strength and functional capacity in female patients with multiple sclerosis. *Asian J. Sports Med.* **2012**, *3*, 279–284. [CrossRef]
103. Learmonth, Y.C.; Paul, L.; Miller, L.; Mattison, P.; McFadyen, A.K. The effects of a 12-week leisure centre-based, group exercise intervention for people moderately affected with multiple sclerosis: A randomized controlled pilot study. *Clin. Rehabil.* **2012**, *26*, 579–593. [CrossRef]
104. Romberg, A.; Virtanen, A.; Ruutiainen, J.; Aunola, S.; Karppi, S.L.; Vaara, M.; Surakka, J.; Pohjolainen, T.; Seppänen, A. Effects of a 6-month exercise program on patients with multiple sclerosis: A randomized study. *Neurology* **2004**, *63*, 2034–2038. [CrossRef]
105. Harvey, L.; Smith, A.D.; Jones, R. The Effect of Weighted Leg Raises on Quadriceps Strength, EMG Parameters and Functional Activities in People with Multiple Sclerosis. *Physiotherapy* **1999**, *85*, 154–161. [CrossRef]
106. Dalgas, U.; Stenager, E.; Jakobsen, J.; Petersen, T.; Hansen, H.J.; Knudsen, C.; Overgaard, K.; Ingemann-Hansen, T. Resistance training improves muscle strength and functional capacity in multiple sclerosis. *Neurology* **2009**, *73*, 1478–1484. [CrossRef] [PubMed]
107. Broekmans, T.; Roelants, M.; Feys, P.; Alders, G.; Gijbels, D.; Hanssen, I.; Stinissen, P.; Eijnde, B. Effects of long-term resistance training and simultaneous electro-stimulation on muscle strength and functional mobility in multiple sclerosis. *Mult. Scler.* **2010**, *17*, 468–477. [CrossRef] [PubMed]
108. Kjølhede, T.; Vissing, K.; de Place, L.; Pedersen, B.G.; Ringgaard, S.; Stenager, E.; Petersen, T.; Dalgas, U. Neuromuscular adaptations to long-term progressive resistance training translates to improved functional capacity for people with multiple sclerosis and is maintained at follow-up. *Mult. Scler.* **2015**, *21*, 599–611. [CrossRef]
109. Manca, A.; Cabboi, M.P.; Dragone, D.; Ginatempo, F.; Ortu, E.; De Natale, E.R.; Mercante, B.; Mureddu, G.; Bua, G.; Deriu, F. Resistance Training for Muscle Weakness in Multiple Sclerosis: Direct Versus Contralateral Approach in Individuals With Ankle Dorsiflexors' Disparity in Strength. *Arch. Phys. Med. Rehabil.* **2017**, *98*, 1348–1356.E1. [CrossRef]
110. Dodd, K.J.; Taylor, N.F.; Shields, N.; Prasad, D.; McDonald, E.; Gillon, A. Progressive resistance training did not improve walking but can improve muscle performance, quality of life and fatigue in adults with multiple sclerosis: A randomized controlled trial. *Mult. Scler.* **2011**, *17*, 1362–1374. [CrossRef]
111. Sangelaji, B.; Kordi, M.; Banihashemi, F.; Nabavi, S.M.; Khodadadeh, S.; Dastoorpoor, M. A combined exercise model for improving muscle strength, balance, walking distance, and motor agility in multiple sclerosis patients: A randomized clinical trial. *Iran. J. Neurol.* **2016**, *15*, 111–120.
112. Savci, S.; Inal-Ince, D.; Arikan, H.; Guclu-Gunduz, A.; Cetisli-Korkmaz, N.; Armutlu, K.; Karabudak, R. Six-minute walk distance as a measure of functional exercise capacity in multiple sclerosis. *Disabil. Rehabil.* **2005**, *27*, 1365–1371. [CrossRef]
113. Xie, X.; Sun, H.; Zeng, Q.; Lu, P.; Zhao, Y.; Fan, T.; Huang, G. Do Patients with Multiple Sclerosis Derive More Benefit from Robot-Assisted Gait Training Compared with Conventional Walking Therapy on Motor Function? A Meta-analysis. *Front. Neurol.* **2017**, *8*, 260. [CrossRef]
114. Colombo, G.; Wirz, M.; Dietz, V. Driven gait orthosis for improvement of locomotor training in paraplegic patients. *Spinal Cord* **2001**, *39*, 252–255. [CrossRef]
115. Karpatkin, H.; Benson, A.; Gardner, N.; Leb, N.; Ramos, N.; Xu, H.; Cohen, E. Pilot trial of speed-intensive gait training on balance and walking in people with multiple sclerosis. *Int. J. Ther. Rehabil.* **2020**, *2020*, 1–10. [CrossRef]
116. Burgomaster, K.A.; Hughes, S.C.; Heigenhauser, G.J.; Bradwell, S.N.; Gibala, M.J. Six sessions of sprint interval training increases muscle oxidative potential and cycle endurance capacity in humans. *J. Appl. Physiol.* **2005**, *98*, 1985–1990. [CrossRef]
117. Protas, E.J.; Tissier, S. Strength and speed training for elders with mobility disability. *J. Aging Phys. Act.* **2009**, *17*, 257–271. [CrossRef]
118. Boyne, P.; Dunning, K.; Carl, D.; Gerson, M.; Khoury, J.; Rockwell, B.; Keeton, G.; Westover, J.; Williams, A.; McCarthy, M.; et al. High-Intensity Interval Training and Moderate-Intensity Continuous Training in Ambulatory Chronic Stroke: Feasibility Study. *Phys. Ther.* **2016**, *96*, 1533–1544. [CrossRef]
119. Rose, M.H.; Løkkegaard, A.; Sonne-Holm, S.; Jensen, B.R. Improved clinical status, quality of life, and walking capacity in Parkinson's disease after body weight-supported high-intensity locomotor training. *Arch. Phys. Med. Rehabil.* **2013**, *94*, 687–692. [CrossRef]
120. Donzé, C. Update on rehabilitation in multiple sclerosis. *Presse Med.* **2015**, *44*, e169–e176. [CrossRef]
121. Wening, J.; Ford, J.; Jouett, L.D. Orthotics and FES for maintenance of walking in patients with MS. *Dis. Mon.* **2013**, *59*, 284–289. [CrossRef]
122. Kelleher, K.J.; Spence, W.D.; Solomonidis, S.; Apatsidis, D. The effect of textured insoles on gait patterns of people with multiple sclerosis. *Gait Posture* **2010**, *32*, 67–71. [CrossRef]
123. Dixon, J.; Hatton, A.L.; Robinson, J.; Gamesby-Iyayi, H.; Hodgson, D.; Rome, K.; Warnett, R.; Martin, D.J. Effect of textured insoles on balance and gait in people with multiple sclerosis: An exploratory trial. *Physiotherapy* **2014**, *100*, 142–149. [CrossRef]
124. Kubsik-Gidlewska, A.M.; Klimkiewicz, P.; Klimkiewicz, R.; Janczewska, K.; Woldańska-Okońska, M. Rehabilitation in multiple sclerosis. *Adv. Clin. Exp. Med.* **2017**, *26*, 709–715. [CrossRef]

125. Loyd, B.J.; Fangman, A.; Peterson, D.S.; Gappmaier, E.; Schubert, M.C.; Thackery, A.; Dibble, L. Rehabilitation to improve gaze and postural stability in people with multiple sclerosis: Study protocol for a prospective randomized clinical trial. *BMC Neurol.* **2019**, *19*, 119. [CrossRef] [PubMed]
126. Cattaneo, D.; Jonsdottir, J.; Zocchi, M.; Regola, A. Effects of balance exercises on people with multiple sclerosis: A pilot study. *Clin. Rehabil.* **2007**, *21*, 771–781. [CrossRef] [PubMed]
127. Muñoz-Lasa, S.; Ferriero, G.; Valero, R.; Gomez-Muñiz, F.; Rabini, A.; Varela, E. Effect of therapeutic horseback riding on balance and gait of people with multiple sclerosis. *G Ital Med Lav Ergon* **2011**, *33*, 462–467. [PubMed]
128. Smedal, T.; Lygren, H.; Myhr, K.M.; Moe-Nilssen, R.; Gjelsvik, B.; Gjelsvik, O.; Strand, L.I. Balance and gait improved in patients with MS after physiotherapy based on the Bobath concept. *Physiother. Res. Int.* **2006**, *11*, 104–116. [CrossRef] [PubMed]
129. Döring, A.; Pfueller, C.F.; Paul, F.; Dörr, J. Exercise in multiple sclerosis—An integral component of disease management. *EPMA J.* **2011**, *3*, 2. [CrossRef]
130. Nguyen, P.T.; Chou, L.-W.; Hsieh, Y.-L. Proprioceptive Neuromuscular Facilitation-Based Physical Therapy on the Improvement of Balance and Gait in Patients with Chronic Stroke: A Systematic Review and Meta-Analysis. *Life* **2022**, *12*, 882. [CrossRef]
131. Shimura, K.; Kasai, T. Effects of proprioceptive neuromuscular facilitation on the initiation of voluntary movement and motor evoked potentials in upper limb muscles. *Hum. Mov. Sci.* **2002**, *21*, 101–113. [CrossRef] [PubMed]
132. Gabriel, D.A.; Kamen, G.; Frost, G. Neural adaptations to resistive exercise: Mechanisms and recommendations for training practices. *Sports Med.* **2006**, *36*, 133–149. [CrossRef]
133. Judica, E.; Boneschi, F.M.; Ungaro, D.; Comola, M.; Gatti, R.; Comi, G.; Rossi, P. Impact of fatigue on the efficacy of rehabilitation in multiple sclerosis. *J. Neurol.* **2011**, *258*, 835–839. [CrossRef]
134. Schwid, S.R.; Covington, M.; Segal, B.M.; Goodman, A.D. Fatigue in multiple sclerosis: Current understanding and future directions. *J. Rehabil. Res. Dev.* **2002**, *39*, 211–224.
135. Mikuľáková, W.; Klímová, E.; Kendrová, L.; Gajdoš, M.; Chmelík, M. Effect of Rehabilitation on Fatigue Level in Patients with Multiple Sclerosis. *Med. Sci. Monit.* **2018**, *24*, 5761–5770. [CrossRef] [PubMed]
136. Schwartz, C.E.; Coulthard-Morris, L.; Zeng, Q. Psychosocial correlates of fatigue in multiple sclerosis. *Arch. Phys. Med. Rehabil.* **1996**, *77*, 165–170. [CrossRef] [PubMed]
137. Rosenberg, J.H.; Shafor, R. Fatigue in multiple sclerosis: A rational approach to evaluation and treatment. *Curr. Neurol. Neurosci. Rep.* **2005**, *5*, 140–146. [CrossRef]
138. Zielińska-Nowak, E.; Włodarczyk, L.; Kostka, J.; Miller, E. New Strategies for Rehabilitation and Pharmacological Treatment of Fatigue Syndrome in Multiple Sclerosis. *J. Clin. Med.* **2020**, *9*, 3592. [CrossRef] [PubMed]
139. Kalb, R.; Brown, T.R.; Coote, S.; Costello, K.; Dalgas, U.; Garmon, E.; Giesser, B.; Halper, J.; Karpatkin, H.; Keller, J.; et al. Exercise and lifestyle physical activity recommendations for people with multiple sclerosis throughout the disease course. *Mult. Scler.* **2020**, *26*, 1459–1469. [CrossRef] [PubMed]
140. Haveman, J.; Van Der Zee, J.; Wondergem, J.; Hoogeveen, J.F.; Hulshof, M.C. Effects of hyperthermia on the peripheral nervous system: A review. *Int. J. Hyperth.* **2004**, *20*, 371–391. [CrossRef]
141. Miller, E.; Kostka, J.; Włodarczyk, T.; Dugué, B. Whole-body cryostimulation (cryotherapy) provides benefits for fatigue and functional status in multiple sclerosis patients. A case-control study. *Acta Neurol. Scand.* **2016**, *134*, 420–426. [CrossRef]
142. Nilsagård, Y.; Denison, E.; Gunnarsson, L.G. Evaluation of a single session with cooling garment for persons with multiple sclerosis—A randomized study. *Disabil. Rehabil. Assist. Technol.* **2006**, *1*, 225–233. [CrossRef]
143. Lappin, M.S.; Lawrie, F.W.; Richards, T.L.; Kramer, E.D. Effects of a pulsed electromagnetic therapy on multiple sclerosis fatigue and quality of life: A double-blind, placebo controlled trial. *Altern. Ther. Health Med.* **2003**, *9*, 38–48.
144. Piatkowski, J.; Kern, S.; Ziemssen, T. Effect of BEMER magnetic field therapy on the level of fatigue in patients with multiple sclerosis: A randomized, double-blind controlled trial. *J. Altern. Complement. Med.* **2009**, *15*, 507–511. [CrossRef]
145. Pilutti, L.A.; Edwards, T.; Motl, R.W.; Sebastião, E. Functional Electrical Stimulation Cycling Exercise in People with Multiple Sclerosis: Secondary Effects on Cognition, Symptoms, and Quality of Life. *Int. J. MS Care* **2019**, *21*, 258–264. [CrossRef] [PubMed]
146. Chang, Y.J.; Hsu, M.J.; Chen, S.M.; Lin, C.H.; Wong, A.M. Decreased central fatigue in multiple sclerosis patients after 8 weeks of surface functional electrical stimulation. *J. Rehabil. Res. Dev.* **2011**, *48*, 555–564. [CrossRef] [PubMed]
147. Shakespeare, D.; Boggild, M.; Young, C.A. Anti-spasticity agents for multiple sclerosis. *Cochrane Database Syst. Rev.* **2003**, *2003*, CD001332. [CrossRef] [PubMed]
148. Galea, M.P. Physical modalities in the treatment of neurological dysfunction. *Clin. Neurol. Neurosurg.* **2012**, *114*, 483–488. [CrossRef]
149. Etoom, M.; Khraiwesh, Y.; Lena, F.; Hawamdeh, M.; Hawamdeh, Z.; Centonze, D.; Foti, C. Effectiveness of Physiotherapy Interventions on Spasticity in People With Multiple Sclerosis: A Systematic Review and Meta-Analysis. *Am. J. Phys. Med. Rehabil.* **2018**, *97*, 793–807. [CrossRef]
150. Barnes, M.; Kocer, S.; Fernandez, M.M.; Balcaitiene, J.; Fheodoroff, K. An international survey of patients living with spasticity. *Disabil. Rehabil.* **2017**, *39*, 1428–1434. [CrossRef]
151. Adams, M.M.; Hicks, A.L. Spasticity after spinal cord injury. *Spinal Cord* **2005**, *43*, 577–586. [CrossRef]
152. Zahraa, F.; Fatima, K.; Ali, F.; Amal, A.; Khodor, H.H.; Hassane, K. PJM and Cryotherapy in a New Approach for Spasticity Management: An Experimental Trial. *Int. J. Pharm. Bio. Med. Sci.* **2022**, *2*, 302–313. [CrossRef]

153. Alcantara, C.C.; Blanco, J.; De Oliveira, L.M.; Ribeiro, P.F.S.; Herrera, E.; Nakagawa, T.H.; Reisman, D.S.; Michaelsen, S.M.; Garcia, L.C.; Russo, T.L. Cryotherapy reduces muscle hypertonia, but does not affect lower limb strength or gait kinematics post-stroke: A randomized controlled crossover study. *Top. Stroke Rehabil.* **2019**, *26*, 267–280. [CrossRef]
154. Sosnoff, J.J.; Shin, S.; Motl, R.W. Multiple sclerosis and postural control: The role of spasticity. *Arch. Phys. Med. Rehabil.* **2010**, *91*, 93–99. [CrossRef]
155. Pau, M.; Coghe, G.; Corona, F.; Marrosu, M.G.; Cocco, E. Effect of spasticity on kinematics of gait and muscular activation in people with Multiple Sclerosis. *J. Neurol. Sci.* **2015**, *358*, 339–344. [CrossRef] [PubMed]
156. Lee, Y.; Chen, K.; Ren, Y.; Son, J.; Cohen, B.A.; Sliwa, J.A.; Zhang, L.Q. Robot-guided ankle sensorimotor rehabilitation of patients with multiple sclerosis. *Mult. Scler. Relat. Disord.* **2017**, *11*, 65–70. [CrossRef] [PubMed]
157. Pompa, A.; Morone, G.; Iosa, M.; Pace, L.; Catani, S.; Casillo, P.; Clemenzi, A.; Troisi, E.; Tonini, A.; Paolucci, S.; et al. Does robot-assisted gait training improve ambulation in highly disabled multiple sclerosis people? A pilot randomized control trial. *Mult. Scler. J.* **2017**, *23*, 696–703. [CrossRef]
158. Etoom, M.; Khraiwesh, Y.; Foti, C. Transcutaneous Electrical Nerve Stimulation for Spasticity. *Am. J. Phys. Med. Rehabil.* **2017**, *96*, e198. [CrossRef]
159. Mills, P.B.; Dossa, F. Transcutaneous Electrical Nerve Stimulation for Management of Limb Spasticity: A Systematic Review. *Am. J. Phys. Med. Rehabil.* **2016**, *95*, 309–318. [CrossRef] [PubMed]
160. Wahls, T.L.; Reese, D.; Kaplan, D.; Darling, W.G. Rehabilitation with neuromuscular electrical stimulation leads to functional gains in ambulation in patients with secondary progressive and primary progressive multiple sclerosis: A case series report. *J. Altern. Complement. Med.* **2010**, *16*, 1343–1349. [CrossRef] [PubMed]
161. McIntyre, A.; Mirkowski, M.; Thompson, S.; Burhan, A.M.; Miller, T.; Teasell, R. A Systematic Review and Meta-Analysis on the Use of Repetitive Transcranial Magnetic Stimulation for Spasticity Poststroke. *PM R* **2018**, *10*, 293–302. [CrossRef]
162. Centonze, D.; Koch, G.; Versace, V.; Mori, F.; Rossi, S.; Brusa, L.; Grossi, K.; Torelli, F.; Prosperetti, C.; Cervellino, A.; et al. Repetitive transcranial magnetic stimulation of the motor cortex ameliorates spasticity in multiple sclerosis. *Neurology* **2007**, *68*, 1045–1050. [CrossRef]
163. Abdollahi, M.; Bahrpeyma, F.; Forogh, B. Investigation of the Effects of Spinal Pulsed Electromagnetic Field on Spasticity of Lower Extremity and Alpha Motoneuron Excitability in Hemiplegic Patients Using Hmax/Mmax ratio. *Cerebrovasc. Dis.* **2013**, *36*, 18–19.
164. Serag, H.; Abdelgawad, D.; Emara, T.; Moustafa, R.; El Nahas, N.; Haroun, M. Effects of Para-Spinal Repetitive Magnetic Stimulation on Multiple Sclerosis Related Spasticity. *Int. J. Phys. Med. Rehabil.* **2014**, *2*, 2. [CrossRef]
165. Ciortea, V.M.; Motoașcă, I.; Borda, I.M.; Ungur, R.A.; Bondor, C.I.; Iliescu, M.G.; Ciubean, A.D.; Lazăr, I.; Bendea, E.; Irsay, L. Effects of High-Intensity Electromagnetic Stimulation on Reducing Upper Limb Spasticity in Post-Stroke Patients. *Appl. Sci.* **2022**, *12*, 2125. [CrossRef]
166. Han, T.R.; Shin, H.I.; Kim, I.S. Magnetic stimulation of the quadriceps femoris muscle: Comparison of pain with electrical stimulation. *Am. J. Phys. Med. Rehabil.* **2006**, *85*, 593–599. [CrossRef] [PubMed]
167. Vinolo-Gil, M.J.; Rodríguez-Huguet, M.; García-Muñoz, C.; Gonzalez-Medina, G.; Martin-Vega, F.J.; Martín-Valero, R. Effects of Peripheral Electromagnetic Fields on Spasticity: A Systematic Review. *J. Clin. Med.* **2022**, *11*, 3739. [CrossRef] [PubMed]
168. Guthrie, T.C.; Nelson, D.A. Influence of temperature changes on multiple sclerosis: Critical review of mechanisms and research potential. *J. Neurol. Sci.* **1995**, *129*, 1–8. [CrossRef] [PubMed]
169. Kargarfard, M.; Etemadifar, M.; Baker, P.; Mehrabi, M.; Hayatbakhsh, R. Effect of aquatic exercise training on fatigue and health-related quality of life in patients with multiple sclerosis. *Arch. Phys. Med. Rehabil.* **2012**, *93*, 1701–1708. [CrossRef]
170. Aghaz, A.; Alidad, A.; Hemmati, E.; Jadidi, H.; Ghelichi, L. Prevalence of dysphagia in multiple sclerosis and its related factors: Systematic review and meta-analysis. *Iran. J. Neurol.* **2018**, *17*, 180–188. [CrossRef]
171. Calcagno, P.; Ruoppolo, G.; Grasso, M.G.; De Vincentiis, M.; Paolucci, S. Dysphagia in multiple sclerosis—Prevalence and prognostic factors. *Acta Neurol. Scand.* **2002**, *105*, 40–43. [CrossRef]
172. Ansari, N.N.; Tarameshlu, M.; Ghelichi, L. Dysphagia In Multiple Sclerosis Patients: Diagnostic And Evaluation Strategies. *Degener. Neurol. Neuromuscul. Dis.* **2020**, *10*, 15–28. [CrossRef]
173. Farazi, M.; Ilkhani, Z.; Jaferi, S.; Haghighi, M. Rehabilitation Strategies of Dysphagia in a Patient with Multiple Sclerosis: A Case Study. *Zahedan J. Res. Med. Sci.* **2019**, *21*, e85783. [CrossRef]
174. D'Amico, E.; Zanghì, A.; Serra, A.; Murabito, P.; Zappia, M.; Patti, F.; Cocuzza, S. Management of dysphagia in multiple sclerosis: Current best practice. *Expert Rev. Gastroenterol. Hepatol.* **2019**, *13*, 47–54. [CrossRef]
175. Kelly, E.A.; Koszewski, I.J.; Jaradeh, S.S.; Merati, A.L.; Blumin, J.H.; Bock, J.M. Botulinum toxin injection for the treatment of upper esophageal sphincter dysfunction. *Ann. Otol. Rhinol. Laryngol.* **2013**, *122*, 100–108. [CrossRef]
176. Schneider, I.; Thumfart, W.F.; Pototschnig, C.; Eckel, H.E. Treatment of dysfunction of the cricopharyngeal muscle with botulinum A toxin: Introduction of a new, noninvasive method. *Ann. Otol. Rhinol. Laryngol.* **1994**, *103*, 31–35. [CrossRef] [PubMed]
177. Murry, T.; Wasserman, T.; Carrau, R.L.; Castillo, B. Injection of botulinum toxin A for the treatment of dysfunction of the upper esophageal sphincter. *Am. J. Otolaryngol.* **2005**, *26*, 157–162. [CrossRef] [PubMed]
178. Cosentino, G.; Gargano, R.; Bonura, G.; Realmuto, S.; Tocco, E.; Ragonese, P.; Gangitano, M.; Alfonsi, E.; Fierro, B.; Brighina, F.; et al. Anodal tDCS of the swallowing motor cortex for treatment of dysphagia in multiple sclerosis: A pilot open-label study. *Neurol. Sci.* **2018**, *39*, 1471–1473. [CrossRef] [PubMed]

179. Al Dandan, H.B.; Coote, S.; McClurg, D. Prevalence of Lower Urinary Tract Symptoms in People with Multiple Sclerosis: A Systematic Review and Meta-analysis. *Int. J. MS Care* **2020**, *22*, 91–99. [CrossRef] [PubMed]
180. Demaagd, G.A.; Davenport, T.C. Management of urinary incontinence. *Pharm. Ther.* **2012**, *37*, 345–361.
181. Lúcio, A.C.; Perissinoto, M.C.; Natalin, R.A.; Prudente, A.; Damasceno, B.P.; D'Ancona, C.A. A comparative study of pelvic floor muscle training in women with multiple sclerosis: Its impact on lower urinary tract symptoms and quality of life. *Clinics* **2011**, *66*, 1563–1568. [CrossRef]
182. Glenn, J. Restorative Nursing Bladder Training program: Recommending a strategy. *Rehabil. Nurs.* **2003**, *28*, 15–22. [CrossRef]
183. Subak, L.L.; Wing, R.; West, D.S.; Franklin, F.; Vittinghoff, E.; Creasman, J.M.; Richter, H.E.; Myers, D.; Burgio, K.L.; Gorin, A.A.; et al. Weight loss to treat urinary incontinence in overweight and obese women. *N. Engl. J. Med.* **2009**, *360*, 481–490. [CrossRef]
184. Cortese, R.; Carotenuto, A.; Di Filippo, M.; Lanzillo, R. Editorial: Cognition in Multiple Sclerosis. *Front. Neurol.* **2021**, *12*, 751687. [CrossRef]
185. Passamonti, L.; Cerasa, A.; Liguori, M.; Gioia, M.C.; Valentino, P.; Nisticò, R.; Quattrone, A.; Fera, F. Neurobiological mechanisms underlying emotional processing in relapsing-remitting multiple sclerosis. *Brain* **2009**, *132*, 3380–3391. [CrossRef]
186. Hung, Y.; Yarmak, P. Neurorehabilitation for Multiple Sclerosis Patients with Emotional Dysfunctions. *Front. Neurol.* **2015**, *6*, 272. [CrossRef] [PubMed]
187. Chalk, H.M. Mind over matter: Cognitive—Behavioral determinants of emotional distress in multiple sclerosis patients. *Psychol. Health Med.* **2007**, *12*, 556–566. [CrossRef] [PubMed]
188. Phillips, L.H.; Henry, J.D.; Nouzova, E.; Cooper, C.; Radlak, B.; Summers, F. Difficulties with emotion regulation in multiple sclerosis: Links to executive function, mood, and quality of life. *J. Clin. Exp. Neuropsychol.* **2014**, *36*, 831–842. [CrossRef]
189. Taylor, P.; Dorstyn, D.S.; Prior, E. Stress management interventions for multiple sclerosis: A meta-analysis of randomized controlled trials. *J. Health Psychol.* **2020**, *25*, 266–279. [CrossRef] [PubMed]
190. Hind, D.; Cotter, J.; Thake, A.; Bradburn, M.; Cooper, C.; Isaac, C.; House, A. Cognitive behavioural therapy for the treatment of depression in people with multiple sclerosis: A systematic review and meta-analysis. *BMC Psychiatry* **2014**, *14*, 5. [CrossRef] [PubMed]
191. Hämäläinen, P.; Rosti-Otajärvi, E. Is neuropsychological rehabilitation effective in multiple sclerosis? *Neurodegen. Dis. Manag.* **2014**, *4*, 147–154. [CrossRef]
192. Crosson, B.; Hampstead, B.M.; Krishnamurthy, L.C.; Krishnamurthy, V.; McGregor, K.M.; Nocera, J.R.; Roberts, S.; Rodriguez, A.D.; Tran, S.M. Advances in neurocognitive rehabilitation research from 1992 to 2017: The ascension of neural plasticity. *Neuropsychology* **2017**, *31*, 900–920. [CrossRef]
193. WHOQOL Group. The World Health Organization Quality of Life assessment (WHOQOL): Position paper from the World Health Organization. *Soc. Sci. Med.* **1995**, *41*, 1403–1409. [CrossRef]
194. Faraclas, E.; Lynn, J.; Lau, J.D.; Merlo, A. Health-Related Quality of Life in people with Multiple Sclerosis: How does this Population Compare to Population-based Norms in Different Health Domains? *J. Patient-Rep. Outcomes* **2022**, *6*, 12. [CrossRef]
195. Berrigan, L.I.; Fisk, J.D.; Patten, S.B.; Tremlett, H.; Wolfson, C.; Warren, S.; Fiest, K.M.; McKay, K.A.; Marrie, R.A. Health-related quality of life in multiple sclerosis: Direct and indirect effects of comorbidity. *Neurology* **2016**, *86*, 1417–1424. [CrossRef]
196. Pérez de Heredia-Torres, M.; Huertas-Hoyas, E.; Sánchez-Camarero, C.; Máximo-Bocanegra, N.; Alegre-Ayala, J.; Sánchez-Herrera-Baeza, P.; Martínez-Piédrola, R.M.; García-Bravo, C.; Mayoral-Martín, A.; Serrada-Tejeda, S. Occupational performance in multiple sclerosis and its relationship with quality of life and fatigue. *Eur. J. Phys. Rehabil. Med.* **2020**, *56*, 148–154. [CrossRef] [PubMed]
197. Ochoa-Morales, A.; Hernández-Mojica, T.; Paz-Rodríguez, F.; Jara-Prado, A.; Trujillo-De Los Santos, Z.; Sánchez-Guzmán, M.A.; Guerrero-Camacho, J.L.; Corona-Vázquez, T.; Flores, J.; Camacho-Molina, A.; et al. Quality of life in patients with multiple sclerosis and its association with depressive symptoms and physical disability. *Mult. Scler. Relat. Disord.* **2019**, *36*, 101386. [CrossRef] [PubMed]
198. Dorstyn, D.S.; Roberts, R.M.; Murphy, G.; Haub, R. Employment and multiple sclerosis: A meta-analytic review of psychological correlates. *J. Health Psychol.* **2019**, *24*, 38–51. [CrossRef]
199. Ysrraelit, M.C.; Fiol, M.P.; Gaitán, M.I.; Correale, J. Quality of Life Assessment in Multiple Sclerosis: Different Perception between Patients and Neurologists. *Front. Neurol.* **2017**, *8*, 729. [CrossRef] [PubMed]
200. Gil-González, I.; Martín-Rodríguez, A.; Conrad, R.; Pérez-San-Gregorio, M. Quality of life in adults with multiple sclerosis: A systematic review. *BMJ Open* **2020**, *10*, e041249. [CrossRef] [PubMed]
201. Ghodspour, Z.; Najafi, M.; Rahimian Boogar, I. Effectiveness of Mindfulness-Based Cognitive Therapy on Psychological Aspects of Quality of Life, Depression, Anxiety, and Stress Among Patients With Multiple Sclerosis. *Pract. Clin. Psychol.* **2018**, *6*, 215–222. [CrossRef]
202. Case, L.K.; Jackson, P.; Kinkel, R.; Mills, P.J. Guided Imagery Improves Mood, Fatigue, and Quality of Life in Individuals With Multiple Sclerosis: An Exploratory Efficacy Trial of Healing Light Guided Imagery. *J. Evid. Based Integr. Med.* **2018**, *23*, 2515690x17748744. [CrossRef]
203. Kikuchi, H.; Niino, M.; Hirotani, M.; Miyazaki, Y.; Kikuchi, S. Pilot study on the effects of cognitive behavioral therapy on depression among Japanese patients with multiple sclerosis. *Clin. Exp. Neuroimmunol.* **2019**, *10*, 180–185. [CrossRef]

204. Thomas, P.W.; Thomas, S.; Kersten, P.; Jones, R.; Slingsby, V.; Nock, A.; Davies Smith, A.; Baker, R.; Galvin, K.T.; Hillier, C. One year follow-up of a pragmatic multi-centre randomised controlled trial of a group-based fatigue management programme (FACETS) for people with multiple sclerosis. *BMC Neurol.* **2014**, *14*, 109. [CrossRef]
205. Jongen, P.J.; Ruimschotel, R.; Heerings, M.; Hussaarts, A.; Duyverman, L.; van der Zande, A.; Valkenburg-Vissers, J.; Wolper, H.; van Droffelaar, M.; Lemmens, W.; et al. Improved self-efficacy in persons with relapsing remitting multiple sclerosis after an intensive social cognitive wellness program with participation of support partners: A 6-months observational study. *Health Qual. Life Outcomes* **2014**, *12*, 40. [CrossRef]
206. Jongen, P.J.; Heerings, M.; Ruimschotel, R.; Hussaarts, A.; Duyverman, L.; van der Zande, A.; Valkenburg-Vissers, J.; van Droffelaar, M.; Lemmens, W.; Donders, R.; et al. Intensive social cognitive treatment (can do treatment) with participation of support partners in persons with relapsing remitting multiple sclerosis: Observation of improved self-efficacy, quality of life, anxiety and depression 1 year later. *BMC Res. Notes* **2016**, *9*, 375. [CrossRef] [PubMed]
207. van Munster, C.E.; D'Souza, M.; Steinheimer, S.; Kamm, C.P.; Burggraaff, J.; Diederich, M.; Kravalis, K.; Dorn, J.; Walsh, L.; Dahlke, F.; et al. Tasks of activities of daily living (ADL) are more valuable than the classical neurological examination to assess upper extremity function and mobility in multiple sclerosis. *Mult. Scler.* **2019**, *25*, 1673–1681. [CrossRef] [PubMed]
208. Goverover, Y. Cognition and activities of daily living in multiple sclerosis. In *Cognition and Behavior in Multiple Sclerosis*; American Psychological Association: Washington, DC, USA, 2018; pp. 171–190. [CrossRef]
209. Freeman, J.A.; Langdon, D.W.; Hobart, J.C.; Thompson, A.J. The impact of inpatient rehabilitation on progressive multiple sclerosis. *Ann. Neurol.* **1997**, *42*, 236–244. [CrossRef] [PubMed]
210. Craig, J.; Young, C.A.; Ennis, M.; Baker, G.; Boggild, M. A randomised controlled trial comparing rehabilitation against standard therapy in multiple sclerosis patients receiving intravenous steroid treatment. *J. Neurol. Neurosurg. Psychiatry* **2003**, *74*, 1225–1230. [CrossRef]
211. Storr, L.K.; Sørensen, P.S.; Ravnborg, M. The efficacy of multidisciplinary rehabilitation in stable multiple sclerosis patients. *Mult. Scler.* **2006**, *12*, 235–242. [CrossRef]
212. Heesen, C.; Böhm, J.; Reich, C.; Kasper, J.; Goebel, M.; Gold, S.M. Patient perception of bodily functions in multiple sclerosis: Gait and visual function are the most valuable. *Mult. Scler.* **2008**, *14*, 988–991. [CrossRef]
213. Motl, R.W.; Sandroff, B.M.; Suh, Y.; Sosnoff, J.J. Energy cost of walking and its association with gait parameters, daily activity, and fatigue in persons with mild multiple sclerosis. *Neurorehabil. Neural Repair* **2012**, *26*, 1015–1021. [CrossRef]
214. Kikkert, L.H.J.; de Groot, M.H.; van Campen, J.P.; Beijnen, J.H.; Hortobágyi, T.; Vuillerme, N.; Lamoth, C.C.J. Gait dynamics to optimize fall risk assessment in geriatric patients admitted to an outpatient diagnostic clinic. *PLoS ONE* **2017**, *12*, e0178615. [CrossRef]
215. Angelini, L.; Hodgkinson, W.; Smith, C.; Dodd, J.M.; Sharrack, B.; Mazzà, C.; Paling, D. Wearable sensors can reliably quantify gait alterations associated with disability in people with progressive multiple sclerosis in a clinical setting. *J. Neurol.* **2020**, *267*, 2897–2909. [CrossRef]
216. van Munster, C.E.; Uitdehaag, B.M. Outcome Measures in Clinical Trials for Multiple Sclerosis. *CNS Drugs* **2017**, *31*, 217–236. [CrossRef]
217. Cofré Lizama, L.E.; Khan, F.; Lee, P.V.; Galea, M.P. The use of laboratory gait analysis for understanding gait deterioration in people with multiple sclerosis. *Mult. Scler.* **2016**, *22*, 1768–1776. [CrossRef] [PubMed]
218. Comber, L.; Galvin, R.; Coote, S. Gait deficits in people with multiple sclerosis: A systematic review and meta-analysis. *Gait Posture* **2017**, *51*, 25–35. [CrossRef] [PubMed]
219. Papagiannis, G.I.; Triantafyllou, A.I.; Roumpelakis, I.M.; Zampeli, F.; Garyfallia Eleni, P.; Koulouvaris, P.; Papadopoulos, E.C.; Papagelopoulos, P.J.; Babis, G.C. Methodology of surface electromyography in gait analysis: Review of the literature. *J. Med. Eng. Technol.* **2019**, *43*, 59–65. [CrossRef] [PubMed]
220. Huang, S.-C.; Guerrieri, S.; Dalla Costa, G.; Pisa, M.; Leccabue, G.; Gregoris, L.; Comi, G.; Leocani, L. Intensive Neurorehabilitation and Gait Improvement in Progressive Multiple Sclerosis: Clinical, Kinematic and Electromyographic Analysis. *Brain Sci.* **2022**, *12*, 258. [CrossRef] [PubMed]
221. Sasaki, J.E.; Bertochi, G.F.A.; Meneguci, J.; Motl, R.W. Pedometers and Accelerometers in Multiple Sclerosis: Current and New Applications. *Int. J. Environ. Res. Public Health* **2022**, *19*, 11839. [CrossRef]
222. Verheyden, G.; Nuyens, G.; Nieuwboer, A.; Van Asch, P.; Ketelaer, P.; De Weerdt, W. Reliability and validity of trunk assessment for people with multiple sclerosis. *Phys. Ther.* **2006**, *86*, 66–76. [CrossRef] [PubMed]
223. Gervasoni, E.; Jonsdottir, J.; Montesano, A.; Cattaneo, D. Minimal Clinically Important Difference of Berg Balance Scale in People With Multiple Sclerosis. *Arch. Phys. Med. Rehabil.* **2017**, *98*, 337–340.e2. [CrossRef]
224. Salcı, Y.; Fil, A.; Keklicek, H.; Çetin, B.; Armutlu, K.; Dolgun, A.; Tuncer, A.; Karabudak, R. Validity and reliability of the International Cooperative Ataxia Rating Scale (ICARS) and the Scale for the Assessment and Rating of Ataxia (SARA) in multiple sclerosis patients with ataxia. *Mult. Scler. Relat. Disord.* **2017**, *18*, 135–140. [CrossRef]
225. Bertoni, R.; Lamers, I.; Chen, C.C.; Feys, P.; Cattaneo, D. Unilateral and bilateral upper limb dysfunction at body functions, activity and participation levels in people with multiple sclerosis. *Mult. Scler.* **2015**, *21*, 1566–1574. [CrossRef]
226. Feys, P.; Lamers, I.; Francis, G.; Benedict, R.; Phillips, G.; LaRocca, N.; Hudson, L.D.; Rudick, R. The Nine-Hole Peg Test as a manual dexterity performance measure for multiple sclerosis. *Mult. Scler.* **2017**, *23*, 711–720. [CrossRef]

227. Keser, I.; Kirdi, N.; Meric, A.; Kurne, A.T.; Karabudak, R. Comparing routine neurorehabilitation program with trunk exercises based on Bobath concept in multiple sclerosis: Pilot study. *J. Rehabil. Res. Dev.* **2013**, *50*, 133–140. [CrossRef]
228. Romaniszyn, P.; Kawa, J.; Stępien, P.; Nawrat-Szołtysik, A. Video-based time assessment in 360 degrees turn Berg balance test. *Comput. Med. Imaging Graph.* **2020**, *80*, 101689. [CrossRef] [PubMed]
229. Kawa, J.; Stępień, P.; Kapko, W.; Niedziela, A.; Derejczyk, J. Leg movement tracking in automatic video-based one-leg stance evaluation. *Comput. Med. Imaging Graph.* **2018**, *65*, 191–199. [CrossRef]
230. Aldenhoven, C.M.; Reimer, L.M.; Jonas, S. mBalance: Detect Postural Imbalance with Mobile Devices. *Stud. Health Technol. Inf.* **2022**, *293*, 30–38. [CrossRef]
231. Vattanasilp, W.; Ada, L.; Crosbie, J. Contribution of thixotropy, spasticity, and contracture to ankle stiffness after stroke. *J. Neurol. Neurosurg. Psychiatry* **2000**, *69*, 34–39. [CrossRef]
232. Tarameshlu, M.; Ghelichi, L.; Azimi, A.R.; Ansari, N.N.; Khatoonabadi, A.R. The effect of traditional dysphagia therapy on the swallowing function in patients with Multiple Sclerosis: A pilot double-blinded randomized controlled trial. *J. Bodyw. Mov. Ther.* **2019**, *23*, 171–176. [CrossRef] [PubMed]
233. Rosenbek, J.C.; Robbins, J.A.; Roecker, E.B.; Coyle, J.L.; Wood, J.L. A penetration-aspiration scale. *Dysphagia* **1996**, *11*, 93–98. [CrossRef]
234. Bergamaschi, R.; Crivelli, P.; Rezzani, C.; Patti, F.; Solaro, C.; Rossi, P.; Restivo, D.; Maimone, D.; Romani, A.; Bastianello, S.; et al. The DYMUS questionnaire for the assessment of dysphagia in multiple sclerosis. *J. Neurol. Sci.* **2008**, *269*, 49–53. [CrossRef]
235. Massetti, T.; Trevizan, I.L.; Arab, C.; Favero, F.M.; Ribeiro-Papa, D.C.; de Mello Monteiro, C.B. Virtual reality in multiple sclerosis—A systematic review. *Mult. Scler. Relat. Disord.* **2016**, *8*, 107–112. [CrossRef]
236. Laver, K.E.; Lange, B.; George, S.; Deutsch, J.E.; Saposnik, G.; Crotty, M. Virtual reality for stroke rehabilitation. *Cochrane Database Syst. Rev.* **2017**, *11*, Cd008349. [CrossRef]
237. Martin, C.L.; Phillips, B.A.; Kilpatrick, T.J.; Butzkueven, H.; Tubridy, N.; McDonald, E.; Galea, M.P. Gait and balance impairment in early multiple sclerosis in the absence of clinical disability. *Mult. Scler.* **2006**, *12*, 620–628. [CrossRef]
238. Erdeo, F.; Salcı, Y.; Uca, A.U.; Armutlu, K. Examination of the effects of coordination and balance problems on gait in ataxic multiple sclerosis patients. *Neurosciences* **2019**, *24*, 269–277. [CrossRef]
239. Eftekharsadat, B.; Babaei-Ghazani, A.; Mohammadzadeh, M.; Talebi, M.; Eslamian, F.; Azari, E. Effect of virtual reality-based balance training in multiple sclerosis. *Neurol. Res.* **2015**, *37*, 539–544. [CrossRef] [PubMed]
240. Berriozabalgoitia, R.; Bidaurrazaga-Letona, I.; Otxoa, E.; Urquiza, M.; Irazusta, J.; Rodriguez-Larrad, A. Overground Robotic Program Preserves Gait in Individuals With Multiple Sclerosis and Moderate to Severe Impairments: A Randomized Controlled Trial. *Arch. Phys. Med. Rehabil.* **2021**, *102*, 932–939. [CrossRef] [PubMed]
241. Verdict. History of Virtual Reality: Timeline. Available online: https://www.verdict.co.uk/history-virtual-reality-timeline/ (accessed on 24 October 2022).
242. Weghorst, S. Augmented reality and Parkinson's disease. *Commun. ACM* **1997**, *40*, 47–48. [CrossRef]
243. Inman, D.P.; Loge, K.; Cram, A.; Peterson, M. Learning to Drive a Wheelchair in Virtual Reality. *J. Spec. Educ. Technol.* **2011**, *26*, 21–34. [CrossRef]
244. Foreman, N.; Wilson, P.; Stanton, D. VR and spatial awareness in disabled children. *Commun. ACM* **1997**, *40*, 76–77. [CrossRef]
245. Baram, Y.; Miller, A. Virtual reality cues for improvement of gait in patients with multiple sclerosis. *Neurology* **2006**, *66*, 178–181. [CrossRef]
246. Sampson, P.; Freeman, C.; Coote, S.; Demain, S.; Feys, P.; Meadmore, K.; Hughes, A.M. Using Functional Electrical Stimulation Mediated by Iterative Learning Control and Robotics to Improve Arm Movement for People With Multiple Sclerosis. *IEEE Trans. Neural. Syst. Rehabil. Eng.* **2016**, *24*, 235–248. [CrossRef]
247. Mahajan, H.; Spaeth, D.; Dicianno, B.; Brown, K.; Cooper, R. Preliminary evaluation of variable compliance joystick for people with multiple sclerosis. *J. Rehabil. Res. Dev.* **2014**, *51*, 951–962. [CrossRef]
248. Australian Institute of Health and Welfare. *How We Manage Stroke in Australia*; AIHW: Canberra, Australian, 2006.
249. Chen, Y.P.; Kang, L.J.; Chuang, T.Y.; Doong, J.L.; Lee, S.J.; Tsai, M.W.; Jeng, S.F.; Sung, W.H. Use of virtual reality to improve upper-extremity control in children with cerebral palsy: A single-subject design. *Phys. Ther.* **2007**, *87*, 1441–1457. [CrossRef]
250. Azulay, J.-P.; Mesure, S.; Blin, O. Influence of visual cues on gait in Parkinson's disease: Contribution to attention or sensory dependence? *J. Neurol. Sci.* **2006**, *248*, 192–195. [CrossRef] [PubMed]
251. Androwis, G.J.; Sandroff, B.M.; Niewrzol, P.; Fakhoury, F.; Wylie, G.R.; Yue, G.; DeLuca, J. A pilot randomized controlled trial of robotic exoskeleton-assisted exercise rehabilitation in multiple sclerosis. *Mult. Scler. Relat. Disord.* **2021**, *51*, 102936. [CrossRef] [PubMed]
252. Androwis, G.J.; Pilkar, R.; Ramanujam, A.; Nolan, K.J. Electromyography Assessment During Gait in a Robotic Exoskeleton for Acute Stroke. *Front. Neurol* **2018**, *9*, 630. [CrossRef] [PubMed]
253. Sandroff, B.M.; Motl, R.W.; Reed, W.R.; Barbey, A.K.; Benedict, R.H.B.; DeLuca, J. Integrative CNS Plasticity With Exercise in MS: The PRIMERS (PRocessing, Integration of Multisensory Exercise-Related Stimuli) Conceptual Framework. *Neurorehabil. Neural Repair* **2018**, *32*, 847–862. [CrossRef]
254. Jensen, S.K.; Yong, V.W. Activity-Dependent and Experience-Driven Myelination Provide New Directions for the Management of Multiple Sclerosis. *Trends Neurosci.* **2016**, *39*, 356–365. [CrossRef]

255. Drużbicki, M.; Guzik, A.; Przysada, G.; Perenc, L.; Brzozowska-Magoń, A.; Cygoń, K.; Boczula, G.; Bartosik-Psujek, H. Effects of Robotic Exoskeleton-Aided Gait Training in the Strength, Body Balance, and Walking Speed in Individuals With Multiple Sclerosis: A Single-Group Preliminary Study. *Arch. Phys. Med. Rehabil.* **2021**, *102*, 175–184. [CrossRef]
256. McGibbon, C.; Sexton, A.; Gryfe, P.; Dutta, T.; Jayaraman, A.; Deems-Dluhy, S.; Novak, A.; Fabara, E.; Adans-Dester, C.; Bonato, P. Effect of using of a lower-extremity exoskeleton on disability of people with multiple sclerosis. *Disabil. Rehabil. Assist. Technol.* **2021**, *16*, 1–8. [CrossRef]
257. De Luca, R.; Russo, M.; Gasparini, S.; Leonardi, S.; Foti Cuzzola, M.; Sciarrone, F.; Zichittella, C.; Sessa, E.; Maggio, M.G.; De Cola, M.C.; et al. Do people with multiple sclerosis benefit from PC-based neurorehabilitation? A pilot study. *Appl. Neuropsychol. Adult* **2021**, *28*, 427–435. [CrossRef]
258. De Luca, R.; Leonardi, S.; Spadaro, L.; Russo, M.; Aragona, B.; Torrisi, M.; Maggio, M.G.; Bramanti, A.; Naro, A.; De Cola, M.C.; et al. Improving Cognitive Function in Patients with Stroke: Can Computerized Training Be the Future? *J. Stroke Cerebrovasc. Dis.* **2018**, *27*, 1055–1060. [CrossRef]
259. De Luca, R.; Calabrò, R.S.; Gervasi, G.; De Salvo, S.; Bonanno, L.; Corallo, F.; De Cola, M.C.; Bramanti, P. Is computer-assisted training effective in improving rehabilitative outcomes after brain injury? A case-control hospital-based study. *Disabil. Health J.* **2014**, *7*, 356–360. [CrossRef] [PubMed]

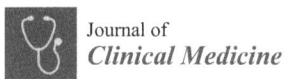

Review

An sEMG-Controlled Forearm Bracelet for Assessing and Training Manual Dexterity in Rehabilitation: A Systematic Review

Selena Marcos-Antón [1], María Dolores Gor-García-Fogeda [2] and Roberto Cano-de-la-Cuerda [2,*]

[1] International Doctorate School, Rey Juan Carlos University, 28008 Madrid, Spain; s.marcosa@alumnos.urjc.es
[2] Department of Physical Therapy, Occupational Therapy, Rehabilitation and Physical Medicine, Rey Juan Carlos University, 28922 Alcorcon, Spain; mariadolores.gor@urjc.es
* Correspondence: roberto.cano@urjc.es; Tel.: +34-914-888-674

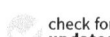

Citation: Marcos-Antón, S.; Gor-García-Fogeda, M.D.; Cano-de-la-Cuerda, R. An sEMG-Controlled Forearm Bracelet for Assessing and Training Manual Dexterity in Rehabilitation: A Systematic Review. *J. Clin. Med.* **2022**, *11*, 3119. https://doi.org/10.3390/jcm11113119

Academic Editors: Hideki Nakano, Akiyoshi Matsugi, Naoki Yoshida and Yohei Okada

Received: 11 March 2022
Accepted: 27 May 2022
Published: 31 May 2022

Publisher's Note: MDPI stays neutral with regard to jurisdictional claims in published maps and institutional affiliations.

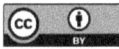

Copyright: © 2022 by the authors. Licensee MDPI, Basel, Switzerland. This article is an open access article distributed under the terms and conditions of the Creative Commons Attribution (CC BY) license (https://creativecommons.org/licenses/by/4.0/).

Abstract: Background: The ability to perform activities of daily living (ADL) is essential to preserving functional independence and quality of life. In recent years, rehabilitation strategies based on new technologies, such as MYO Armband®, have been implemented to improve dexterity in people with upper limb impairment. Over the last few years, many studies have been published focusing on the accuracy of the MYO Armband® to capture electromyographic and inertial data, as well as the clinical effects of using it as a rehabilitation tool in people with loss of upper limb function. Nevertheless, to our knowledge, there has been no systematic review of this subject. Methods: A systematically comprehensive literature search was conducted in order to identify original studies that answered the PICO question (patient/population, intervention, comparison, and outcome): What is the accuracy level and the clinical effects of the MYO Armband® in people with motor impairment of the upper limb compared with other assessment techniques or interventions or no intervention whatsoever? The following data sources were used: Pubmed, Scopus, Web of Science, ScienceDirect, Physiotherapy Evidence Database, and the Cochrane Library. After identifying the eligible articles, a cross-search of their references was also completed for additional studies. The following data were extracted from the papers: study design, disease or condition, intervention, sample, dosage, outcome measures or data collection procedure and data analysis and results. The authors independently collected these data following the CONSORT 2010 statement when possible, and eventually reached a consensus on the extracted data, resolving disagreements through discussion. To assess the methodological quality of papers included, the tool for the critical appraisal of epidemiological cross-sectional studies was used, since only case series studies were identified after the search. Additionally, the articles were classified according to the levels of evidence and grades of recommendation for diagnosis studies established by the Oxford Center for Evidence-Based Medicine. Also, The Cochrane Handbook for Systematic Reviews of Interventions was used by two independent reviewers to assess risk of bias, assessing the six different domains. The Preferred Reporting Items for Systematic Reviews and Meta-Analyses (PRISMA) was followed to carry out this review. Results: 10 articles with a total 180 participants were included in the review. The characteristics of included studies, sample and intervention characteristics, outcome measures, the accuracy of the system and effects of the interventions and the assessment of methodological quality of the studies and risk of bias are shown. Conclusions: Therapy with the MYO Armband® has shown clinical changes in range of motion, dexterity, performance, functionality and satisfaction. It has also proven to be an accurate system to capture signals from the forearm muscles in people with motor impairment of the upper limb. However, further research should be conducted using bigger samples, well-defined protocols, comparing with control groups or comparing with other assessment or therapeutic tools, since the studies published so far present a high risk of bias and low level of evidence and grade of recommendation.

Keywords: activities of daily living; dexterity; functional independence; MYO armband; rehabilitation; semi-immersive virtual reality; technologies; upper limb impairment; virtual reality

1. Introduction

The ability to perform activities of daily living (ADL) is essential to preserve functional independence and quality of life [1]. This ADL performance can be severely restricted in people with neurological disorders such as children with congenital disorders or developmental disabilities and adults with acquired injuries or neurodegenerative diseases, due to upper limb motor impairment [1]. These functional disorders are often related to loss of dexterity, which is defined as "fine, voluntary movements used to manipulate small objects during a specific task" [2]. Also, dexterity is associated with two related concepts: manual dexterity (ability to handle objects with the hand) and fine motor dexterity (in-hand manipulations as separate skills from the gross motor grasp and release skills associated with manual dexterity) [2]. Hence, rehabilitation processes should enable patients to restore their functional capacity by training dexterity [3].

In recent years, rehabilitation strategies based on new technologies have been implemented to improve dexterity in people with upper limb impairment, enhancing patient comfort [3]. Virtual reality (VR) seems to have the potential to improve upper limb rehabilitation [4], since it creates virtual environments similar to the real world where the user can interact with appealing surroundings and perform significant, high repetition, high transfer capacity, and motivating tasks, maximizing neuroplasticity and motor learning thanks to the provided feedback [5,6]. Also, these motivating and appealing environments created by VR could help recover health conditions and community integration [7]. Furthermore, these devices achieve higher intensity at a sustainable cost [5,6,8].

The MYO Armband® is a semi-immersive VR device that captures forearm movements [9]. It consists of an accelerometer, a gyroscope, a magnetometer (inertial measure unit (IMU)) and eight surface electromyography (sEMG) sensors [9,10]. The electromyographic signal is streamed wirelessly at a frequency of 200 Hz and the orientation and position data from the inertial sensor is transmitted at a frequency of 50 Hz. This system, which integrates motion tracking and electromyography with VR, provides quantitative data on muscle activity that can be used not only for objective assessment but also as a semi-immersive VR therapeutic tool [9,10].

Over the last few years, many studies have been published focusing on the accuracy of the MYO Armband® to capture electromyographic and inertial data [4,11], as well as the clinical effects of using it as a rehabilitation tool in people with loss of upper limb function [8–10]. Nevertheless, to our knowledge, there has been no systematic review of this subject. Therefore, we conducted a systematic review with the aim of analyzing the accuracy and the clinical effects of using the MYO Armband® in people with motor impairment of the upper extremity.

2. Materials and Methods

2.1. Design

The Preferred Reporting Items for Systematic Reviews and Meta-Analyses (PRISMA) [12] was used to carry out this systematic review, starting with a PICO (patient/population, intervention, comparison, and outcome) question: Which is the accuracy level and the clinical effects of the MYO Armband® in people with motor impairment of the upper limb as compared with other assessment techniques or interventions or no intervention whatsoever?

2.2. Search Strategy

A systematically comprehensive literature search was conducted from June to November 2021 in order to identify original studies that answered the PICO question, using the following data sources: Pubmed, Scopus, Web Of Science (WOS), ScienceDirect, Physiotherapy Evidence Database (PEDro) and the Cochrane Library. After identifying the eligible articles, a cross-search of their references was also completed for additional studies.

The combinations of keywords were: *"MYO Armband" AND (rehabilitation OR "manual dexterity" OR "upper limb" OR disability)*. The detailed search strategy for each database is shown in Table 1.

Table 1. Search filters in databases.

Database	Search Filter
PubMed	- Availability: full text - Publication date: last 5 years
Scopus	- Year: 2016, 2017, 2018, 2019, 2020, 2021 - Language: English - Document type: any article
Web of Science	- Year: 2016, 2017, 2018, 2019, 2020, 2021 - Language: English - Document type: any article
ScienceDirect	- Year: 2016, 2017, 2018, 2019, 2020, 2021 - Language: English - Article type: research article - Subject area: engineering, computer science, neuroscience
PEDro	No filter
Cochrane Library	- Year: from 2016 until 2021

Two authors independently searched and screened titles and abstracts to identify studies meeting inclusion criteria. Duplicates were removed and disagreements regarding the selection of studies were resolved by a third author.

2.3. Study Selection

Studies published in Spanish and English between January 2016 and November 2021 were considered for inclusion in this review, regardless of their methodological design.

The exclusion criteria were: no access to full-text, poster communications, congress or symposium reports, and technical analysis studies with no clinical application or perspective.

2.4. Participants

This review considered studies that included subjects with motor impairment of the upper limb. Studies that included healthy subjects as the control group (CG) and studies that analyzed the accuracy of the device comparing healthy subjects with affected subjects were also taken into consideration.

2.5. Interventions

For the clinical trials, the intervention group had to follow a rehabilitation program using the MYO Armband® either isolated or combined with other therapeutic strategies, in any dosage and provided in any setting (inpatient, outpatient, or domicile).

For the case studies, they had to analyze the accuracy of the MYO Armband® or assess and/or carry out an intervention using sEMG in people with motor impairment of the upper limb.

2.6. Outcome Measures

Studies that analyzed parameters related to the accuracy to capture signals and the functioning of the system were included. Additionally, studies that analyzed outcomes that measure mobility, dexterity, and upper limb function, as well as outcomes related to these parameters were also included.

2.7. Data Extraction and Analysis

The following data were extracted from the papers: study design, disease or condition, intervention, sample, dosage, outcome measures or data collection procedure, and data analysis and results. The authors independently collected these data following the CONSORT 2010 statement [13] when possible, and eventually reached a consensus on the extracted data, resolving disagreements through discussion.

2.8. Assessment of Methodological Quality of the Studies and Risk of Bias

To assess methodological quality, we used the tool for the critical appraisal of epidemiological cross-sectional studies adapted by Ciaponni [14] from the work of Berra et al. [15], since only case series studies were identified after the search. This tool contains 31 items divided into 6 dimensions: (a) research question or aim of the research, (b) participants, (c) comparability between groups, (d) definition and measurement of the primary variables, (e) statistical analysis and confusion, (f) results, (g) conclusions, external validity and applicability of the results, (h) conflict of interests and (i) follow-up. Dimensions "b" to "e" assess internal validity and items 25 and 26 assess external validity. Methodological quality is considered high when most of the dimensions are rated as "good" or "very good"; medium when most of the dimensions are rated as "good" or "fair" or internal validity is rated as "medium"; and low when most of the dimensions are rated as "fair" or "bad" or internal validity is rated as "low".

Additionally, the articles were classified according to the levels of evidence and grades of recommendation for diagnosis studies established by the Oxford Center for Evidence-Based Medicine [16].

The Cochrane Handbook for Systematic Reviews of Interventions [17] was used by two independent reviewers to assess the risk of bias, assessing the six different domains:

(a) Selection bias: relates to recruiting process and participant allocation. To analyze it, randomization and allocation concealing must be considered.
(b) Performance bias: refers to systematic differences between groups in the care that is provided, or in exposure to factors other than the interventions of interest. To analyze it, blinding procedures must be examined.
(c) Detection bias: refers to systematic differences between groups in how outcomes are determined and may occur during intervention and follow-up. Blinding of outcome assessors must be considered when analyzing it, since it may reduce the risk.
(d) Attrition bias: systematic differences between groups in withdrawals from a study. It occurs when there are withdrawals that lead to incomplete outcome data or when withdrawals in both groups differ significantly.
(e) Reporting bias: refers to systematic differences between reported and unreported findings. This can occur once the study is finished and it is due to the selective report of results, reporting only statistically significant data.
(f) Other biases: occur when reviewers include methodological aspects that are not assessed in the domains described before. They relate mainly to certain trial designs, such as crossover trials.

Each study was assessed independently and was considered a "low risk of bias" when each domain was addressed properly. Otherwise, it was considered a "high risk of bias". If a study did not provide enough information, it was considered "dubious". Disagreement was resolved through discussion with a third reviewer.

3. Results

The literature search and the article selection process are detailed in Figure 1. The initial search yielded 108 articles. Once the duplicates were removed and eligibility criteria were applied, 10 articles with a total of 180 participants were included in the review [4,7,9–11,18–22]. The characteristics of included studies are shown in Tables 2 and 3.

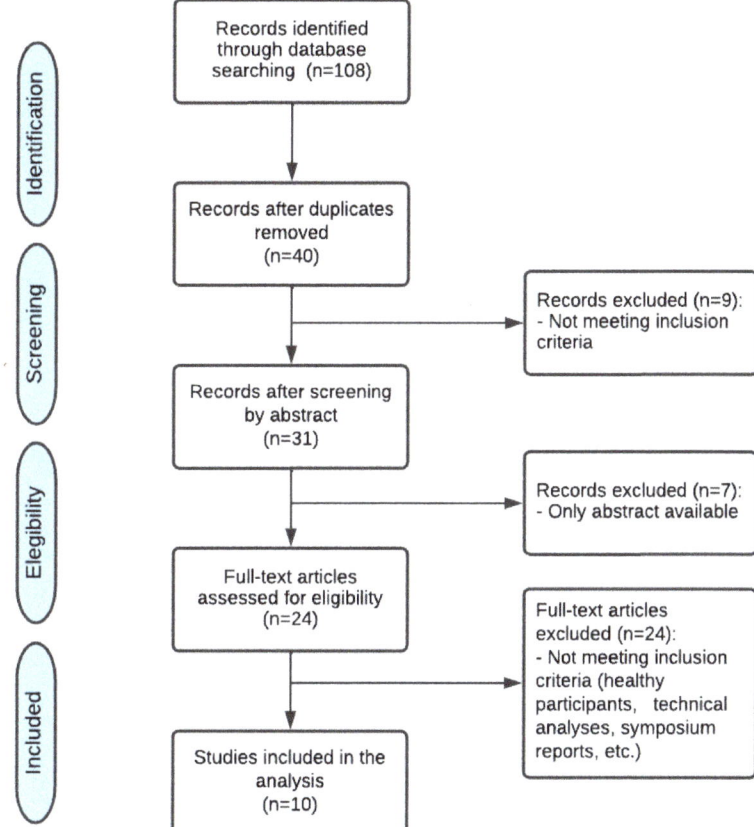

Figure 1. PRISMA Flow chart for identifying studies for systematic review.

Table 2. Characteristics of the studies focused on the accuracy of the device as an assessment tool.

Study	Participants (Disease and Sample Size)	Protocol	Data Collection Process	Outcome Measures	Results
Melero et al. [4]	Disease: amputation n: 3	Dance game with visual feedback using Kinect® + MYO Armband®	10 game trials for each patient	Detection time, reaction time and operating time. O = R + D	D = 0.24 s/R = 0.92 s/O = 1.15 s MD = 2.6 s Operating time (R + MD) = 3.56 s Initial expected operating time = 6 s
Ryser et al. [11]	Disease: stroke n: 3	Assessing the accuracy of the MYO® to detect movement intention in order to control a dynamic hand orthosis device	Performing three gestures, each for 60 s	Classification algorithm	Accuracy for five gestures for all samples: 98%. Accuracy for three gestures related to ADL: 94.3%. Accuracy in people with stroke: 78–99%. The system is suitable for stroke rehabilitation
Lyu et al. [18]	Disease: stroke n: 6 healthy + 2 stroke	Visuomotor training task using the MYO Armband®	Accuracy: four gestures, 25 repetitions per gesture, 4 s contraction, 2 s relaxation, 30 s rest Validation: 36 blocks of exercises, four trials per block	sEMG signals captured via MYO®	Accuracy: 99.3% for wrist extension, 82% for radial deviation, 100% for flexion Accuracy in healthy subjects: 92.5% Validation: task performance improves through training Stroke patients: no event was reported regarding calibration, donning, or executing tasks with the device. Lower accuracy than healthy subjects
Gaetani et al. [19]	Disease: transradial amputation n: 9 (8 healthy + 1 congenital amelia)	performing three different gestures with hand fingers to collect sEMG data with the MYO® and analyze accuracy and response time	10 s of flexion, 10 s of extension, and 10 s of rest	Learning algorithm, analysis of sEMG signal	Average accuracy of gesture recognition: 90.4% Accuracy in subject with amputation: 93.3% Response time: <1 s The system works also on subjects with small not-trained muscles
Sattar et al. [20]	Disease: transhumeral amputation n: 18 (15 healthy + 3 amputees)	Creation of BCI to control upper limb prostheses: sEMG (MYO Armband®) + fNIRS The armband acquired the sEMG signals for four-arm motions: elbow extension, elbow flexion, wrist pronation, and wrist supination	Training session: resting period of 3 min to establish a data baseline. Data acquisition: initial 5-sec rest followed by a 20-sec task period	Data processing from sEMG and fNIRS using MATLAB®	The hybrid sEMG and fNIRS system is a feasible approach to improve the CA for transhumeral amputees, improving the control performances of multifunctional upper-limb prostheses. The average accuracy of 94.6% and 74% was achieved for elbow and wrist motions by sEMG for healthy and amputated subjects, respectively Simultaneously, the fNIRS modality showed an average accuracy of 96.9% and 94.5% for hand motions of healthy and amputated subjects
Castiblanco et al. [21]	Disease: stroke n: 10 (6 healthy + 4 stroke)	Healthy: collection of six sEMG signals (four from right arm and two from left). One trial. Stroke: 12 sEMG signals (eight from impaired side, two from non-impaired). Three trials. All with visual feedback	Maintaining each movement 3–5 s (open-close the hand, flexion-extension of the wrist, spread the fingers, and pinch-grip each finger)	Classification algorithms	Exercises with best performance: opening-closing hand Exercises with worst performance: pinch-grip finger it was possible to identify the hand movements from sEMG signals for subjects who had a motor disability due to stroke with a correct classification rate of 85%

ADL: activities of daily living; BCI: Brain-computer interface; D: detection time; fNIRS: Functional near-infrared spectroscopy; MD: maximum detection time; O: operating time; R: reaction time; sEMG: Surface electromyography.

Table 3. Characteristics of the studies focused on the clinical effects of the device as a rehabilitation tool.

Study	Participants (Disease and Sample Size)	Intervention or Protocol	Dosage	Outcome Measures	Results
Esfahlani et al. [7]	Disease: stroke n: 20	3D games controlled with Kinect® and MYO®	8 weeks 1 h/day, (days per week not specified)	EQ (Rasch Analysis), MAS, angular velocity, acceleration, ROM	Flow, presence, and absorption EQ: participants enjoyed the sessions the activities covered a good ROM for the upper body Suggest audio feedback
Esfahlani et al. [9]	Disease: stroke, MA and TBI n: 23 (10 healthy CG; 2 stroke, 2 TBI and 9 MA IG)	Serious game controlled by Kinect® + MYO® + pedal	45-minute sessions, no further information	ROM response time, electromyographic data, velocity, orientation, and inertial information	Improvement in performance reflected in response time and ROM High interest and engagement The combination of MYO® and Kinect® increase the accuracy to detect gestures
Esfahlani et al. [10]	Disease: MS n: 52 (40 MS IG; 12 healthy CG)	IG: video games using Kinect + MYO + Pedal GC: not specified	10 weeks 5 days/week 1 h/day	MAS, ROM	Statistically significant differences in performance and ROM. High interest and engagement
MacIntosh et al. [22]	Disease: CP n: 19	Video game controlled by completing therapeutic gestures detected via electromyography and inertial sensors on the forearm via the MYO® and custom software	4 weeks 17 min/day	AHA, BBT, wrist extension, grip strength, COPM, SEAS	Moderate improvements in active wrists extension, grip strength, COPM and BBT, small improvement in AHA Positive results in SEAS No adverse effects

AHA: Assisting Hand Assessment; BBT: Box & Blocks Test; COPM: Canadian Occupational Performance Measure; CP: Cerebral Palsy; EQ: Engagement Questionnaire; MS: multiple sclerosis, CG: control group; IG: intervention group; TBI: traumatic brain injury; ROM: range of movement; SEAS: Self-Reported Experiences of Activity Settings.

3.1. Sample Characteristics

One study (n = 19) included a sample of children with cerebral palsy (CP) with ages ranging from 8 to 18 years [22]. Three studies (n = 7) included patients with upper limb amputation: one of them did not specify the amputation level [4], another included transradial amputees [19] and the other transhumeral amputees [20]. Five studies (n = 31) examined patients with stroke [7,9,11,18,21]: three of them did not specify the characteristics of the impairment, one included people (n = 3) with mildly to severely impaired hand function [11], and the other included people (n = 4) with different levels of impairment [21]. Two studies examined people (n = 49) with multiple sclerosis (MS) [9,10] but did not specify the level of disability in the Expanded Disability Status Scale (EDSS) and one study included patients with traumatic brain injury (TBI) without specifying cause or severity [9]. Combined, these articles included 57 healthy subjects to compare their results with those of the patients who presented some condition or disease.

3.2. Intervention Characteristics

All studies used semi-immersive VR. Six of them [4,11,18–21] implemented protocols designed to analyze the accuracy of the sEMG system. One of these used a protocol based on a dance game and added the Kinect® sensor to track position in amputees, with the aim of knowing the time taken for each hand gesture to be detected by the system as well as its total operating time [4]. Another compared the accuracy of the information captured by the MYO Armband® with functional near-infrared spectroscopy (fNIRS) and evaluated the effectiveness of the combination of both systems to obtain information about motor intention in patients with transhumeral amputation, which may be useful to improve the control of upper limb prostheses [20]. The other four studies [11,18,19,21] used different upper limb exercise protocols with or without visual feedback that allowed to calculate the accuracy of the MYO Armaband®.

The rest of the articles included in this review [7,9,10,22] analyzed the clinical effects of video game-based therapy with the MYO Armband®. Three of them [7,9,10] combined the use of the MYO Armband® with other devices such as the Kinect® sensor or a foot pedal for gaming.

The studies were heterogeneous regarding dosage. Processes to obtain data in those studies analyzing the sensor's accuracy differed significantly. In the studies evaluating the clinical effects of the MYO Armband® combined with semi-immersive VR, the mean session duration was 45.66 ± 24.82 min (range 17–60 min) [7,9,10,22]; only one study specified the number of sessions (50 sessions) [10]; and the mean number of weeks was 7.33 ± 3.05 (range 4–10 weeks) [7,10,22].

3.3. Outcome Measures

The studies that examined the accuracy to capture sEMG signals used different classification and data processing algorithms, as well as the information provided by the sEMG in Hz. Melero et al. [4] evaluated the operating time, which is the time taken for each hand gesture to be detected by the system from the moment it appears on the screen. It can be broken down into detection time (the time it takes for each specific gesture to be recognized by the system) and reaction time (the time it takes the subject to perform a hand gesture from the moment it appears on the screen). In addition, three studies [11,19,21] analyzed the accuracy of the MYO Armband® by using classification algorithms in people with stroke and in transradial amputees. They used a software to apply mathematical formulations to the data collected from the sEMG, calculating the percentages of the accuracy of the system. Finally, two studies [18,20] used the sEMG signal to know the characteristics of the forearm muscle contraction performed by the participants. The second [20] also compared this signal with the data collected from another motion capture device and analyzed the effectiveness of combining both devices as an assessment approach.

The studies were also heterogeneous regarding outcome measures. Those articles analyzing clinical effects used physical evaluation tools, as well as functional and cognitive.

One of the articles [22] used the Assisting Hand Assessment (AHA) to assess spontaneous bimanual performance and the Box and Blocks Test (BBT) to assess unilateral hand dexterity. Two articles [7,10] used the Motor Assessment Scale (MAS), a scale to assess motor function in people with stroke. They also evaluated wrist extension, grip strength, and angular velocity [7,22]. Range of motion (ROM) was also assessed in most of the studies. In relation to functional and cognitive assessment, one study [22] used the Canadian Occupational Performance Measure (COPM) to assess self-perception of performance in everyday living and the Self-Reported Experiences of Activity Settings (SEAS) to assess participation experiences. Finally, another study [7] assessed the patient's engagement during therapy with the Engagement Questionnaire (EQ).

3.4. Accuracy of the System and Effects of the Interventions

In regard to the accuracy of the system to assess motor control of the upper limb, we found values that varied between 78% and 99% in mildly to severely impaired subjects after stroke [11,21], and the accuracy for three gestures involved in ADL (rest, close, open, key pinch and precision pinch) was 94% [11]. On the other hand, no event was reported regarding calibration, donning, or executing tasks with the device [18]. In patients with amputation, the results showed that it takes less than 3 s on average for each gesture to be detected and an overall operating time below 4 s. Since the authors expected the operating time to be below 6 s, they concluded that the MYO Armband® was suitable for accurately detecting gestures in people with amputations of the upper limb [4]. Additionally, the study that included transradial amputees [19] found a percentage of accuracy of 93.3% whereas the one that included transhumeral amputees [20] reported an accurfor of 94.6% and 74% for elbow and wrist movements respectively. This accuracy increased significantly by combining sEMG with fNIRS, which demonstrates the feasibility of a hybrid sEMG and fNIRS system to improve the control performances of multifunctional upper-limb prostheses.

Secondly, those studies that examined clinical effects showed improvements after intervention with the MYO Armband®. One study found improvements in functionality related to ROM [10], whereas another showed a moderate increase in grip strength and dexterity as well as higher scores in the COPM and SEAS [22]. Also, some studies reported that the participants showed high interest and engagement during the activities due to a good feeling of immersion in the game, as well as a feeling of enjoyment and motivation [7,8,10].

3.5. Assessment of Methodological Quality of the Studies and Risk of Bias

Table 4 shows the results obtained after analyzing the quality of the studies using the tool for the critical appraisal of epidemiological cross-sectional studies [14]. Internal validity was rated as low for 60% of the articles, medium in 30%, and high in 10% of them. External validity was poor for 100% of the studies. Overall methodological quality was rated as low for 60% of the articles, medium for 30%, and high for 10%.

Table 4. Scores for each article after evaluation with the tool for the critical appraisal of epidemiological cross-sectional studies.

	Tool item	Melero et al. [4]	Esfahlani et al. [7]	Esfahlani et al. [9]	Esfahlani et al. [10]	Ryser et al. [11]	Lyu et al. [18]	Gaetani et al. [19]	Sattar et al. [20]	Castiblanco et al. [21]	MacIntosh et al. [22]
Methodological analysis	1	VG	F	F	F	F	VG	F	VG	VG	VG
	2	NS	B	B	NS	B	NS	B	F	B	G
	3	NS	B	B	F	B	NS	B	F	F	G
	4	NS	B	B	G	B	B	B	B	B	F
	5	NS	NS	B	NS	B	NS	B	B	B	G
	6	B	NS	NS	NS	B	G	F	NS	F	VG
	7	NA	NA	B	G	NA	F	NA	B	F	G
	8	NA	NA	F	B	NA	B	NA	G	F	G
	9	NA	NA	G	G	NA	B	NA	G	B	G
	10	NA	NA	NS	NS	NA	F	NA	NS	NS	G
	11	G	G	F	G	F	F	F	F	F	VG
	12	F	G	B	F	F	F	NS	F	F	VG
	13	NS	G	B	F	B	NS	G	F	NS	VG
	14	B	F	F	F	F	F	B	F	F	G
	15	F	B	VG	F	NS	F	B	B	G	F
	16	F	F	G	G	NS	G	NS	B	G	F
	17	G	NS	NS	NS	NS	NS	NS	B	NS	NS
	18	F	NS	NS	NS	NS	F	G	B	NS	NS
	19	VG	B	F	F	F	F	F	G	G	G
	20	F	F	G	G	G	G	F	G	G	VG
	21	F	B	F	G	F	F	B	G	G	VG
	22	NA	B	VG	G	B	F	G	NS	F	G
	23	G	F	G	G	VG	G	G	F	NS	G
	24	G	F	G	VG	VG	G	B	F	NS	G
	25	B	B	B	B	B	B	B	B	B	F
	26	NS	B	F	B	F	F	B	B	NS	B
	27	VG	VG	VG	NS	B	NS	F	NS	F	F
	28	NS	G	NS	G	NS	NS	NS	NS	NS	VG
	29	NS	NS	NS	NS	NS	NS	NS	NS	NS	VG
	30	NS	NS	NS	NS	NS	NS	NS	NS	NS	VG
	31	NS	NS	NS	NS	NS	NS	NS	NS	NS	NS
	Internal validity	LOW	LOW	LOW	MEDIUM	LOW	MEDIUM	LOW	LOW	MEDIUM	HIGH
	External validity	LOW	LOW	LOW	LOW	LOW	LOW	LOW	LOW	LOW	LOW
	Overall quality	LOW	LOW	LOW	MEDIUM	LOW	MEDIUM	LOW	LOW	MEDIUM	HIGH

VG: very good; G: good; F: fair; B: bad; NA: not applicable; NS: not specified.

The levels of evidence and grades of recommendation are detailed in Table 5. All articles were classified as level of evidence 4, with a grade of recommendation of C.

Table 5. Levels of evidence and grades of recommendation established by the Oxford Center for Evidence-based Medicine.

Study	Level of Evidence	Grade of Recommendation
Melero et al. [4]	4	C
Esfahlani et al. [7]	4	C
Esfahlani et al. [9]	4	C
Esfahlani et al. [10]	4	C
Ryser et al. [11]	4	C
Lyu et al. [18]	4	C
Gaetani et al. [19]	4	C
Sattar et al. [20]	4	C
Castiblanco et al. [21]	4	C
MacIntosh et al. [22]	4	C

Figure 2 summarizes the results of the assessment of the risk of bias sorted by article.

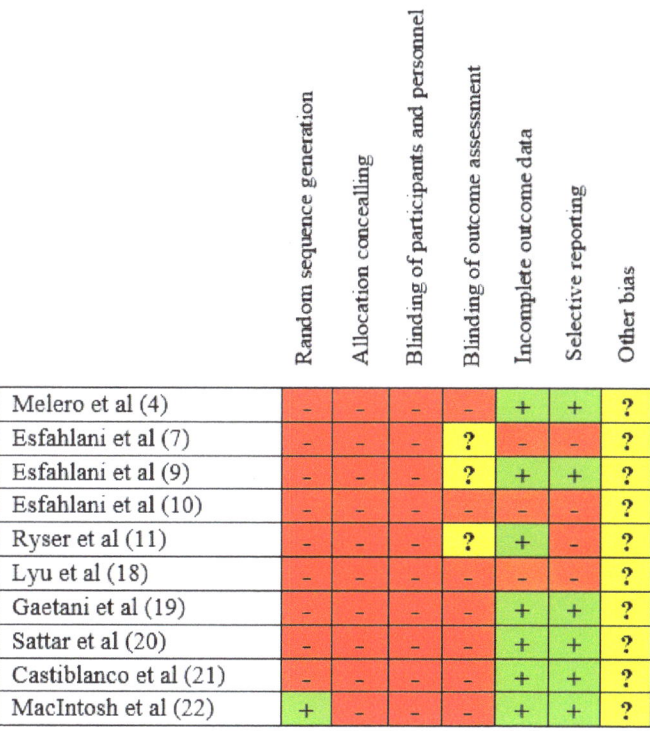

"+" Meets criteria.
"-" Does not meet criteria.
"?" Dubious.

Figure 2. Assessment of risk of bias. Assessments by the reviewers for each risk sorted by article.

4. Discussion

For years, information and communication technologies have been used as an assessment and therapeutic tool in the field of rehabilitation [23,24]. VR-based therapy has been increasingly implemented to complement conventional therapy in people with motor control disorders [25,26]. This is, to our knowledge, the first systematic review that summarizes the available evidence on the use of the MYO Armband® as an assessment and rehabilitation tool in people with motor impairment of the upper limb. Our results suggest that the use of the MYO Armband® as a therapeutic tool in people with motor impairment of the upper limb improves ROM, grip strength, dexterity, functionality, and ADL performance. They also show good satisfaction and feeling of immersion reported by users. Furthermore, the MYO Armband® could be considered an assessment tool suitable to detect small changes during the rehabilitation progress, since the accuracy of the system proved to be high.

Semi-immersive VR combined with the MYO Armaband® provide opportunities for motor and cognitive tasks recreating real-life scenarios and simulations of activities by capturing human motion [27]. Also, semi-immersive VR has shown to have fewer side effects, such as "cybersickness", compared to immersive VR [27,28]. For these reasons, together with the wide availability of these systems and their sustainable cost, semi-immersive VR is recommended to complement conventional therapy in the rehabilitation of upper limb impairment [27].

In the articles included in this review, the MYO Armband® was combined with different devices. On one hand, some studies used these combinations in order to obtain more information about the orientation, position, and movement of the upper limb. For instance, Esfalahni et al. [7,9,10] combined the MYO Armband® with the Kinect® sensor to increase the number of movements detected, providing a better feeling of representation, connection, and control of the game in real-time [10]. The cited studies found statistically significant improvements in strength and dexterity of the upper limb, as well as high user satisfaction. On the other hand, Sattar et al. [20] combined the MYO Armaband® with fNIRS to increase the accuracy to obtain information about muscle activity and motor intention, achieving an accuracy of over 90%. These findings suggest that using the MYO Armband® in combination with other VR devices could improve data collection regarding muscle activity, movement, usability, and interaction, which could translate into better clinical effects. Sattar et al., also examined the use of these two devices combined to collect data about motor intention in order to improve control of upper limb prostheses in transhumeral amputees. While the MYO Armband® predicted flexion, extension, pronation, and supination of the elbow, the fNIRS obtained signals for hand opening and closing. For this reason, this approach can be useful to enhance the control performances of multifunctional prostheses with a high level of accuracy. However, and even though this is an innovative approach since it is the first time that someone combines these devices pursuing this goal, further research is required to learn if this strategy is more efficient, comfortable, and beneficial than the ones currently implemented.

In regard to the data concerning the accuracy of the device, although the articles examined reported high percentages of the accuracy of the sEMG system of the MYO Armband® [4,11,18–21], these results cannot be generalized due to their small sample size. Only one study analyzed the operating time [4], reporting positive results on the speed of the system to detect gestures in upper limb amputees, and opening the possibility of introducing more complex movements in future research. This study showed that the average time for a gesture to be detected was 2.62 s, which the authors considered suitable for gaming. Additionally, three studies analyzed the accuracy of the device to obtain information about electromyography, orientation, and position in people with stroke, finding heterogeneous results. Lyu et al. [18] found an accuracy below 92.5%, which was the accuracy found in a sample of healthy subjects; although they did not report any problem regarding calibration, donning, or executing tasks with the device. Ryser et al. [11] found an accuracy of 78–99% in a sample of people with mildly to severely impaired hand function, whereas Castiblanco et al. [21] reported an accuracy of 85%. These results should be interpreted with caution, since the sample size was very small (n = 9), and the participants presented different levels of disability and upper limb impairment. We observe the same situation when examining the articles by Gaetani et al. [19] and Sattar et al. [20]: they reported an accuracy over 73% in transhumeral amputees and over 93% in transradial amputees, with a response time below 1 s, but their sample size was very small in both studies (n = 1 and n = 4 respectively). Anyhow, an accuracy over 75% provides an argument in favor of the MYO Armband®.

Regarding the studies focused on the clinical effects of interventions with the MYO Armband®, those with samples of people with stroke and MS found improvements in upper limb ROM and function [7,9,10]. These results are consistent with the meta-analysis published by Cortés-Pérez et al. [29] who reported that the Leap Motion Capture System (LMCS), another semi-immersive VR commercial device, improved upper limb function and ROM in people with neurological disease. They also observed that these clinical effects were higher when the VR-based therapy was combined with conventional therapy. In addition, Avcil et al. [30] conducted a randomized clinical trial and found that video game-based therapy using Nintendo® Wii and LMCS enhanced significantly dexterity, grip strength, and functional ability in people with CP. In our study, the only article that included a sample with CP [22] also found significant changes in grip strength, bimanual activities, dexterity, function, functional performance, and participation. However, we must note that, in our view, the heterogeneity of the interventions, the small sample size, the short duration of the protocols, and the lack of a control group may have diminished the effect of the interventions.

The dosage of therapy was very heterogeneous between studies. While the study by Esfahlani et al. [10] on people with MS implemented a 10-week protocol with 1-h sessions five days per week, the same research team implemented an 8-week protocol with 1-h sessions in a different study with people with stroke, although in this case, they did not specify the number of sessions per week [7]. Lamers et al. [31] concluded that there is no consensus on the optimum dosage of upper limb rehabilitation in people with MS. However, most of the studies included in their systematic review had an intervention duration of 8 weeks or more, with 30–60-min sessions 2–5 days per week. Also, it should be noted that the systematic review by Laver et al. [32] published by the Cochrane Library suggested that RV protocols that provided more than 15 h of therapy resulted in greater benefits in people with stroke than those providing a smaller dose.

Another advantage of VR observed in the studies included in this review is that it can improve user's motivation, interest, adherence, and satisfaction towards therapy [7,9,10], and this is common to other studies that examine semi-immersive VR-based therapy in different disorders, such as cardiovascular diseases [33,34], brain damage [35,36], children and adults with CP [37–39], neurodegenerative diseases [40,41] or chronic pain [42].

Only one study included in this review analyzed the adverse effects of the interventions with the MYO Armband®, reporting no adverse events during or after therapy [22].

Nevertheless, the risk of bias was high for all the articles, so the results should be interpreted with caution. Only 10% of the studies randomized the sample, in most of them the assessors and/or therapists were not blind and in at least 30% the results were incomplete. Also, the level of evidence and grade of recommendation were low since all studies were case series.

Limitations

There are some limitations to this review that are important to highlight. First, due to the heterogeneity of the interventions, outcome measures, and dosage, it was impossible to conduct a meta-analysis of the results. Also, we only selected articles published in English or Spanish in the last 5 years and the search was limited to a few databases, which may have reduced the number of articles included. In addition, the low methodological quality of the studies, the small and heterogeneous samples, the high risk of bias, and low level of evidence and grade of recommendation are factors that may limit the extrapolation of our results to all patients with motor impairment of the upper limb.

5. Conclusions

VR systems appear to be an effective rehabilitation approach when combined with conventional therapy in people with motor impairment of the upper limb. Specifically, therapy with the MYO Armband® has shown clinical changes in ROM, dexterity, performance, functionality and satisfaction. It has also proven to be an accurate system to capture signals from the forearm muscles in people with motor impairment of the upper limb. However, further research should be conducted using bigger samples, well-defined protocols, comparing with control groups or comparing with other assessment or therapeutic tools, since the studies published so far present a high risk of bias and low level of evidence and grade of recommendation.

Author Contributions: Conceptualization, S.M.-A. and R.C.-d.-l.-C.; formal analysis, S.M.-A. and R.C.-d.-l.-C.; investigation, S.M.-A., M.D.G.-G.-F. and R.C.-d.-l.-C.; resources, S.M.-A., M.D.G.-G.-F. and R.C.-d.-l.-C.; data curation, S.M.-A., M.D.G.-G.-F. and R.C.-d.-l.-C.; writing—original draft preparation, S.M.-A. and R.C.-d.-l.-C.; writing—review and editing, S.M.-A., M.D.G.-G.-F. and R.C.-d.-l.-C.; supervision, R.C.-d.-l.-C. All authors have read and agreed to the published version of the manuscript.

Funding: This research received no external funding.

Institutional Review Board Statement: Not applicable.

Informed Consent Statement: Not applicable.

Data Availability Statement: Not applicable.

Conflicts of Interest: The authors declare no conflict of interest.

References

1. Totty, M.S.; Wade, E. Muscle Activation and Inertial Motion Data for Noninvasive Classification of Activities of Daily Living. *IEEE Trans. Biomed. Eng.* **2018**, *65*, 1069–1076. [CrossRef] [PubMed]
2. Yancosek, K.E.; Howell, D. A narrative review of dexterity assessments. *J. Hand Ther.* **2009**, *22*, 258–269. [CrossRef] [PubMed]
3. Nasri, N.; Orts-Escolano, S.; Cazorla, M. An sEMG-Controlled 3D Game for Rehabilitation Therapies: Real-Time Time Hand Gesture Recognition Using Deep Learning Techniques. *Sensors* **2020**, *20*, 6451. [CrossRef] [PubMed]
4. Melero, M.; Hou, A.; Cheng, E.; Tayade, A.; Lee, S.C.; Unbearth, M.; Navab, N. Upbeat: Augmented Reality-Guided Dancing for Prosthetic Rehabilitation of Upper Limb Amputees. *J. Healthc. Eng.* **2019**, *2019*, 2163705. [CrossRef] [PubMed]
5. Waliño-Paniagua, C.N.; Gomez-Calero, C.; Jiménez-Trujillo, M.I.; Aguirre-Tejedor, L.; Bermejo-Franco, A.; Ortiz-Gutiérrez, R.M.; Cano-de-la-Cuerda, R. Effects of a Game-Based Virtual Reality Video Capture Training Program Plus Occupational Therapy on Manual Dexterity in Patients with Multiple Sclerosis: A Randomized Controlled Trial. *J. Healthc. Eng.* **2019**, *2019*, 2163705. [CrossRef]
6. Perrochon, A.; Borel, B.; Istrate, D.; Compagnat, M.; Daviet, J.C. Exercise-based Games Interventions at Home in Individuals with a Neurological Disease: A Systematic Review and Meta-Analysis. *Ann. Phys. Rehabil Med.* **2019**, *62*, 366–378. [CrossRef]
7. Esfahlani, S.S.; Thompson, T.; Parsa, A.D.; Brown, I.; Cirstea, S. ReHabgame: A non-immersive virtual reality rehabilitation system with applications in neuroscience. *Heliyon* **2018**, *4*, e00526. [CrossRef]
8. Rutkowski, S.; Kiper, P.; Cacciante, L.; Cieślik, B.; Mazurek, J.; Turolla, A.; Szczepańska-Gieracha, J. Use of virtual reality-based training in different fields of rehabilitation: A systematic review and meta-analysis. *J. Rehabil. Med.* **2020**, *52*, jrm00121. [CrossRef]
9. Esfahlani, S.S.; Muresan, B.; Sanaei, A.; Wilson, G. Validity of the Kinect and Myo armband in a serious game for assessing upper limb movement. *Entertain. Comput.* **2018**, *27*, 150–156. [CrossRef]
10. Esfahlani, S.S.; Butt, J.; Shirvani, H. Fusion of Artificial Intelligence in Neuro-Rehabilitation Video Games. *IEEE Access* **2019**, *7*, 102617–102627. [CrossRef]
11. Ryser, F.; Butzer, T.; Held, J.P.; Lambercy, O.; Gassert, R. Fully embedded myoelectric control for a wearable robotic hand orthosis. In Proceedings of the 2017 International Conference on Rehabilitation Robotics (ICORR), London, UK, 17–20 July 2017; pp. 615–621. [CrossRef]
12. Moher, D.; Liberati, A.; Tetzlaff, J.; Altman, D.G.; PRISMA Group. Preferred reporting items for systematic reviews and meta-analyses: The PRISMA statement. *PLoS Med.* **2009**, *6*, e1000097. [CrossRef] [PubMed]
13. Schulz, K.F.; Altman, D.G.; Moher, D.; for the CONSORT Group. CONSORT 2010 Statement: Updated guidelines for reporting parallel group randomised trials. *BMJ* **2010**, *340*, 698–702. [CrossRef] [PubMed]

14. Ciapponi, A. Guía de lectura crítica de estudios observacionales en epidemiología. *Evid. Actual. Práct. Ambul.* **2010**, *13*, 135–140. [CrossRef]
15. Berra, S.; Elorza-Ricart, J.M.; Estrada, M.D.; Sánchez, E. Instrumento para la lectura crítica y la evaluación de estudios epidemiológicos transversales. *Gac. Sanit.* **2008**, *22*, 492–497. [CrossRef]
16. Oxford CEBM. Oxford Centre for Evidence-Based Medicine: Levels of Evidence (March 2009). Available online: https://www.cebm.ox.ac.uk/resources/levels-of-evidence/oxford-centre-for-evidence-based-medicine-levels-of-evidence-march-2009 (accessed on 10 March 2022).
17. Higgins, J.P.T.; Thomas, J. Assessing risk of bias in a randomized trial. In *Cochrane Handbook for Systematic Reviews of Interventions*, 2nd ed.; Higgins, J.P.T., Savović, J., Page, M.J., Elbers, R.G., Sterne, J.A.C., Eds.; The Cochrane Collaboration; John Wiley & Sons, Ltd.: Oxford, UK, 2019; pp. 205–228. [CrossRef]
18. Lyu, M.; Lambelet, C.; Woolley, D.; Zhang, X.; Chen, W.; Ding, X.; Gassert, R.; Wenderoth, N. Training wrist extensor function and detecting unwanted movement strategies in an EMG-controlled visuomotor task. In Proceedings of the 2017 International Conference on Rehabilitation Robotics (ICORR), London, UK, 17–20 July 2017; pp. 1549–1555. [CrossRef]
19. Gaetani, F.; de Fazio, R.; Zappatore, G.A.; Visconti, P. A prosthetic limb managed by sensors-based electronic system: Experimental results on amputees. *Bull. Electr. Eng. Inform.* **2020**, *9*, 514–524. [CrossRef]
20. Sattar, N.Y.; Kausar, Z.; Usama, S.A.; Naseer, N.; Farooq, U.; Abdullah, A.; Mirtaheri, P. Enhancing Classification Accuracy of Transhumeral Prosthesis: A Hybrid sEMG and fNIRS Approach. *IEEE Access.* **2021**, *9*, 113246–113257. [CrossRef]
21. Castiblanco, J.C.; Ortmann, S.; Mondragon, I.F.; Alvarado-Rojas, C. Myoelectric pattern recognition of hand motions for stroke rehabilitation. *Biomed. Signal Process. Control* **2020**, *57*, 101737. [CrossRef]
22. MacIntosh, A.; Desailly, E.; Vignais, N.; Vigneron, V.; Biddiss, E. A biofeedback-enhanced therapeutic exercise video game intervention for young people with cerebral palsy: A randomized single-case experimental design feasibility study. *PLoS ONE* **2020**, *15*, e0234767. [CrossRef]
23. Zasadzka, E.; Trzmiel, T.; Pieczyńska, A.; Hojan, K. Modern Technologies in the Rehabilitation of Patients with Multiple Sclerosis and Their Potential Application in Times of COVID-19. *Medicina* **2021**, *57*, 549. [CrossRef]
24. Nizamis, K.; Athanasiou, A.; Almpani, S.; Dimitrousis, C.; Astaras, A. Converging Robotic Technologies in Targeted Neural Rehabilitation: A Review of Emerging Solutions and Challenges. *Sensors* **2021**, *21*, 2084. [CrossRef]
25. Lopes, J.B.P.; Duarte, N.A.C.; Lazzari, R.D.; Oliveira, C.S. Virtual reality in the rehabilitation process for individuals with cerebral palsy and Down syndrome: A systematic review. *J. Bodyw. Mov. Ther.* **2020**, *24*, 479–483. [CrossRef] [PubMed]
26. Norouzi, E.; Gerber, M.; Pühse, U.; Vaezmosavi, M.; Brand, S. Combined virtual reality and physical training improved the bimanual coordination of women with multiple sclerosis. *Neuropsychol. Rehabil.* **2021**, *31*, 552–569. [CrossRef] [PubMed]
27. Hwang, N.K.; Choi, J.B.; Choi, D.K.; Park, J.M.; Hong, C.W.; Park, J.S.; Yoon, T.H. Effects of Semi-Immersive Virtual Reality-Based Cognitive Training Combined with Locomotor Activity on Cognitive Function and Gait Ability in Community-Dwelling Older Adults. *Healthcare* **2021**, *9*, 814. [CrossRef] [PubMed]
28. Luque-Moreno, C.; Ferragut-Garcías, A.; Rodríguez-Blanco, C.; Heredia-Rizo, A.M.; Oliva-Pascual-Vaca, J.; Kiper, P.; Oliva-Pascual-Vaca, A. A Decade of Progress Using Virtual Reality for Poststroke Lower Extremity Rehabilitation: Systematic Review of the Intervention Methods. *BioMed Res. Int.* **2015**, *2015*, 342529. [CrossRef] [PubMed]
29. Cortés-Pérez, I.; Zagalaz-Anula, N.; Montoro-Cárdenas, D.; Lomas-Vega, R.; Obrero-Gaitán, E.; Osuna-Pérez, M.C. Leap Motion Controller Video Game-Based Therapy for Upper Extremity Motor Recovery in Patients with Central Nervous System Diseases. A Systematic Review with Meta-Analysis. *Sensors* **2021**, *21*, 2065. [CrossRef] [PubMed]
30. Avcil, E.; Tarakci, D.; Arman, N.; Tarakci, E. Upper extremity rehabilitation using video games in cerebral palsy: A randomized clinical trial. *Acta Neurol. Belg.* **2021**, *121*, 1053–1060. [CrossRef]
31. Lamers, I.; Maris, A.; Severijns, D.; Dielkens, W.; Geurts, S.; van Wijmeersch, B.; Feys, P. Upper Limb Rehabilitation in People with Multiple Sclerosis: A Systematic Review. *Neurorehabil. Neural Repair* **2016**, *30*, 773–793. [CrossRef]
32. Laver, K.E.; Lange, B.; George, S.; Deutsch, J.E.; Saposnik, G.; Crotty, M. Virtual reality for stroke rehabilitation. *Cochrane Database Syst. Rev.* **2017**, *11*, CD008349. [CrossRef]
33. García-Bravo, S.; Cuesta-Gómez, A.; Campuzano-Ruiz, R.; López-Navas, M.J.; Domínguez-Paniagua, J.; Araújo-Narváez, A.; Barreñada-Copete, E.; García-Bravo, C.; Flórez-García, M.T.; Botas-Rodríguez, J.; et al. Virtual reality and video games in cardiac rehabilitation programs. A systematic review. *Disabil. Rehabil.* **2021**, *43*, 448–457. [CrossRef]
34. Da Cruz, M.M.A.; Ricci-Vitor, A.L.; Borges, G.L.B.; da Silva, P.F.; Turri-Silva, N.; Takahashi, C.; Grace, S.L.; Vanderlei, L.C.M. A Randomized, Controlled, Crossover Trial of Virtual Reality in Maintenance Cardiovascular Rehabilitation in a Low-Resource Setting: Impact on Adherence, Motivation, and Engagement. *Phys. Ther.* **2021**, *101*, pzab071. [CrossRef]
35. Cano-Mañas, M.J.; Collado-Vázquez, S.; Cano-de la Cuerda, R. Videojuegos comerciales en la rehabilitación de pacientes con ictus subagudo: Estudio piloto. *Rev. Neurol.* **2017**, *65*, 337–347. [CrossRef] [PubMed]
36. Cano-Mañas, M.J.; Collado-Vázquez, S.; Cano-de la Cuerda, R. Realidad Virtual Semi-Inmersiva en el Paciente con Accidente Cerebrovascular Subagudo. Ph.D. Thesis, Department of Physical Therapy, Occupational Therapy, Rehabilitation and Physical Medicine, Rey Juan Carlos University, Alcorcón, Spain, 2021.
37. Fandim, J.V.; Saragiotto, B.T.; Porfírio, G.J.M.; Santana, R.F. Effectiveness of virtual reality in children and young adults with cerebral palsy: A systematic review of randomized controlled trial. *Braz. J. Phys. Ther.* **2021**, *25*, 369–386. [CrossRef] [PubMed]

38. Luna-Oliva, L.; Ortiz-Gutiérrez, R.M.; Cano-de la Cuerda, R.; Piédrola, R.M.; Alguacil-Diego, I.M.; Sánchez-Camarero, C.; Martínez Culebras, M.C. Kinect Xbox 360 as a therapeutic modality for children with cerebral palsy in a school environment: A preliminary study. *NeuroRehabilitation* **2013**, *33*, 513–521. [CrossRef] [PubMed]
39. Diez-Alegre, M.I.; Cano-de la Cuerda, R. Empleo de un video juego como herramienta terapéutica en adultos con parálisis cerebral tipo tetraparesia espástica: Estudio piloto. *Fisioterapia* **2012**, *34*, 23–30. [CrossRef]
40. Oña, E.D.; Balaguer, C.; Cano-de la Cuerda, R.; Collado-Vázquez, S.; Jardón, A. Effectiveness of Serious Games for Leap Motion on the Functionality of the Upper Limb in Parkinson's Disease: A Feasibility Study. *Comput. Intell. Neurosci.* **2018**, *2018*, 7148427. [CrossRef]
41. Moreno-Verdú, M.; Ferreira-Sánchez, M.R.; Cano-de la Cuerda, R.; Jiménez-Antona, C. Eficacia de la realidad virtual sobre el equilibrio y la marcha en esclerosis múltiple. Revisión sistemática de ensayos controlados aleatorizados. *Rev. Neurol.* **2019**, *68*, 357–368. [CrossRef]
42. Garcia, L.M.; Birckhead, B.J.; Krishnamurthy, P.; Sackman, J.; Mackey, I.G.; Louis, R.G.; Salmasi, V.; Maddox, T.; Darnall, B.D. An 8-Week Self-Administered At-Home Behavioral Skills-Based Virtual Reality Program for Chronic Low Back Pain: Double-Blind, Randomized, Placebo-Controlled Trial Conducted During COVID-19. *J. Med. Internet Res.* **2021**, *23*, e26292. [CrossRef]

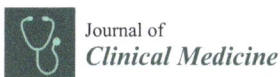

Review

Therapeutic Effects of the Pilates Method in Patients with Multiple Sclerosis: A Systematic Review

Gustavo Rodríguez-Fuentes [1,*], Lucía Silveira-Pereira [2], Pedro Ferradáns-Rodríguez [2] and Pablo Campo-Prieto [1]

1. HealthyFit Research Group, Department of Functional Biology and Health Sciences, Faculty of Physiotherapy, Galicia Sur Health Research Institute (IISGS), University of Vigo, 36005 Pontevedra, Spain; pcampo@uvigo.es
2. Physiotherapist, Private Clinic, 36210 Vigo, Spain; luciasilveirapereira@hotmail.com (L.S.-P.); pedroferradans@gmail.com (P.F.-R.)
* Correspondence: gfuentes@uvigo.es; Tel.: +34-986-801-750

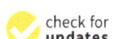

Citation: Rodríguez-Fuentes, G.; Silveira-Pereira, L.; Ferradáns-Rodríguez, P.; Campo-Prieto, P. Therapeutic Effects of the Pilates Method in Patients with Multiple Sclerosis: A Systematic Review. *J. Clin. Med.* **2022**, *11*, 683. https://doi.org/10.3390/jcm11030683

Academic Editor: Akiyoshi Matsugi

Received: 2 December 2021
Accepted: 26 January 2022
Published: 28 January 2022

Publisher's Note: MDPI stays neutral with regard to jurisdictional claims in published maps and institutional affiliations.

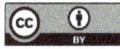

Copyright: © 2022 by the authors. Licensee MDPI, Basel, Switzerland. This article is an open access article distributed under the terms and conditions of the Creative Commons Attribution (CC BY) license (https://creativecommons.org/licenses/by/4.0/).

Abstract: The Pilates Method is a rehabilitation tool with verified benefits in pain management, physical function, and quality of life in many different physiotherapy areas. It could be beneficial for patients with multiple sclerosis (pwMS). The aim of the study was to summarize current evidence for the effectiveness of Pilates in pwMS. A comprehensive search of Cinahl, Scopus, Web of Science, PEDro, and PubMed (including PubMed Central and Medline) was conducted to examine randomized controlled trials (RCT) that included Pilates intervention in multiple sclerosis. The PEDro scale and the Cochrane risk-of-bias tool, RoB-2, were used to evaluate risk of bias for RCT. Twenty RCT (999 patients) were included. Ten were of good quality (PEDro), and seven had low risk of bias (RoB-2). Pilates improves balance, gait, physical-functional conditions (muscular strength, core stability, aerobic capacity, and body composition), and cognitive functions. Fatigue, quality of life, and psychological function did not show clear improvement. There was good adherence to Pilates intervention (average adherence ≥ 80%). Cumulative data suggest that Pilates can be a rehabilitation tool for pwMS. High adherence and few adverse effects were reported. Future research is needed to develop clinical protocols that could maximize therapeutic effects of Pilates for pwMS.

Keywords: multiple sclerosis; pilates-based exercise; exercise therapy; neurorehabilitation; physical therapy modalities

1. Introduction

Multiple sclerosis (MS) is a chronic autoimmune and inflammatory neurological disease that affects the myelinated axons in the central nervous system, characterized by neurological deterioration over time [1]. MS is the most common non-traumatic disabling disease in young adults [2]. It usually starts in early adult life, typically in the third decade [3], with most patients presenting with periodic neurological relapses [4], but the disease course is unpredictable [5].

MS is one of the most common diseases of the central nervous system (2.2 million people worldwide in 2016 data) [4]. MS cases are twice as high in women as in men [1], and it is more prevalent in North America, Western Europe, and Australasia [4].

MS shows several patterns: 80% of all cases are "relapsing-remitting" MS (RRMS), characterized by exacerbations and remissions, which can turn into "secondary-progressive" MS (SPMS), with progressive disability between attacks; 15% are cases of "primary-progressive" MS (PPMS), where there is a progressive disability from the beginning; and 5% are "progressive-relapsing" MS (PRMS), where the disease worsens gradually, but also presents outbreaks [5]. However, Lublin et al. [6] recommended reviewing these descriptions of the clinical course or phenotype of MS in 2014, suggested defining phenotypes based on disease activity (based on clinical relapse rate and imaging findings) and disease progression, and recommended removing the PRMS phenotype.

MS is characterized by a wide spectrum of symptoms, including cognitive dysfunction, optic neuritis, diplopia, sensory loss, muscle weakness, gait ataxia, loss of bladder control, spasticity, and excessive fatigue [1,4,7]. In addition, patients with multiple sclerosis (pwMS) present high risk of falling (fall rate of 56%) [8].

Physical exercise has been postulated as one of the non-pharmacological strategies of interest, due to its low cost and positive effects on the physical and mental health of the MS population [9–11]. Although historically, exercise was not recommended for pwMS due to fear of aggravating the disease [12], current evidence indicates that physical exercise is positive for managing symptoms, restoring function, optimizing quality of life, and facilitating activities of daily living [13–18]. Tallner et al. [19] and Pilutti et al. [20] suggest that physical activity has no significant influence on clinical disease activity.

Pilates is a method of physical exercise that focuses on core stability, strength, flexibility, posture, muscle control, breathing, and mind–body connection [21]. Nowadays, the method is an accepted rehabilitation tool, with verified benefits in pain management, physical function, and quality of life when used as an intervention in many different physiotherapy areas [22,23]. This therapeutic modality of the Pilates Method could provide improvement of functional impairment to pwMS.

This systematic review aims to provide an overview of the literature, and to analyse the therapeutic effects of Pilates in pwMS.

2. Materials and Methods

2.1. Search Process

This study was carried out according to the PRISMA (Preferred Reporting Items for Systematic Reviews and Meta-Analyses) guidelines [24]. The search strategy was designed to find research studies providing information on the therapeutic effects of Pilates in pwMS. Seven electronic databases were used for the search (Cinahl, Scopus, Web of Science, PEDro, and PubMed (including PubMed Central and Medline)), up to July 2021, using the key words and Boolean operators "Multiple Sclerosis" AND "Pilates" OR "Pilates-based exercises" OR "Pilates exercise" OR "Pilates training".

2.2. Selection Procedure and Eligibility Criteria

Two reviewers (G.R.-F. and L.S.-P.) independently selected trials for inclusion using predetermined inclusion criteria. First, we screened by titles and abstracts. Second, we acquired the full text of the remaining citations, and read each one to determine eligibility. In all cases, we resolved any disagreements about trial inclusions by consensus among reviewers, and consulted a third reviewer (P.F.-R.) if disagreements persisted.

The selection criteria included randomised controlled clinical trials (RCTs) written in English, Portuguese, or Spanish up to July 2021.

2.3. Data Extraction

The information in each study regarding purpose, characteristics of the sample, type of intervention and characteristics of Pilates intervention, dropouts, adherence/attendance, study variables, assessments, findings, and adverse effects of the Pilates intervention was recorded in a data log grid by one author (G.R.-F.). The information was subsequently independently revised by another three authors.

2.4. Assessment of Methodological Quality

To assess the methodological quality of the RCTs, the PEDro scale [25] was applied by two authors independently (G.R.-F. and P.C.-P.). Whenever discrepancies emerged, a third author was requested (P.F.-R.). The suggested cut-off points for categorizing studies by quality with the PEDro scale were as follows: excellent (9–10), good (6–8), fair (4–5), and poor (<3) [26].

In addition, an assessment of the risk of bias was carried out with the Cochrane risk-of-bias tool for randomized trials, RoB 2 [27]. This tool is structured into five bias domains: bias arising from the randomisation process, bias due to deviations from intended interventions, bias due to missing outcome data, bias in measurement of the outcome, and bias in selection of the reported result. In addition, there is an overall risk-of-bias judgment that generally corresponds to the worst risk of bias in any of the domains. Risk-of-bias judgment for each domain and overall can be "low", "some concerns", or "high".

3. Results

There were 204 articles initially identified through database searches. After duplicate titles were removed, 138 studies remained. Another 93 potential articles were removed after the title and abstract review. Forty-five full texts were reviewed, and twenty articles [28–47] were used in the analysis based on inclusion and exclusion criteria. Figure 1 shows the PRISMA selection process flow chart [24].

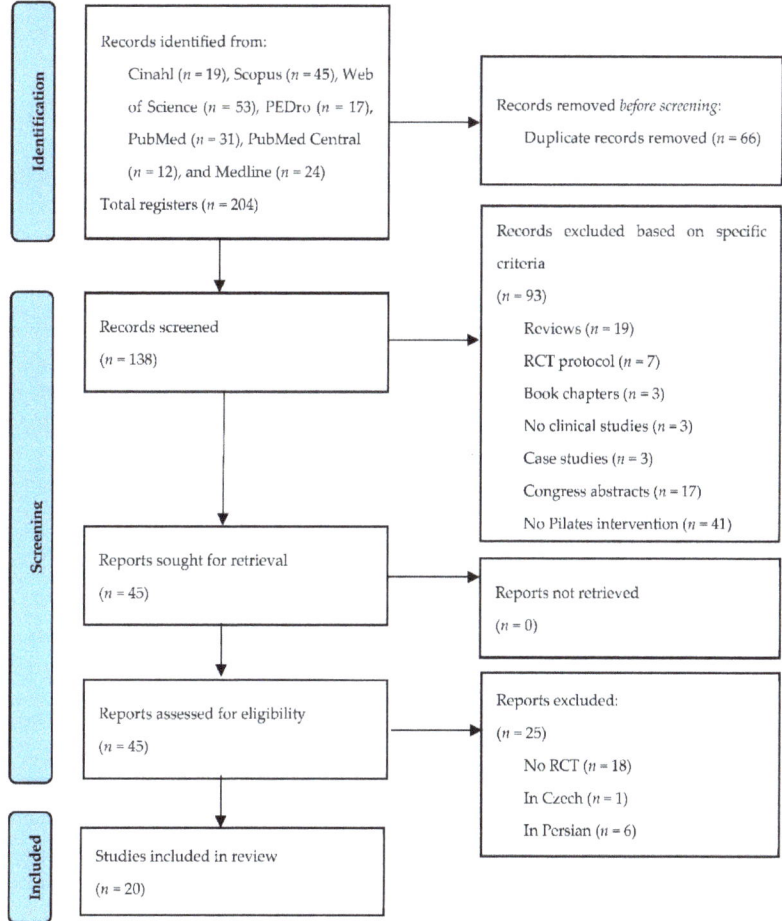

Figure 1. PRISMA flow chart of the study selection.

Table 1 shows a summary of the main findings of the reviewed studies, and more extensive information is presented in Supplementary Materials (Table S1). Table 2 summarizes the main features of the Pilates intervention, and Table 3 describes the methodological characteristics of the studies (PEDro scale and sample size calculation). Finally, Figure 2 shows risk of bias of the reviewed studies.

Table 1. Main findings of the reviewed studies.

Variables	Main Findings with Pilates Method	Other Findings
Balance	• Significant improvement [28,30,34,36–38,40–47] • Significant improvement compared with physician care [30] or with 1-h massage [38]	• No significant differences between Pilates and rebound therapy [45] or aquatic therapy [47]
Gait	• Significant improvement [28,31,32,34,36–38,40,43,44] • Significant improvement compared with standard physiotherapy care [31] or with home relaxation exercises [32]	• No significant improvement [42] • Significant improvement in standardized exercises group compared to Pilates group [43]
Physical-functional conditions	• Significant improvement in muscle strength [28,33,41,42,46] • Significant improvement in core stability [28,34,41] • Significant improvement in physical performance [42,44] • Significant improvement in aerobic capacity [33] • Significant improvement in body composition [36]	
Fatigue	• Significant improvement [28,29,32,35–37,41,42,44]	• No significant improvement in post-intervention Pilates group, but there was in aerobic exercise group [42] (no difference between groups)
Quality of life	• Significant improvement [32,41,44] • Significant improvement compared with traditional exercises group [44]	• No difference between Pilates + a 1-h massage therapy group and a 1-h massage therapy group [38]
Cognitive function	• Significant improvement [32,34,42,44] • Significant improvement compared with home relaxation exercises group [32] and with home exercises group [34]	
Psychological function	• Significant improvement in depression symptoms [29] • Significant improvement in anxiety [29] • Significant improvement in depression symptoms and anxiety compared with wait-list group [29]	• Significant improvement in home-based Pilates group compared with supervised Pilates group in anxiety symptoms [35] • No significant improvement in depression symptoms [44]
Adherence	• Average adherence to the treatment above 80–85% [31,32,34,35,37,38,46]	• Lack of compliance values [28–30,33,36,39–42,44,45,47] • Higher compliance in standardized exercises group or relaxation group than Pilates group [43]

Table 1. Cont.

Variables	Main Findings with Pilates Method	Other Findings
Adverse effects and dropouts	• 9 cases of adverse effects [28,31,37,42] • 62 dropouts in Pilates groups [28,29,32–36,38,39,41,46]	• 3 cases of adverse effects in no-Pilates groups [34,42] • 45 dropouts in no-Pilates groups [29,31,34–37,39,40,42,43,47] • 24 dropouts in unspecified group [41,44] • Don't know the dropouts [45] • Don't know the adverse effects cases [33,36,39,41,44,45,47]

Table 2. Pilates intervention characteristics of reviewed studies.

Study and Year	MS Type (Patients in Pilates Group)	Mean EDSS Score ± sd (Range)	Weeks	Session per Week	Session Duration (min)	Type of Pilates	Pilates Session (Number When Conducted in Group)	Professional	Adverse Events (Case)	Pilates Training Program
Güngör et al. [28], 2021	RRMS (34)/SPMS (8)	(1–5.5)	8	2	60–75	Floor mat work	Individual	Physiotherapist	No	Yes (in Supplementary Material)
Fleming et al. [29], 2021	NA	<3 (PDDS)	8	2	60	Floor mat work	Individual	Certified Pilates instructor	No	Yes (in a previous study)
Gheitasi et al. [30], 2021	NA	4.6 ± 1.6 (3–5)	12	3	60	Floor mat work	Unclear	NA	No	No
Arntzen et al. [31], 2020	RRMS (32)/PPMS (5)/SPMS (2)	2.45 ± 1.65 (1–6.5)	6	3	60	Floor mat work	Group (3)	Neurological physiotherapists	Yes (1)	Yes (in a previous study)
Ozkul et al. [32], 2020	RRMS (17)	1.50 ± 0.77 (<4)	8	3	60	Floor mat work	NA	Physiotherapist	No	Yes
Banitalebi et al. [33], 2020	RRMS (47)	23 (0–4) + 13 (4.5–6) + 11 (6.5–8)	12	3	15/100	NA	NA	NA	NA	No
Abasiyanik et al. [34], 2020	RRMS (14)/SPMS (2)	3.06 ± 1.65 (<6)	8	1 (+2 at home)	55–60	Floor mat work	Group (2–3)	Certified Pilates physiotherapist	No	Yes
Fleming et al. [35], 2019	NA	<3 (PDDS)	8	2	60	Floor mat work	Individual	Certified Pilates instructor	No	Yes
Eftekhari and Etemadifar [36], 2018	RRMS (13)	2–6	8	3	50–60	Floor mat work	NA	NA	NA	Yes
Ozkul tel al. [37], 2018	RRMS	1 (0.87–2.12)	8	3	60	Floor mat work	NA	Physiotherapist	Yes (3)	Yes
Duff et al. [38], 2018	RRMS (14)/PPMS (1)	2.1 ± 1.8 (range 0–5, PDDS)	12	2	50	Apparatus work and floor mat work	Group (5–10)	Certified Pilates instructor	No	No
Eftekhari and Etemadifar [39], 2018	RRMS(13)	2–6	8	3	40–50	Floor mat work	NA	NA	NA	Yes
Kalron et al. [40], 2017	RRMS (22)	4.3 ± 1.3 (3–6)	12	1	30	NA	Individual	Certified Pilates physiotherapist	No	No
Bulguroglu et al. [41], 2017	NA	<4.5	8	2	60–90	Floor mat work or Reformer work	Individual	Certified Pilates physiotherapist	NA	No
Kara et al. [42], 2017	RRMS (9)	2.85 ± 1.57 (<6)	8	2	45–60	Floor mat work	NA	Physiotherapist	Yes (4)	Yes
Fox et al. [43], 2016	RRMS (13)/PPMS (12)/SPMS (8)	4–6.5	12	1	30	Floor mat work	Individual	Certified Pilates physiotherapist	No	Yes (in a previous study)
Küçük et al. [44], 2016	NA	3.2 ± 2.2 (≤6)	8	2	45–60	Floor mat work	Group	Physiotherapist	NA	Yes
Hosseini Sisi et al. [45], 2014	NA	0–4	8	3	60	NA	NA	NA	NA	No
Guclu-Cunduz et al. [46], 2014	NA	2 (0–4)	8	2	60	NA	Group	Certified Pilates physiotherapist	No	No
Marandi et al. [47], 2013	NA	<4.5	12	3	60	NA	NA	NA	NA	No

EDSS: Expanded Disability Status Scale; **min**: minute; **MS**: multiple sclerosis; **NA**: not available; **PDDS**: Patient-Determined Disease Steps; **PPMS**: primary progressive multiple sclerosis; **RRMS**: relapsing-remitting multiple sclerosis; **sd**: standard deviation; **SPMS**: secondary progressive multiple sclerosis.

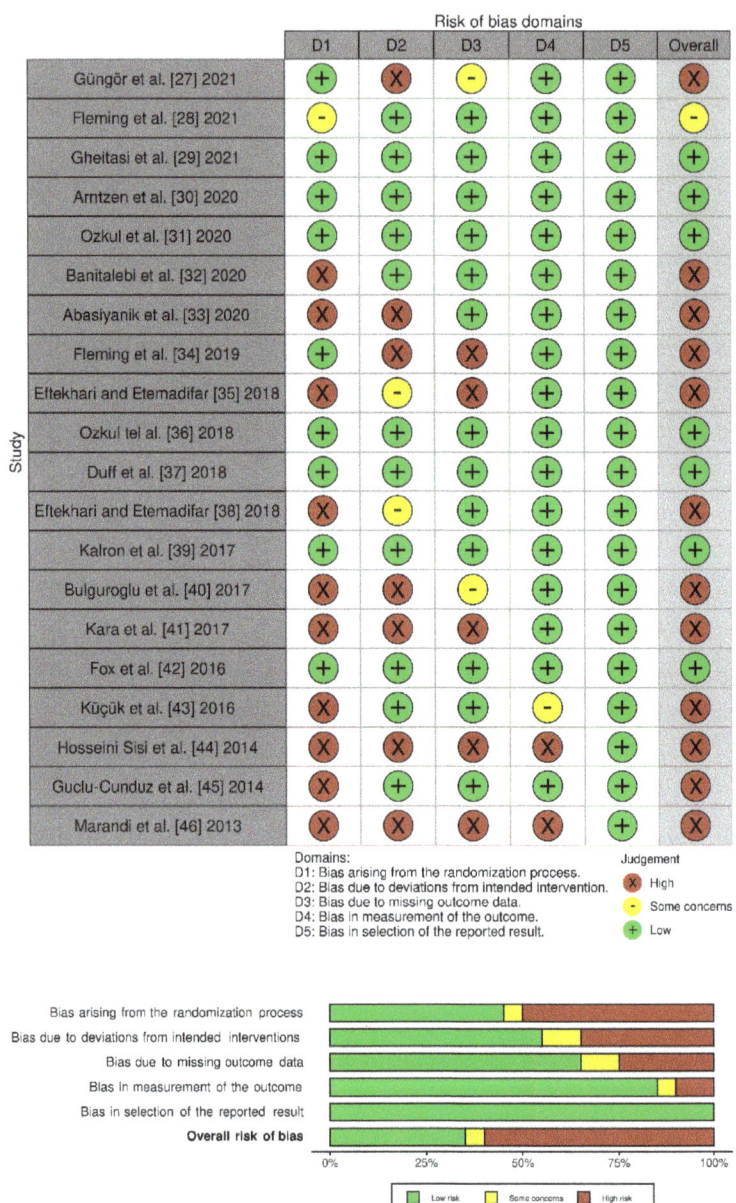

Figure 2. Risk of bias of the reviewed studies: (**up**) for each domain, (**down**) overall judgement.

Table 3. Methodological quality assessment of the reviewed studies using PEDro scale, and sample size calculation.

Study and Year	Sample Size Calculation	#1	#2	#3	#4	#5	#6	#7	#8	#9	#10	#11	Total
Güngör et al. [28], 2021	Yes	1	1	1	1	1	0	0	0	0	1	1	6/10
Fleming et al. [29], 2021	Yes	1	1	0	1	0	0	1	1	1	1	1	7/10
Gheitasi et al. [30], 2021	Yes	1	1	1	1	0	0	0	1	1	1	1	7/10
Arntzen et al. [31], 2020	Yes	1	1	1	1	0	0	1	1	1	1	1	8/10
Ozkul et al. [32], 2020	Yes	0	1	1	1	0	0	1	1	1	1	1	8/10
Banitalebi et al. [33], 2020	No	1	1	1	1	0	0	1	1	0	1	0	6/10
Abasiyanik et al. [34], 2020	Yes	1	1	0	1	0	0	0	0	0	1	1	4/10
Fleming et al. [35], 2019	No	1	1	1	1	0	0	0	0	0	0	1	4/10
Eftekhari and Etemadifar [36], 2018	No	1	1	0	1	0	0	1	0	0	1	1	5/10
Ozkul tel al. [37], 2018	Yes	1	1	1	1	0	0	1	1	0	0	1	6/10
Duff et al. [38], 2018	Yes	1	1	0	1	0	0	1	1	1	1	1	7/10
Eftekhari and Etemadifar [39], 2018	No	1	1	0	1	0	0	0	0	0	1	1	4/10
Kalron et al. [40], 2017	No	1	1	1	1	0	0	1	0	0	1	1	7/10
Bulguroglu et al. [41], 2017	No	1	1	0	1	0	0	1	0	0	1	1	5/10
Kara et al. [42], 2017	No	1	0	0	0	0	0	1	0	0	1	1	3/10
Fox et al. [43], 2016	Yes	1	1	1	1	0	0	1	1	1	1	1	8/10
Küçük et al. [44], 2016	No	1	1	0	1	0	0	0	1	0	1	1	5/10
Hosseini Sisi et al. [45], 2014	No	1	1	0	0	0	0	0	0	0	1	1	3/10
Guclu-Cunduz et al. [46], 2014	No	1	0	0	1	0	0	1	1	1	0	1	5/10
Marandi et al. [47], 2013	No	1	1	0	0	0	0	0	0	0	1	1	3/10
		17	16	9	15	1	0	10	10	6	15	17	

#1, eligibility criteria (not included in the total score); #2, random allocation; #3, concealed allocation; #4, baseline comparability; #5, participant blinding; #6, therapist blinding; #7, assessor blinding; #8, outcomes were obtained from more than 85%; #9, intention to treat analysis; #10, between-group difference; #11, point estimates and variability.

4. Discussion

The purpose of this review was to identify the possible therapeutic effects of Pilates for pwMS. These were the main variables studied, as well as the influence of Pilates on each of them.

4.1. Balance

Balance was studied in 14 papers [28,30,34,36–38,40–47]. In each of these, one of the following scales or assessment methods was used: Timed Up and Go Test [28,30,34,38,40–42,44–46], Berg Balance Scale [29,36,40,42,44–46], Activities-Specific Balance Confidence Scale [34,41,43,46], Functional Reach Test [30,40], Balance Platform [28,37], Falls Efficacy Scale International [34], Fullerton Advanced Balance Scale [38], Four Square Step Test [40], Single-leg Stance [41], Trunk Impairment Scale [44], and Six-and-Spot Step Test [47]. In all 14, Pilates yielded significant improvements post-intervention. The studies of Hosseini Sisi et al. [45] and Marandi et al. [47] only compared the results for this parameter with other therapies (rebound therapy [45] and aquatic therapy [47]), and did not report significant differences between interventions. In contrast, the study by Gheitasi et al. [30], with solid methodological quality (7 on PEDro scale), found significant improvement from Pilates compared with usual physician care; and Duff et al. [38] (7 on PEDro scale), which compared Pilates with 1-h of massage per week, found significant improvement from Pilates in balance and gait.

These findings are in line with other reviews [48]. As such, balance seems to be an important issue in pwMS that can benefit from Pilates interventions.

4.2. Gait/Walking

This variable was assessed in 11 studies [28,31,32,34,36–38,40,42–44] using: 6 Minute Walk Test [32,34,36–38,40], 12-Item Multiple Sclerosis Walking Scale [31,34,40,43], 10 Meter Walk Test [31,36,43], Timed 25-Foot Walk [34,42,44], 2 Minute Walk Test (2MWT) [28,31,40], the walking section of the Patients' Global Impression of Change Scale [31], and Rivermead Visual Gait Assessment [31]. Ten studies found significant improvements in gait post-intervention [28,31,32,34,36–38,40,43,44]. Of note are the studies by Arntzen et al. [31] (8 on PEDro scale), where there were significant differences in favour of Pilates with respect to standard physiotherapy care; and by Ozkul et al. [32] (8 on PEDro scale), where Pilates presented significant improvements in gait quality when compared with relaxation exercises carried out at home. Also of interest is the significant 2MWT improvement found by Güngör et al. [28], both for patients in the Pilates group under the supervision of a physiotherapist and those doing home-based Pilates training.

Gait is a variable intimately related to balance. Two papers focused on studying both parameters combined: Kalron et al. [40] and Fox et al. [43]. The two studies compared the results obtained with the Pilates intervention with those from standard physical exercise. In Kalron et al. [40], both groups improved, although no significant differences were found between them. In contrast, in Fox et al. [43], the group doing standardised exercises obtained significant post-intervention improvements compared with those undergoing the Pilates intervention. Therefore, although Pilates has positive effects on gait and balance in pwMS, it seems that they are no better than other modes of physical exercise.

4.3. Physical-Functional Conditions

Within this variable, we include those studies which assess muscle strength: (leg extension 1 RM [38], sit-ups test [41], modified push-ups test [28,41], quadriceps and hamstrings isokinetic strength [28], and hand held dynamometer [46]), core stability (curl-up test [28,34], plank hold test [38], side bridge test [28,41], trunk flexion test [28,41], prone bridge test [41], and Biering-Sorensen test [28]), physical performance (9-Hole Peg test [42,44]; and time to roll from right to left, lie/sit, sit/stand, and repeated sit/stand [42,44]), aerobic capacity (consumption of VO_2 on treadmill, and Physiological Cost Index [33]), physical activity (accelerometer monitoring activity [31,38], Godin Leisure-Time Exercise Questionnaire [29,35]), and body composition [36]. The reported results suggest that intervention with Pilates could be a valid tool for improving strength [33,46], core stability [34,41], physical performance [42,44], aerobic capacity [33], and body composition [36] in pwMS. However, the heterogeneity of the assessment tests employed hampers data aggregation and direct comparison of the results.

4.4. Fatigue

Pilates improved fatigue significantly in pwMS in nine studies [28,29,32,35–37,41,42,44] of the ten that evaluated it [28,29,32,35–37,40–42,44]. Nevertheless, none of these found significant differences when compared with other interventions. Once again, different scales were used to evaluate fatigue: Modified Fatigue Scale [29,35,36,40,44], Fatigue Impact Scale [32,42], and Fatigue Severity Scale [28,37,41]. Pilates provides positive results, but whether it is better than other treatments remain unclear. Specifically, in the study by Kara et al. [42], the group doing aerobic exercises did obtain significant post-intervention improvements in fatigue, but the Pilates group did not. Nonetheless, this result needs to be interpreted with caution, because there were not significant differences between the groups, the sample size was small, and there were a lot of losses in the Pilates group post-intervention. Güngör et al. [28] also obtained significant improvements in fatigue in both the supervised Pilates training group and the home-based Pilates training group, but without differences between the groups, although there was a loss of 20% from the latter group, which could have altered the findings.

In summary, fatigue remains a poorly studied variable [4,7] despite being a widespread alteration in pwMS.

4.5. Quality of Life

Four of the studies evaluated this parameter [32,38,41,44]. Two scales were used: the Multiple Sclerosis Quality of Life-54 instrument [32,38,41], and the Multiple Sclerosis

International Quality of Life Questionnaire [44]. Significant improvements were obtained for this variable in three of the four studies [32,41,44] in both the physical and mental sections of the scales; in one of which [44], the results were significantly better in the Pilates group than in the control group.

4.6. Cognitive/Psychological Function

Cognitive functions were analysed in four studies [32,34,42,44], using the following scales: Brief Repeatable Battery of Neuropsychological Tests [32], Brief International Cognitive Assessment for MS [34], and Paced Auditory Serial Addition Test [42,44]. All of them obtained significant post-intervention improvements in this parameter. Of interest are the studies by Ozkul et al. [32] and Abasiyanik et al. [34], which compared the Pilates intervention with doing exercises at home (relaxation in the case of Ozkul et al. [32]), and obtained significantly better results in this variable with the Pilates intervention. Although somewhat surprising, the results in these studies open the door to incorporating measurements of cognitive parameters in future work using Pilates, as has been done in others where exercise was also the base of the intervention [49–53].

On the other hand, Fleming et al. [29,35] assessed depression and anxiety in pwMS, and Küçük et al. [44] assessed depression. The results do not offer any clear direction: although in Fleming et al. [29], the home-based Pilates group obtained significant improvement in comparison with the control group with regard to depression and anxiety, in earlier work [35], the same author stated that the supervised Pilates group presented a significant worsening of anxiety symptoms with respect to the home-based Pilates group. In addition, Küçük et al. [44] did not find significant improvements in depression following the Pilates intervention. It is possible that these results are due to other factors, such as the comorbidities or severity of MS, as Kara et al. [42] report that both the Pilates and aerobic exercise groups, despite the improvement in depression experienced, did not present values significantly better than healthy adults.

4.7. Attendance/Adherence

In general, for the studies presenting data on compliance by patients with the Pilates sessions, there is an average adherence to the treatment above 80–85% [31,32,34,35,37,38,46]. The outstanding levels of adherence, in addition to the clinical results, are one of the highlights of using Pilates interventions in pwMS. Nevertheless, in the study by Fox et al. [43], the Pilates exercise group only had 66% adherence compared with 84% and 92% in the groups doing standardized exercises or relaxation, respectively. Most of the papers do not state values for compliance [28–30,33,36,39–42,44,45,47], which is an important limitation. Adherence is usually linked to the patient's motivation for the treatment offered [54]; hence, it is a relevant issue in a disease such as MS, a long-duration chronic illness requiring physical-functional conditions to be as stable as possible over time, to maintain the independence and autonomy of patients. Lack of adherence may reflect a deterioration in the fitness of pwMS, and greater expense in terms of healthcare and personnel resources.

4.8. Sample Characteristics

The population analysed in these studies comprised 999 pwMS, and 868 finished them (131 dropouts, 13.11%). In terms of age, patients in their third and fourth decades predominated [28–30,32,34,36–42,45,46] (only three of the studies [31,43,44] include patients aged over 60), and this is in line with the epidemiological data [3]. With regard to sex, the majority are women (602), compared with 226 men, which also matches the epidemiological data for the disease (3:1 women to men ratio [2,3]). Dropout rates may vary between sexes, as in the study by Bulguroglu et al. [41]. Surprisingly, in some of the studies, the sample consists exclusively of women [33,35,36,39,46,47] or men [30,45], which complicates cross-sex validation of the results.

The majority of the samples include MS of the RRMS type (86.76%), this being the most common form of MS [5]. In eight studies [29,30,35,41,44–47], the clinical state of the disease in the participants is unfortunately not specified.

The degree of disability in the samples was quantified in most cases using the Expanded Disability Status Scale [28,30–34,36,37,39–47], with the average scores on this questionnaire being highly variable, tending normally to an average score of 4.5 [28,31,32,34,37,40–42,44–47]. Only the study by Banitalebi et al. [33] included patients with a score of up to 8 on this scale: patients need to use aids for walking once their score reaches 6. Three studies employed the Patient-Determined Disease Steps Scale [29,35,38] to measure the degree of disability. The lack of standard evaluations, combined with the fact that some studies do not specify the clinical type of MS [29,30,35,41,44–47], leads to important knowledge gaps that ought to be addressed in future research. The performance of participants in Pilates programs will determine the design of the exercises, and the therapeutic objectives intended for each type of MS. Amatya et al. [5] agree that it is key to analyse these aspects to offer more effective and specific multidisciplinary treatment for each pwMS.

4.9. Characteristics of the Pilates Interventions

The type of Pilates intervention is specified in the majority of the cases, with mat work being the preferred modality [28–32,34–39,41–44]. In Duff et al. [38], the Pilates group did sessions of mat work and fitness equipment, whereas in Bulguroglu et al. [41], a mat work group was compared with one using Pilates exercise machines, and with a control group doing relaxation and respiration exercises at home. The Pilates intervention on the mat is likely preferred for economy and space reasons, as well as for its convenience for group therapy sessions. However, in Bulguroglu et al. [41], although both modalities achieved significant post-intervention improvements, there is significantly greater improvement in the exercise machine group when looking at vertebral mobility using the Trunk Flexion Test. It would be useful for future studies to analyse whether working with machines offers greater benefits than mat work, in both therapeutic and cost-effectiveness terms.

It is also challenging to evaluate the benefits offered by at-home video-guided Pilates interventions for pwMS. The studies [29,35] that presented this intervention offer encouraging results. The Pilates intervention guided by DVD obtained good results in relation to symptoms of anxiety, depression, and fatigue. It is unclear whether the DVD modality is a better choice than the supervised intervention, from both the therapeutic and cost-effectiveness points of view. It would be helpful to analyse DVD-guided Pilates intervention as a sole treatment, or as a complement to the work of health professionals, as well as the requirements necessary (for instance, workload recommended), or the potential options for tracking the workload or motivation of pwMS to continue with the Pilates program.

In the majority of the studies, the session duration ranges from 45 to 60 min [29–32,34–38,42,44–47], with weekly frequency mainly established at two [28,29,35,38,41,42,44,46] or three [30–33,36,37,39,45,47] sessions per week, except for three with one session/week [34,40,43]. Most interventions lasted 8 [28,29,34–37,39,41,42,44–46] or 12 weeks [30,33,38,40,43,47]. Because in most of the studies there was no long-term monitoring after the intervention, it is unclear whether the outcomes attained are maintained. Only the study by Arntzen et al. [31], the one with the shortest intervention (6 weeks), tracked outcomes up to 30 weeks. These results point to sustained benefits for gait in the Pilates group after 18 (walking speed, perceived limitations, and distance walked) and 30 weeks (distance walked). We propose to schedule follow-up assessments in order to define whether the effects of the Pilates persist, in addition to establishing, in cases where the treatment is suspended (such as for vacation), after how long the treatment ought to be resumed to avert a significant loss of the benefits achieved.

The sessions took place for individuals in six studies [28,29,35,40,41,43], and for groups in five studies [31,34,38,44,46], whereas in nine studies, was not specified [30,32,33,36,37,39,42,45,47]. Eight studies [30,33,38,40,41,45–47] do not provide details regarding the Pilates program applied. Future research should be more precise in how the interventions are described, as this would facilitate replication, comparison, and evolution of the protocols.

With regard to the session supervision, the professional in charge was a physiotherapist in 11 studies [29,31,32,34,37,40–44,46], 5 of which specified that a Pilates certification was held [34,40,41,43,46]. In six studies [30,33,36,39,45,47], the professional responsible for directing the sessions is not specified. From our point of view, the physiotherapist is the ideal person for conducting these interventions in patients, optimally with a Pilates specialisation, to guarantee more effective and safer sessions while following the guidelines of the method properly.

4.10. Adverse Effects and Dropouts

Whether the intervention had adverse effects is relevant for pwMS. Adverse effects during the intervention were specified in four studies [28,31,37,42], with a total of nine cases (five for exacerbation of symptoms, two for relapse, and two due to the work intensity). In seven studies [33,36,39,41,44,45,47], it is not specified whether there were any adverse effects, although there were some dropouts. Adverse effects should be reported, and the cause of dropping out should be clarified, as well as the possible link with undesired effects of the treatment, to provide assurance in future research with Pilates in pwMS. It is also relevant for the validity of the outcomes to be verified. As shown in Table 3, in nine studies [28,34–36,41,42,45–47], one key result could not be obtained in at least 85% of the initial sample, hindering attribution of the results to the intervention.

4.11. Methodological Quality of the Studies

Table 3 shows that the average score obtained by the studies was 5.5/10 on the PEDro scale. Following Foley et al. [26], a score of 9–10 means excellent quality, 6–8 is good, 4–5 is acceptable, and <4 points is poor. In our review, 10 studies [28–33,37,38,40,43] have a value ≥ 6 points (3 reach 8 points [31,32,43], and only 3 [42,45,47] have a score <4 points on this scale). Given the PEDro scale design, the principal limitation is that none of the studies were double-blind. It also seems important for future studies to include appropriate randomization of the sample (as reflected in domain 1 of Figure 2), and an analysis of the results by treatment intention, which would help to control the detection biases (domain 3, Figure 2). All these issues would enhance the internal validity of the studies and their bias control.

Table 3 shows that only nine studies [28–32,34,37,38,43] have incorporated a sample size calculation, thus facilitating extrapolation of their results. Future investigations should take this into account in their design, as this would bring external validity to the results, and enhance their ecological value. According to the present review, this issue can eminently be improved.

4.12. Limitations

The main limitation is the methodological quality of the studies: although acceptable in most cases, greater control over biases and larger population samples are required.

Furthermore, the lack of data about adverse effects, whether these are related to some of the dropouts, and the type of MS should be clarified, and could limit the scope of our conclusions if the disease status could be related to a higher number of dropouts. The tendency to analyse the influence of Pilates in pwMS with mild to moderate degree of disability is also relevant, so the studies included show limited information on the effects of Pilates in pwMS who are already starting to have significant problems with ADL and walking. Further, studies have often included patients with different types of MS or with different degrees of disability, and no systematic information is collected on drug treatment.

Another limitation is the lack of an adequate blind allocation, with masked assessors and intention-to-treat analyses.

Overall, the need for standardisation is obvious, as it would allow future researchers to compare different studies, their results, and the effectiveness of the Pilates to choose the best approach for clinical use. Furthermore, the heterogeneity of the evaluation scales does not allow a reliable comparison between studies, or aggregation of the results to support the findings.

We suggest follow-up assessments in future studies to explore how long improvements last, and to propose suitable guidelines for the dichotomy between treatment period and pause period between treatment programs.

Finally, the exclusion of grey literature due to our study selection criteria could have led us to omit certain papers referring to our area of study, and whose results might have been of interest for this review.

5. Conclusions

The outcomes support the therapeutic use of Pilates in MS management. Our findings suggest that Pilates is a safe active treatment method for pwMS (few adverse effects), with high adherence (low dropout rate), and which can improve important parameters in the target population, such as balance, gait, physical-functional capacities, and even cognitive functions. Findings are fairly limited for other variables, as in the case of fatigue, quality of life, and psychiatric conditions such as depression or anxiety.

Additional high-quality RCTs with large enough population samples are needed to substantiate the advantages of Pilates as a tool for rehabilitation in pwMS.

Supplementary Materials: The following are available online at https://www.mdpi.com/article/10.3390/jcm11030683/s1, Table S1: Characteristics of the included studies.

Author Contributions: Conceptualization, G.R.-F. and L.S.-P.; database searches, G.R.-F. and L.S.-P.; data extraction, G.R.-F.; data extraction supervision, L.S.-P., P.F.-R. and P.C.-P.; methodological quality assessment, G.R.-F., P.C.-P. and P.F.-R.; writing—original draft preparation, L.S.-P. and G.R.-F.; all authors contributed to the critical revision of manuscript. All authors have read and agreed to the published version of the manuscript.

Funding: This research received no external funding.

Institutional Review Board Statement: Not applicable.

Informed Consent Statement: Not applicable.

Data Availability Statement: All relevant data are included in the paper.

Acknowledgments: The authors would like to thank Adrian Mariño Enriquez for useful comments and contributions on the article.

Conflicts of Interest: The authors declare no conflict of interest.

References

1. Goldenberg, M.M. Multiple sclerosis review. *Pharm. Ther.* **2012**, *37*, 175–184.
2. Dobson, R.; Giovannoni, G. Multiple sclerosis—A review. *Eur. J. Neurol.* **2018**, *26*, 27–40. [CrossRef] [PubMed]
3. Reich, D.S.; Lucchinetti, C.F.; Calabresi, P.A. Multiple Sclerosis. *N. Engl. J. Med.* **2018**, *378*, 169–180. [CrossRef] [PubMed]
4. Wallin, M.T.; Culpepper, W.J.; Nichols, E.; Bhutta, Z.A.; Gebrehiwot, T.T.; Hay, S.I.; Khalil, I.A.; Krohn, K.J.; Liang, X.; Naghavi, M.; et al. Global, regional, and national burden of multiple sclerosis 1990–2016: A systematic analysis for the Global Burden of Disease Study 2016. *Lancet Neurol.* **2019**, *18*, 269–285. [CrossRef]
5. Amatya, B.; Khan, F.; Galea, M. Rehabilitation for people with multiple sclerosis: An overview of Cochrane Reviews. *Cochrane Database Syst. Rev.* **2019**, *1*, CD012732. [CrossRef] [PubMed]
6. Lublin, F.D.; Reingold, S.C.; Cohen, J.A.; Cutter, G.R.; Sørensen, P.S.; Thompson, A.J.; Wolinsky, J.S.; Balcer, L.J.; Banwell, B.; Barkhof, F.; et al. Defining the clinical course of multiple sclerosis: The 2013 revisions. *Neurology* **2014**, *83*, 278–286. [CrossRef] [PubMed]
7. Heine, M.; Van De Port, I.; Rietberg, M.B.; van Wegen, E.E.H.; Kwakkel, G. Exercise therapy for fatigue in multiple sclerosis. *Cochrane Database Syst. Rev.* **2015**, *9*, CD009956. [CrossRef]

8. Nilsagård, Y.; Gunn, H.; Freeman, J.; Hoang, P.; Lord, S.; Mazumder, R.; Cameron, M. Falls in people with MS—an individual data meta-analysis from studies from Australia, Sweden, United Kingdom and the United States. *Mult. Scler. J.* **2014**, *21*, 92–100. [CrossRef]
9. Rietberg, M.B.; Brooks, D.; Uitdehaag, B.M.; Kwakkel, G. Exercise therapy for multiple sclerosis. *Cochrane Database Syst. Rev.* **2005**, *2005*, CD003980. [CrossRef]
10. Dalgas, U.; Stenager, E.; Ingemann-Hansen, T. Review: Multiple sclerosis and physical exercise: Recommendations for the application of resistance-, endurance- and combined training. *Mult. Scler. J.* **2008**, *14*, 35–53. [CrossRef]
11. Motl, R.W.; Sandroff, B. Benefits of Exercise Training in Multiple Sclerosis. *Curr. Neurol. Neurosci. Rep.* **2015**, *15*, 62. [CrossRef] [PubMed]
12. Petajan, J.H.; White, A.T. Recommendations for physical activity in patients with multiple sclerosis. *Sports Med.* **1999**, *27*, 179–191. [CrossRef] [PubMed]
13. Snook, E.M.; Motl, R.W. Effect of Exercise Training on Walking Mobility in Multiple Sclerosis: A Meta-Analysis. *Neurorehabilit. Neural Repair* **2008**, *23*, 108–116. [CrossRef] [PubMed]
14. Padgett, P.K.; Kasser, S.L. Exercise for Managing the Symptoms of Multiple Sclerosis. *Phys. Ther.* **2013**, *93*, 723–728. [CrossRef] [PubMed]
15. Pearson, M.; Dieberg, G.; Smart, N. Exercise as a Therapy for Improvement of Walking Ability in Adults with Multiple Sclerosis: A Meta-Analysis. *Arch. Phys. Med. Rehabil.* **2015**, *96*, 1339–1348.e7. [CrossRef] [PubMed]
16. Motl, R.W.; Sandroff, B.; Kwakkel, G.; Dalgas, U.; Feinstein, A.; Heesen, C.; Feys, P.; Thompson, A. Exercise in patients with multiple sclerosis. *Lancet Neurol.* **2017**, *16*, 848–856. [CrossRef]
17. Khan, F.; Amatya, B. Rehabilitation in Multiple Sclerosis: A Systematic Review of Systematic Reviews. *Arch. Phys. Med. Rehabil.* **2016**, *98*, 353–367. [CrossRef]
18. Demaneuf, T.; Aitken, Z.; Karahalios, A.; Leong, T.I.; De Livera, A.M.; Jelinek, G.A.; Weiland, T.; Marck, C.H. Effectiveness of Exercise Interventions for Pain Reduction in People with Multiple Sclerosis: A Systematic Review and Meta-analysis of Randomized Controlled Trials. *Arch. Phys. Med. Rehabil.* **2018**, *100*, 128–139. [CrossRef]
19. Tallner, A.; Waschbisch, A.; Wenny, I.; Schwab, S.; Hentschke, C.; Pfeifer, K.; Mäurer, M. Multiple sclerosis relapses are not associated with exercise. *Mult. Scler. J.* **2011**, *18*, 232–235. [CrossRef]
20. Pilutti, L.A.; Platta, M.E.; Motl, R.W.; Latimer, A. The safety of exercise training in multiple sclerosis: A systematic review. *J. Neurol. Sci.* **2014**, *343*, 3–7. [CrossRef]
21. Wells, C.; Kolt, G.; Bialocerkowski, A. Defining Pilates exercise: A systematic review. *Complement. Ther. Med.* **2012**, *20*, 253–262. [CrossRef] [PubMed]
22. Cruz-Ferreira, A.; Fernandes, J.; Laranjo, L.; Bernardo, L.M.; Silva, A. A Systematic Review of the Effects of Pilates Method of Exercise in Healthy People. *Arch. Phys. Med. Rehabil.* **2011**, *92*, 2071–2081. [CrossRef] [PubMed]
23. Byrnes, K.; Wu, P.-J.; Whillier, S. Is Pilates an effective rehabilitation tool? A systematic review. *J. Bodyw. Mov. Ther.* **2017**, *22*, 192–202. [CrossRef] [PubMed]
24. Page, M.J.; McKenzie, J.E.; Bossuyt, P.M.; Boutron, I.; Hoffmann, T.C.; Mulrow, C.D.; Shamseer, L.; Tetzlaff, J.M.; Akl, E.A.; Brennan, S.E.; et al. The PRISMA 2020 statement: An updated guideline for reporting systematic reviews. *BMJ* **2021**, *372*, n71. [CrossRef]
25. Maher, C.G.; Sherrington, C.; Herbert, R.D.; Moseley, A.M.; Elkins, M. Reliability of the PEDro Scale for Rating Quality of Randomized Controlled Trials. *Phys. Ther.* **2003**, *83*, 713–721. [CrossRef]
26. Foley, N.C.; Teasell, R.W.; Bhogal, S.K.; Speechley, M.R. Stroke Rehabilitation Evidence-Based Review: Methodology. *Top. Stroke Rehabil.* **2003**, *10*, 1–7. [CrossRef]
27. Sterne, J.A.C.; Savović, J.; Page, M.J.; Elbers, R.G.; Blencowe, N.S.; Boutron, I.; Cates, C.J.; Cheng, H.Y.; Corbett, M.S.; Eldridge, S.M.; et al. RoB 2: A revised tool for assessing risk of bias in randomised trials. *BMJ* **2019**, *366*, l4898. [CrossRef]
28. Güngör, F.; Tarakci, E.; Özdemir-Acar, Z.; Soysal, A. The effects of supervised versus home Pilates-based core stability training on lower extremity muscle strength and postural sway in people with multiple sclerosis. *Mult. Scler. J.* **2021**, *28*. [CrossRef]
29. Fleming, K.M.; Coote, S.B.; Herring, M.P. Home-based Pilates for symptoms of anxiety, depression and fatigue among persons with multiple sclerosis: An 8-week randomized controlled trial. *Mult. Scler. J.* **2021**, *27*, 2267–2279. [CrossRef]
30. Gheitasi, M.; Bayattork, M.; Andersen, L.L.; Imani, S.; Daneshfar, A. Effect of twelve weeks pilates training on functional balance of male patients with multiple sclerosis: Randomized controlled trial. *J. Bodyw. Mov. Ther.* **2020**, *25*, 41–45. [CrossRef]
31. Arntzen, E.C.; Straume, B.; Odeh, F.; Feys, P.; Normann, B. Group-based, individualized, comprehensive core stability and balance intervention provides immediate and long-term improvements in walking in individuals with multiple sclerosis: A randomized controlled trial. *Physiother. Res. Int.* **2019**, *25*, e1798. [CrossRef] [PubMed]
32. Ozkul, C.; Guclu-Gunduz, A.; Eldemir, K.; Apaydin, Y.; Yazici, G.; Irkec, C. Combined exercise training improves cognitive functions in multiple sclerosis patients with cognitive impairment: A single-blinded randomized controlled trial. *Mult. Scler. Relat. Disord.* **2020**, *45*, 102419. [CrossRef] [PubMed]
33. Banitalebi, E.; Ghahfarrokhi, M.M.; Negaresh, R.; Kazemi, A.; Faramarzi, M.; Motl, R.W.; Zimmer, P. Exercise improves neurotrophins in multiple sclerosis independent of disability status. *Mult. Scler. Relat. Disord.* **2020**, *43*, 102143. [CrossRef] [PubMed]

34. Abasıyanık, Z.; Ertekin, Ö.; Kahraman, T.; Yigit, P.; Özakbaş, S. The effects of Clinical Pilates training on walking, balance, fall risk, respiratory, and cognitive functions in persons with multiple sclerosis: A randomized controlled trial. *Explore* **2020**, *16*, 12–20. [CrossRef] [PubMed]
35. Fleming, K.; Coote, S.; Herring, M. The feasibility of Pilates to improve symptoms of anxiety, depression, and fatigue among people with Multiple Sclerosis: An eight-week randomized controlled pilot trial. *Psychol. Sport Exerc.* **2019**, *45*, 101573. [CrossRef]
36. Eftekhari, E.; Etemadifar, M. Impact of Clinical Mat Pilates on Body Composition and Functional Indices in Female Patients with Multiple Sclerosis. *Crescent J. Med. Biol. Sci.* **2018**, *5*, 297–305.
37. Ozkul, C.; Guclu-Gunduz, A.; Irkec, C.; Fidan, I.; Aydin, Y.; Ozkan, T.; Yazici, G. Effect of combined exercise training on serum brain-derived neurotrophic factor, suppressors of cytokine signaling 1 and 3 in patients with multiple sclerosis. *J. Neuroimmunol.* **2018**, *316*, 121–129. [CrossRef]
38. Duff, W.R.; Andrushko, J.; Renshaw, D.W.; Chilibeck, P.D.; Farthing, J.P.; Danielson, J.; Evans, C.D. Impact of Pilates Exercise in Multiple Sclerosis. *Int. J. MS Care* **2018**, *20*, 92–100. [CrossRef]
39. Eftekhari, E.; Etemadifar, M. Interleukin-10 and brain-derived neurotrophic factor responses to the Mat Pilates training in women with multiple sclerosis. *Sci. Med.* **2018**, *28*, 31668. [CrossRef]
40. Kalron, A.; Rosenblum, U.; Frid, L.; Achiron, A. Pilates exercise training vs. physical therapy for improving walking and balance in people with multiple sclerosis: A randomized controlled trial. *Clin. Rehabilitation* **2016**, *31*, 319–328. [CrossRef]
41. Bulguroglu, I.; Guclu-Gunduz, A.; Yazici, G.; Ozkul, C.; Irkec, C.; Nazliel, B.; Batur-Caglayan, H. The effects of Mat Pilates and Reformer Pilates in patients with Multiple Sclerosis: A randomized controlled study. *NeuroRehabilitation* **2017**, *41*, 413–422. [CrossRef] [PubMed]
42. Kara, B.; Küçük, F.; Poyraz, E.C.; Tomruk, M.S.; Idıman, E. Different types of exercise in Multiple Sclerosis: Aerobic exercise or Pilates, a single-blind clinical study. *J. Back Musculoskelet. Rehabilitation* **2017**, *30*, 565–573. [CrossRef] [PubMed]
43. Fox, E.E.; Hough, A.D.; Creanor, S.; Gear, M.; Freeman, J.A. Effects of Pilates-Based Core Stability Training in Ambulant People with Multiple Sclerosis: Multicenter, Assessor-Blinded, Randomized Controlled Trial. *Phys. Ther.* **2016**, *96*, 1170–1178. [CrossRef] [PubMed]
44. Kucuk, F.; Kara, B.; Poyraz, E.C.; Idiman, E. Improvements in cognition, quality of life, and physical performance with clinical Pilates in multiple sclerosis: A randomized controlled trial. *J. Phys. Ther. Sci.* **2016**, *28*, 761–768. [CrossRef]
45. Hosseini Sisi, S.Z.; Sadeghi, H.; Massood Nabavi, S. The effects of 8 weeks of rebound therapy and Pilates practices on static and dynamic balances in males with multiple sclerosis. *Adv. Environ. Biol.* **2014**, *7*, 4290–4293.
46. Guclu-Gunduz, A.; Citaker, S.; Irkec, C.; Nazliel, B.; Batur-Caglayan, H.Z. The effects of pilates on balance, mobility and strength in patients with multiple sclerosis. *NeuroRehabilitation* **2014**, *34*, 337–342. [CrossRef]
47. Marandi, S.M.; Nejad, V.S.; Shanazari, Z.; Zolaktaf, V. A Comparison of 12 Weeks of Pilates and Aquatic Training on the Dynamic Balance of Women with Mulitple Sclerosis. *Int. J. Prev. Med.* **2013**, *4*, S110–S117.
48. Sánchez-Lastra, M.A.; Martínez-Aldao, D.; Molina, A.J.; Ayán, C. Pilates for people with multiple sclerosis: A systematic review and meta-analysis. *Mult. Scler. Relat. Disord.* **2019**, *28*, 199–212. [CrossRef]
49. Middleton, L.E.; Barnes, D.E.; Lui, L.-Y.; Yaffe, K. Physical Activity over the Life Course and Its Association with Cognitive Performance and Impairment in Old Age. *J. Am. Geriatr. Soc.* **2010**, *58*, 1322–1326. [CrossRef]
50. Giesser, B.S. Exercise in the management of persons with multiple sclerosis. *Ther. Adv. Neurol. Disord.* **2015**, *8*, 123–130. [CrossRef]
51. Willey, J.Z.; Gardener, H.; Caunca, M.R.; Moon, Y.P.; Dong, C.; Cheung, Y.K.; Sacco, R.L.; Elkind, M.S.; Wright, C.B. Leisure-time physical activity associates with cognitive decline. *Neurology* **2016**, *86*, 1897–1903. [CrossRef] [PubMed]
52. Vanderbeken, I.; Kerckhofs, E. A systematic review of the effect of physical exercise on cognition in stroke and traumatic brain injury patients: The Northern Manhattan Study. *NeuroRehabilitation* **2017**, *40*, 33–48. [CrossRef] [PubMed]
53. Marques, K.A.P.; Trindade, C.B.B.; Almeida, M.C.V.; Bento-Torres, N.V.O. Pilates for rehabilitation in patients with multiple sclerosis: A systematic review of effects on cognition, health-related physical fitness, general symptoms and quality of life. *J. Bodyw. Mov. Ther.* **2020**, *24*, 26–36. [CrossRef] [PubMed]
54. Washington, F.; Langdon, D. Factors affecting adherence to disease-modifying therapies in multiple sclerosis: Systematic review. *J. Neurol.* **2021**, 1–12. [CrossRef] [PubMed]

MDPI
St. Alban-Anlage 66
4052 Basel
Switzerland
www.mdpi.com

Journal of Clinical Medicine Editorial Office
E-mail: jcm@mdpi.com
www.mdpi.com/journal/jcm

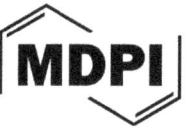

Disclaimer/Publisher's Note: The statements, opinions and data contained in all publications are solely those of the individual author(s) and contributor(s) and not of MDPI and/or the editor(s). MDPI and/or the editor(s) disclaim responsibility for any injury to people or property resulting from any ideas, methods, instructions or products referred to in the content.

www.ingramcontent.com/pod-product-compliance
Lightning Source LLC
LaVergne TN
LVHW070151120526
838202LV00013BA/912